MEDICAL SCREENING

and the

Employee Health Cost Crisis

MEDICAL SCREENING

and the

Employee Health Cost Crisis

Mark A. Rothstein

The Bureau of National Affairs, Inc., Washington, D.C.

Library of Congress Cataloging-in-Publication Data

Rothstein, Mark A.
  Medical screening and the employee health cost crisis/Mark A. Rothstein. p.   cm.
  Sequel to: Medical screening of workers/Mark A. Rothstein. © 1984.
  "BNA books."
  Includes index.
  ISBN 0-87179-628-7
  1. Medical screening—Law and legislation—United States. 2. Industrial hygiene—Law
and legislation—United States. 3. Insurance, Health—Law and legislation—United States.
4. Medical screening—United States. 5. Industrial hygiene—United States. 6. Insurance,
Health—United States. I. Rothstein, Mark A. Medical screening of workers. II. Title.
  [DNLM: 1. Civil Rights—United States—legislation. 2. Employment—United States—
legislation. 3. Insurance, Health—economics—United States. 4. Mass Screening. WA 245
R847ma] KF3570.R663 1989
344.73'0465—dc19
[347.304465]
DNLM/DLC
for Library of Congress   89-977
                                                                                        CIP

Published by BNA Books
1231 25th Street, N.W., Washington, D.C. 20037

International Standard Book Number: 0-87179-628-7
Printed in the United States of America

To the memory of
Leah and Jack Rosenfeld

Foreword

In 1989, occupational health professionals must be almost as familiar with laws relating to medical screening as with medical issues such as test selection and interpretation of results. Those who employ such professionals and those who receive their services should also be familiar with the legal requirements affecting screening programs. Further, as government agencies and legislative bodies develop policies or laws in this area, others will benefit from a deeper knowledge of current requirements and legal trends. This book is of interest to all those groups.

In the five years since the publication of Professor Rothstein's book, *Medical Screening of Workers*, worksite medical screening has been advocated as part of the response to two major national health problems—AIDS and drug abuse. In these instances, screening to identify and exclude positive individuals has occurred. The extent and acceptability of screening has varied between these two situations. Generally, policies have been developed to discourage use of screening for human immunodeficiency virus (HIV) infection in workers, including even health care and public safety workers whose jobs entail a risk of HIV exposure. In contrast, drug screening has been more widely accepted. The disparity in these practices relate both to legal and political forces as well as to medical considerations. All aspects are discussed in detail in this book.

To a large extent, medical screening in the workplace borrows techniques, guiding scientific principles, and its rationale from screening which occurs in the broader realm of public health. In turn, public health screening programs borrow from the clinical practice of medicine. Although some of this transferral is appropriate, much is lost in this translation process—particularly in regard to the rationale which specifies the benefits of screening to the individual, to the workplace, and to society. Thus, screening in the workplace must be evaluated by considering the scientific, legal, and ethical basis for this common practice.

Why are screening programs performed? Often, screening programs are initiated in response to an ill-defined feeling that more information will lead to a simple solution to a difficult problem. Similarly, in clinical medicine, patients with vague complaints often receive multiple tests in an attempt to identify a treatable condition.

Preferably, screening programs are designed to identify a specific outcome, the detection of which leads to individual benefit. As such, screening represents a tool in disease prevention. However, as pointed out by Professor Rothstein, screening programs are now being developed to predict who will develop certain diseases. By identifying such individuals and excluding them from employment, employers may avoid the higher costs of health care to these "high-risk" persons.

The use of screening to predict which individuals are at high risk for disease has increased in the last five years. In some ways, this use derives from the contributions of epidemiology to our understanding of disease causation. Epidemiologic studies typically evaluate multiple causes for a particular disease and quantify their relative importance. Such studies investigate the relative importance of environmental exposures and personal behaviors and identify other traits (i.e., risk modifiers) which alter the efficacy of a causal factor. In identifying specific associations and in altering our conceptualization of disease causation, epidemiologic research has provided much of the scientific justification for screening.

In view of this history, we should examine the degree to which epidemiologic thought and findings have been misapplied to justify screening programs. Epidemiologic studies consider associations in a group of persons; screening programs focus on individuals. Often, group results cannot be used to support action directed at the individual. Due to the variability of cause and effect relationships, the presence of a risk factor in an individual does not indicate with certainty that the individual will develop the disease with which the factor has been associated in an epidemiologic study. For example, most people who drink alcohol heavily don't die of liver disease. Most workers exposed to asbestos will not die of lung cancer or mesothelioma. Most individuals excluded from a job following detection of a risk factor, such as alcohol use or prior asbestos exposure, will not go on to develop the disease to which the factor relates. Thus, due to the inherent limitations in the application of epidemiologic findings, screening programs may generate actions which are inappropriate for the majority of those individuals being screened.

In summary, I find this book both informative and unsettling. For the practicing occupational physician, this book provides both factual information, useful as a guide to practice, and legal cases in which certain common practices are called into question. In addressing the potential for misuse of screening tests to "predict" disease, Professor Rothstein raises important concerns and goes beyond his previous book in providing recommendations for policy development. Of particular importance is his discussion of the relationship of workplace medical screening to employer-provided health insurance and access to health care and to national health policy. Clearly, his thoughts will be of value in the months ahead as increased attention is paid to the role of screening in the workplace.

EDWARD L. BAKER, M.D., M.P.H.
Deputy Director
National Institute for Occupational
        Safety and Health

Atlanta
April 1989

Preface

In *Medical Screening of Workers* (1984), I described the increasing use by many employers of x-rays, laboratory tests, and other medical procedures in an effort to identify whether certain applicants and employees were at increased risk of developing occupational injuries and illnesses. The testing at issue was designed to prevent injuries and illnesses through better job placement, thereby relieving the physical and financial hardships from employees and reducing the economic costs to employers of absenteeism, turnover, disability claims, workers' compensation, and lost productivity.

Although appropriate job placement is a laudable goal, I expressed concern about the potential for discrimination that would exist with widespread medical screening. There were clear indications that some inappropriate medical procedures already were being used despite a lack of medical efficacy or, in some cases, in disregard of the health risks to the individual. Moreover, even where the tests were accurate, they were often being used without due regard for the legal, ethical, social, and economic consequences of their use.

In that book, I predicted that medical screening of workers was likely to increase. I was half right. In only five years, medical screening of workers has grown tremendously in prevalence and in importance. It has gone from an obscure and esoteric issue to front page news and one of the most controversial of contemporary concerns. Drug testing, AIDS testing, and other measures are widely debated. Frequently, the only area of agreement is an acknowledgment that employee medical screening involves important societal interests.

The medical screening which has grown so rapidly in the last five years, however, is different in kind than I predicted. Unlike the measures I described in *Medical Screening of Workers*, the new medical screening is concerned mostly with screening for nonoccupational illness. With health insurance and related benefits costs increasing dramatically, growing numbers of employers have embraced detailed medical screening as a method of cost containment. Inasmuch as millions of Americans depend upon employer-provided health insurance, any changes in employee selection or health benefits could have significant effects on access to health care and American health care policy.

This book has been written as a sequel to *Medical Screening of Workers*. It is intended both to "stand alone" and to follow up on themes raised in the first book. Except for some essential background information, substantially all of the material in this book is new. The book raises many questions, but provides only some of the possible answers. For many of the questions, including the overarching one of what roles individuals, employers, insurers, and the government should play in funding health care, the answer will depend on the forging of a political consensus through public debate. It is hoped that *Medical Screening and the Employee Health Cost Crisis* will help to shape and to stimulate this important debate.

MARK A. ROTHSTEIN

Houston, Texas
April 1989

Acknowledgments

Writing an interdisciplinary book for a varied audience on a complex and controversial topic is either extremely bold or extremely imprudent, or maybe a little of each. It certainly would be foolhardy to write a book on the broad ramifications of workplace medical screening without consulting with a panel of experts from various disciplines, including bioethics, economics, employee benefits, employment law, epidemiology, genetics, health care finance, health law, health policy, and occupational medicine. I have been extremely fortunate to receive the wisdom and guidance of an incomparable group of experts: Les Boden, Bob Bolton, Pat Buffler, Carroll Curtis, Gail David, Andria Knapp, Tom Murray, Laura Rothstein, Marge Shaw, and Bill Winslade.

The book contains excerpts from various books, periodicals, and scholarly journals. I am indebted to the following publishers for granting permission to reprint portions of their copyrighted materials: American College of Occupational Medicine, American Medical Association, Dr. Bruce Ames, Center for Work Performance Problems, *Fortune*, A. Foster Higgins & Co., Inc., Hanley & Belfus Publishers, Hewitt Associates, *Hippocrates*, Institute for Social Research, Kelly Communications, *Medical World News*, Random House, Inc., *Science*, Thieme Medical Publishers, Inc., *Wall Street Journal*.

The research involved in such a wide-ranging book presented a difficult challenge, but my student assistants were equal to the task. I am grateful to Barbara Bessette-Henderson and Becky Martin for their scientific and health policy research assistance and to Elizabeth Cook, Esther Cortez, Jackie Hollabaugh, Steve Lovelady, Etheldra Scoggin, and Linda Wilson for their legal research assistance.

I want to give special thanks to Dean Robert L. Knauss of the University of Houston Law Center for his encouragement and support.

I also want to thank Linda Grier for her cheerful and tireless word processing of this manuscript through its numerous revisions.

Finally, I want to thank my family, Laura, Julia, and Lisa, for their love, patience, and understanding as I completed "just one more project."

Contents

Foreword   vii

Preface   xi

Acknowledgments   xiii

1. **The Growing Importance of Medical Screening**   1

   Medical Screening and Cost Containment   1
   The Occupational Physician   6
   Medical Screening and Employee Selection   12
   Medical Records   18

2. **Diagnostic Screening**   21

   Impairment, Disability, and Handicap   21
   History, Physical, and Diagnostic Procedures   22
   Psychological Screening   31
   Mandatory Examinations   36

3. **Predictive Screening**   44

   Medical Screening and Occupational Illness   44
   Reproductive Hazards   47
   Medical Screening and Nonoccupational Illness   55
   Cigarette Smoking   59
   The Limits of Predictive Screening   65

4. **Genetic Testing**   70

   Biochemical Genetics: 1963–1983   70
   Recombinant DNA Technology: 1983–1993   72
   Applied Genetics: 1993 and Beyond   76

5. AIDS   81

Background   81
AIDS and the Workplace   84
AIDS and Cost Containment   89
Employer Policies   91

6. Drug Testing   95

Drugs and the Workplace   95
Drug Testing in the Public and Private Sectors   100
Drug Testing Technology   104
Legal Challenges   110
Developing a Sound Policy   117

7. Handicap Discrimination Law   125

Medical Information and "Handicaps"   125
A Framework for Medico-Legal Decisionmaking   132
Employer Defenses: Safety and Cost   140
Specific Medical Conditions   144

8. Labor and Employment Law   160

Constitutional Law   160
Common Law Actions for Wrongful Discharge   163
Occupational Safety and Health Act   166
National Labor Relations Act and Collective
        Bargaining   170
Title VII and the ADEA   174

9. Employee Benefits and Tort Law   180

Workers' Compensation and Unemployment
        Insurance   180
Regulation of Benefits   184
Dignitary Torts   187
Personal Injury Litigation   191

10. Health Insurance   195

Employers and Health Insurance   195
Health Care Cost Containment   198

Health Insurance Underwriting   205
Health Promotion and Wellness Programs   210
Mandated Benefits   213

11.   In Search of Medical Screening Policy   218

Medical Screening and Employment Policy   218
Medical Screening and Social Policy   222
Medical Screening and Health Policy   224
Some Final Thoughts   229

Notes   231

Glossary of Medical, Scientific, and Health Care Terms   275

Glossary of Legal Terms   281

Table of Cases Mentioned in Text   285

Index   291

1

The Growing Importance of Medical Screening

Medical Screening and Cost Containment

Medical screening of workers has become an established practice in many industries. It involves the use of medical criteria in the selection and maintenance of a work force and is sometimes referred to as "selection screening." Medical screening, of course, is not new. Since the turn of the century large industrial companies have employed "factory surgeons" to determine whether applicants and employees were free of disease and had the necessary strength, stamina, vision, hearing, and other physical attributes to perform the job. For example, in 1909 Dr. Harry E. Mock began a program of physical examinations at Sears, Roebuck and Company to discover and isolate individuals with tuberculosis.[1]

In recent years, medical screening has changed both qualitatively and quantitatively. The purpose of screening no longer is simply "diagnostic," that is, to decide whether an individual is free of contagious diseases and capable of performing the job. Increasingly, "predictive screening" attempts to identify whether currently capable individuals are at risk of developing a medical impairment at some future time. This newer form of medical screening is greatly affected by technological advancements and is likely to become an increasingly important part of the employee selection process.

Each year American companies require their employees to submit to millions of blood tests, urine tests, x-rays, pulmonary function tests, and other medical and laboratory procedures. In fact, with the exception of typing and similar skills tests for office and clerical employees, medical screening is the most widely used preemployment test in all major employment categories.[2] Merely looking at the increasing number of tests performed each year,

1

however, does not convey the sense of change in medical screening—changes that already have occurred and that are likely to occur in the future.

The National Institute for Occupational Safety and Health (NIOSH), a part of the Department of Health and Human Services, has conducted the most extensive studies on the frequency of medical screening in industry. A comparison of data from its 1972-1974 *National Occupational Hazard Survey* with data from the 1981-1983 follow-up *National Occupational Exposure Survey* indicates that there has been a substantial increase in medical screening in just a nine-year period.

As exhibited in Table 1–1, medical screening by both periodic and preplacement examinations has increased. Although medical screening continues to be much more common in large plants, the largest percentage increase has been in preplacement examinations in small plants. Consistent with Table 1–1 is a 1988 study by A. Foster Higgins & Co., which found that 55 percent of companies with fewer than 500 employees required preemployment physical examinations, with the percentage increasing each year.[3]

Table 1–2 shows that, by percentage, blood and urine testing increased more than other kinds of tests.

Table 1–3 indicates that the largest increases were in the services and wholesale/retail trade sectors.

Other forms of medical screening, not specifically covered by the NIOSH studies, also have become much more common. For example, among *Fortune* 500 corporations, only ten percent performed drug testing in 1982; by 1985 the figure had reached 25 percent;[4] and by 1987 nearly 50 percent of these largest corporations performed drug testing.[5] A 1988 survey of the chief executive officers of large corporations showed that three percent of the companies tested job applicants or current employees for antibodies to the human immunodeficiency virus (HIV), eight percent favored testing current employees in the future, and 39 percent said they would not hire individuals testing HIV positive—all despite the fact that such policies are illegal.[6]

The increase in the various types of medical screening may be attributable to a number of factors. First, for employees exposed to toxic substances such as asbestos, lead, and ethylene oxide, Occupational Safety and Health Administration (OSHA) standards require preplacement and periodic medical examinations. This would

Table 1–1

Percentage of Workers With Screening Examinations by Plant Size

Type of Examination	Estimated % of Workers	
	1972–1974	1981–1983
Total Sample		
Preplacement	47.7	58.8
Periodic	33.7	40.2
Small Plants		
(<100 Workers)		
Preplacement	19.2	26.6
Periodic	12.2	13.4
Medium Plants		
(100–499 Workers)		
Preplacement	48.9	56.4
Periodic	29.3	38.1
Large Plants		
(>500 Workers)		
Preplacement	83.3	87.8
Periodic	65.4	68.8

Source: National Institute for Occupational Safety and Health (NIOSH) National Occupational Hazard Survey 1972–1974; NIOSH National Occupational Exposure Survey 1981–1983 (preliminary data), *reported in* Ratcliffe, Halperin, Frazier, et al., *The Prevalence of Screening in Industry: Report from the National Institute for Occupational Safety and Health National Occupational Hazard Survey*, 28 J. Occup. Med. 906, 907–908 (1986). Reprinted by permission.

account for increases in periodic pulmonary function tests, for example. Second, some employees working under a collective bargaining agreement may be subject to periodic medical examinations pursuant to a safety and health provision in the agreement. Approximately one-third of all union contracts contain a provision relating to medical examinations.[7]

These two factors may explain the increased medical screening by large employers (which are more likely to be unionized), in certain industries (e.g., where there is exposure to toxic substances), and in the use of certain procedures (e.g., chest x-rays,

Table 1–2

Relative Frequency of Specific Periodic Examinations

Test	Estimated % of Workers	
	1972–1974	1981–1983
Chest radiograph	25.0	33.0
Ophthalmologic	22.3	31.4
Audiometric	21.4	40.2
Blood	14.7	36.0
Urine	14.4	34.9
Pulmonary function	13.5	28.9
Allergies	—*	7.4
Immunizations	24.2	19.0

Source: National Institute for Occupational Safety and Health (NIOSH) National Occupational Hazard Survey 1972–1974; NIOSH National Occupational Exposure Survey 1981–1983 (preliminary data), *reported in* Ratcliffe, Halperin, Frazier, et al., *The Prevalence of Screening in Industry: Report from the National Institute for Occupational Safety and Health National Occupational Hazard Survey*, 28 J. Occup. Med. 906, 908 (1986). Reprinted by permission.
*Information not recorded.

pulmonary function tests). Other medical screening procedures may be required of federal government contractors. Nevertheless, Tables 1–1 to 1–3 demonstrate that the largest percentage increases occurred in categories less likely to be affected by OSHA requirements, collective bargaining, or government contracts: preplacement examinations in small plants, blood and urine tests, and testing in the service sector. In other categories there was actually a decline. The reasons behind the increases offer the best evidence of the future direction of medical screening.

It has become increasingly clear that the newer forms of medical screening are not concerned with employee susceptibility to workplace hazards so much as with employee health in general. Simply stated, some medical procedures have been instituted as a cost-containment measure. A healthy work force means lower workers' compensation costs, reduced absenteeism, less turnover, lower disability and health insurance costs, reduced tort liability (such as

Table 1–3

Changes in Frequency of Screening Examinations by Industry Type

Industry Sector	Estimated % of Workers					
	Preplacement		Blood (Periodic)		Chest Radiograph (Periodic)	
	1972–1974	1981–1983	1972–1974	1981–1983	1972–1974	1981–1983
Transportation/public utilities	81.6	72.7	12.2	32.6	32.7	28.5
Manufacturing	67.0	61.8	24.1	35.0	35.9	33.6
Services	40.9	69.0	13.7	59.5	30.5	53.7
Wholesale/retail trade	22.0	34.6	5.9	17.3	13.9	13.0
Finance/insurance	33.2	—*	1.0	—*	7.3	—*
Contract construction	8.0	12.0	11.0	9.3	4.0	8.3

Source: National Institute for Occupational Safety and Health (NIOSH) National Occupational Hazard Survey 1972–1974; NIOSH National Occupational Exposure Survey 1981–1983 (preliminary data), reported in Ratcliffe, Halperin, Frazier, et al., The Prevalence of Screening in Industry: Report from the National Institute for Occupational Safety and Health National Occupational Hazard Survey, 28 J. Occup. Med. 906, 908 (1986). Reprinted by permission.
*Not surveyed in National Occupational Exposure Survey.

asbestos products liability suits), and higher productivity. Of course, some medical screening is performed because of altruistic concerns with having a safe and healthy work force.

Of all the costs associated with employee illness, the largest and most rapidly increasing cost is health insurance. According to a recent study, 97 percent of medium and large companies offer health insurance as an employee benefit.[8] Employee health benefits costs increased from 8.9 percent in 1986 to 9.7 percent in 1987 of total payroll costs—about $1,985 per employee.[9] Both self-insured companies and experience-rated, privately insured companies had substantial increases in health benefits costs. Despite celebrated efforts at corporate cost containment,[10] in 1988 health costs soared 18.6 percent to $2,354 per employee. The largest employers (40,000 or more employees) had costs of $2,605, and self-funded plans had increases of 24.8 percent.[11]

Increased health care costs also have led to more medical screening by small employers. According to Dr. Dominick S. Zito, medical director of Preventive Plus, a company that performs medical examinations for industry: "Small companies find their liability insurance and benefits packages are getting so expensive that they are looking for any way to cut costs."[12] If the per incident cost of employee and retiree health care cannot be controlled, there will be increasing pressure on companies of all sizes to use medical screening to avoid hiring people who are likely to be extensive users of health care resources.

The Occupational Physician

The task of evaluating the medical fitness of applicants and employees is the responsibility of the occupational physician. Indeed, it is the primary *raison d'etre* of the occupational physician. According to one estimate, "[p]erhaps 90% of all visits to occupational health specialists involve the medical determination of employability."[13] Although the actual hiring and firing is done by human resources or personnel departments, the occupational physician serves as "investment analyst in the human capital market."[14] It is therefore important to understand the role of the occupational physician, including the physician's training, loyalties, and legal and ethical duties.

During the last two decades, the importance of occupational medicine has been bolstered by a series of events. There has been a steady stream of scientific discoveries linking certain occupational exposures with cancer, lung disease, reproductive disorders, and other medical conditions. The Occupational Safety and Health Act, passed in 1970, mandates preplacement and periodic medical examinations and biological monitoring of workers exposed to substances such as asbestos, benzene, and lead. Health care cost containment, wellness programs, and employee assistance programs have grown tremendously. New technological advances, such as immunoassays used in drug urinalysis, have boosted the use of laboratory procedures.

Occupational medicine, a branch of preventive medicine, deals with environmental sources of illness. Scientifically, it is grounded more in epidemiology than pathology. It considers both the worker and the work. Although most occupational medicine is practiced by general practitioners and internists, the recent developments discussed above suggest a greater need for trained occupational medicine specialists. Nevertheless, from 1970 to 1982, while the number of physicians specializing in diagnostic radiology (up 447 percent), gastroenterology (up 164 percent), therapeutic radiology (up 149 percent), neurology (up 139 percent), and plastic surgery (up 137 percent) all increased dramatically, the number of occupational medicine specialists actually decreased by five percent.[15] From 1985 to 1995, the number of preventive medicine specialists, which includes occupational medicine, is expected to decrease another 5.8 percent—the only decrease of any specialty.[16]

As of September 1, 1987, there were 81,410 residents in 6,319 approved programs in the United States, but there were only 118 residents in occupational medicine in 25 approved programs.[17] A major reason is the lack of financial support for residency programs in occupational medicine. As of May 1988, the American Occupational Medical Association (AOMA), had about 4,100 members.[18] (In October 1988, AOMA joined with the American Academy of Occupational Medicine, an association of 400 full-time occupational physicians, to form the new American College of Occupational Medicine.) In all, there are estimated to be from about 10,000 to 15,000 physicians practicing occupational medicine full or part time.[19] Between 1955 and 1988 only 1,257 physicians were certified as occupational medicine specialists by the American Board of Preventive Medicine and it is not known how many of these 1,257 individuals are still in practice.[20] About the only growth in occupational medicine recently is a burgeoning number of "industrial medicine" clinics. In many instances, these are little more than trauma centers staffed by physicians with little knowledge of the "occupational" component of occupational medicine.

The problems of untrained physicians providing acute care and performing occupational health screening are illustrated by a 1986 study of an asbestos disease screening program offered to New York City sheet metal workers by a corporate medical service. In reviewing the medical records of more than 800 workers who were examined, the study found, among other things, inadequate recordkeeping procedures, a lack of comprehensive occupational histories, and "an extreme lack of concordance" between the staff radiologist and certified specialist readers in the interpretation of x-rays.[21]

The fact that relatively few physicians practicing occupational medicine have formal training in occupational medicine contributes not only to problems of technical competence, but also to questions of ethical commitment.

> "The subspecialty of occupational medicine is unique in that most of its practitioners have not received years of specialized education, but simply adopt the field as an alternative career. The sense of commitment to ethical practice, which is usually instilled during formal residency training, is largely missing from occupational medicine. Never having resolved difficult situations under the guidance of professors, the occupational physician has no teaching role models and most often has never gone through the transition to subspecialty status."[22]

Equally disturbing, but not as widely discussed, is the lack of training in occupational medicine received by all physicians. A 1988 report by the National Academy of Sciences' Institute of Medicine concluded that most physicians in the United States had a poor grasp of occupational disease.[23] It is not surprising. The average medical school curriculum only devotes a total of four hours to the subject of occupational medicine.[24] This shortcoming will become increasingly apparent when, through recent efforts to disseminate occupational exposure and medical records to workers, family practitioners will be forced to confront occupational medical problems.

A number of recent regulatory initiatives in occupational health have been based, at least in part, on the assumption that employee health will be improved by sharing with employees all relevant occupational health information. In 1980 the Occupational Safety and Health Administration (OSHA) promulgated a standard giving employees a right of access to their exposure and medical records. The declared purpose of the standard was "to enable workers to play a meaningful role in their own health management."[25] From 1980 to 1985, 25 states passed "right to know" laws and OSHA issued a Hazard Communication Standard requiring employers to disclose the identities, properties, and hazards of toxic substances used in the workplace.[26] In 1988 the House of Representatives passed and the Senate barely defeated the High Risk Occupational Disease Notification and Prevention Act.[27] The proposed legislation would have required that workers and former workers be notified if prior exposures in the workplace placed them in a "population at risk" for an occupationally related disease.

If workers receive more information about the risks and symptoms of occupational disease, theoretically many occupational illnesses that otherwise would not have been diagnosed correctly will be diagnosed and proper treatment and efforts at prevention will be facilitated. The responsibility for making these diagnoses, however, will fall mostly on primary care physicians who have had little training or experience in occupational medicine. Referral of these numerous cases to a few occupational health centers is impossible. A greater emphasis on occupational medicine in medical school curricula and in continuing medical education courses is therefore essential if the "access" and "notice" approach is going to lead to real improvement in worker health.

Historically, occupational medicine has not been considered a favored specialty by physicians because of, among other reasons, a perceived lack of independence, insufficient challenge, and inadequate rewards. There is also the widely noted conflict of interest of employer-retained physicians examining, assessing, and even treating individuals who are not their "patients" in the traditional sense.[28] Such conflicts are epitomized when the company physician's medical opinion results in a refusal to hire or the physician testifies on behalf of the company (and against the employee) in a workers' compensation case. Despite some attempts to make company physicians more independent, the physician's conflict of interest, real or perceived, still pervades the occupational physician-employee relationship and casts a shadow on the medical and legal duties of both parties.

"Physicians often find themselves in conflicting roles among the requirements of professional ethics; the obligations to the patient; the demands of the employer, government agencies, or other third parties; and their responsibilities to public health. These conflicting loyalties have clouded the scientific and social perspective on such evaluations and have been responsible for much of the criticism expressed about occupational medicine by the medical community in the past."[29]

The conflict of interest problem seemingly exists because of the unusual status of the company-retained examining physician. According to Dr. Saul Milles, Corporate Medical Director of General Electric Corporation: "We walk the tight line between being a patient-advocate and an employee of the company charged with protecting health in the work place."[30] Nevertheless, the notion of an individual being required to submit to a medical examination by a physician selected and compensated by a third party is not unique to the workplace setting. Millions of "third-party examinations" are performed each year upon applicants for insurance, personal injury litigants, claimants of benefits (e.g., Social Security, veterans' benefits, workers' compensation), and individuals entering or already within institutions (e.g., prisons, military).[31] Indeed, with the compartmentalization of medical functions, the typical hospital patient is likely to be examined by a number of physicians, nurses, and other health care professionals who were not selected by the patient and whose precise role is neither understood nor questioned.

The traditional legal view remains that there is no physician-patient relationship between an individual and a third-party physician. According to one theory, if only an examination is performed and no treatment is contemplated, there is no physician-patient relationship.[32] Also, if the examination is for the benefit of the third party rather than the examinee, there is no physician-patient relationship.[33] Both approaches, the "treatment" rule and the "benefit" rule, however, are overly simplistic and ill-serve the myriad of relationships common in third-party examinations. Occupational physicians often examine *and* treat, and the benefit of their services often goes to both employer *and* employee. Therefore, to determine if there is a physician-patient relationship, other factors also must be considered, including whether there is an ongoing medical relationship between the parties or merely a single examination, what the reasonable expectations of the physician and patient are regarding the nature of the examination, and the nature of the patient's consent to the examination.

If a physician-patient relationship is established, a physician is required to use "that degree of care, skill and proficiency which is commonly exercised by the ordinary skillful, careful and prudent physician engaged in similar practice under the same or similar circumstances."[34] The standard of care required of a specialist is higher. It is the degree of care, skill, and proficiency commonly exercised by a specialist in good standing.[35] Where there is no physician-patient relationship, some courts hold that the physician has no duty except to avoid injuring the individual during the course of the examination.[36] Other courts hold that the physician owes the individual some degree of reasonable care[37] or, if the physician undertakes to give some medical advice during the course of the examination, to exercise the same degree of care as one who renders services gratuitously.[38]

Besides these broad legal duties, the hybrid nature of the physician-employee relationship would seem to demand some affirmative disclosures on the part of the physician. At a minimum, the following three disclosures should be a part of every third-party occupational medical examination.

First, the physician should indicate to the examinee the purpose of the examination and who has retained the physician's services. Many examinees are unclear, mistaken, or misled about the role of the physician.

Second, the physician should advise the examinee of the limited scope of the examination. This disclosure prevents examinees from erroneously assuming that the third-party assessment is the equivalent of a patient-retained physician's comprehensive examination. The AOMA's *Guidelines for Employee Health Services in Hospitals, Clinics and Medical Research Institutions* is instructive: "New employees should be advised that the preplacement health evaluation is not intended to take the place of private medical attention, and they should not be given the impression that they had undergone a complete health assessment."[39]

Third, where appropriate, the physician should advise the examinee of the need for additional medical consultation and treatment. This is especially important where the physician discovers a serious medical condition about which the examinee may be unaware.[40]

A similar set of affirmative disclosure duties has been urged by Dr. Patrick G. Derr of the Department of Philosophy of Clark University:

"[W]orkers or applicants . . . [should] be told who will have access to such information, how long it will be retained, and whether it will be divulged to other agencies or parties. And they should be given such information before they are evaluated and before they provide health histories or submit to preliminary lab studies. They should be told these things because, in point of fact, ordinary reasonable persons would *want* to know these things."[41]

Making these disclosures is not likely to be time-consuming, to undermine the examination or "relationship," or to affect the potential liability of the physician. It is, however, likely to improve the health of some examinees, to ensure the integrity of the examination, and to raise the esteem in which occupational medicine practitioners are held.

Medical Screening and Employee Selection

Medical screening of workers is comprised of two elements. First, there is the purely medical evaluation of the health of the individual. Second, the medical information is used in making a personnel decision. It is important to consider both elements and the ways in which they interrelate.

Medical screening may take place at any of several stages in the employment relationship, including: preemployment (to determine whether an applicant is medically fit for employment); preplacement (to determine the most appropriate job assignment); periodic (to assess the employee's ongoing health status, including any occupationally induced changes); return to work (such as after a leave of absence or medical leave); and disability evaluation (to determine eligibility for private or public benefits or to reassign a disabled worker). From a broad policy standpoint, preemployment medical screening is most important because of its critical gatekeeping function and its potential for discrimination.

Theoretically, the medical assessment part of medical screening consists of the physician evaluating the task demands and physical requirements of a particular job, evaluating the physical condition of the applicant or employee, and determining whether the individual is able to perform the job safely and efficiently. Dr. Richard Ilka, former Corporate Medical Director of Marathon Oil Company, has questioned whether many of the physicians engaged in the practice of occupational medicine have the training or inclination to undertake such job-specific inquiries. His discussion focused on Principle 6 of the AOMA Code of Ethics:

> "6. Physicians should strive conscientiously to become familiar with the medical fitness requirements, the environment, and the hazards of the work done by those they serve, and with the health and safety aspects of the products and operations involved."[42]

In his view, this principle, and the concept of job-specific pre-employment examinations is unrealistic.

> "Although this is a fundamental function of occupational medicine, it is enshrined more in principle than in practice. Efforts to do more than casually observe work practices can be seen as provoking worker anxiety. As a contracting physician, there is usually no incentive for this activity. The daily pressure of cases and examinations keeps the industrial physician in the clinic. Most lack the training in the fundamental scientific disciplines to be able to follow this principle effectively or understand what is seen if chance finds them on the plant floor."[43]

An important question is whether the preceding observation can be reconciled with data showing that applicants and employees in large plants,[44] in certain industries,[45] or with certain exposures[46] are more likely to be given an examination or a more detailed examination. One possible explanation is that while whether an examination is required and the nature of the examination tend to vary by industry, the examinations within an industry or at a particular workplace tend to be uniform and not hazard specific. The use of "generic" examinations raises both medical and legal concerns. From a medical standpoint, "the administration of the same standard preplacement physical examination to a variety of employees with different job descriptions leads to a loss of utility."[47] According to Dr. E. Carroll Curtis, Corporate Medical Director of Westinghouse Electric Corporation: "To do a preplacement exam without knowing what a person does is like listening to one side of a phone conversation. You miss a lot of information and can distort things."[48]

From a legal standpoint, if more generic, industry-wide examinations are used, it may be more difficult for an employer to establish the job relatedness of any particular medical criterion in a legal action alleging discrimination in employment on the basis of handicap. (For a further discussion, see Chapter 7.)

In evaluating the medical conditions of individual applicants and employees, occupational physicians commonly use medical questionnaires, a history and physical examination, and laboratory and other diagnostic procedures. The specifics and the comprehensiveness of the assessment may vary, but one thing is clear: Much of what is done in the course of a preemployment medical examination is irrelevant to occupational health. Physicians often "test employees across a broad cross section of medically relevant, but occupationally specious, categories, ie, categories unrelated to a person's ability to perform the job in question."[49] Indeed, virtually *all* chest x-rays,[50] back x-rays,[51] psychological testing,[52] and other procedures widely in use are not medically indicated for screening asymptomatic individuals in the workplace setting.

There are at least four possible reasons why medically unindicated procedures continue to be used in the medical screening of workers. First, even if a procedure has a low predictive value (postive) for individual screening, it may be considered cost effective in screening an entire worker population. (For a further discussion, see Chapter 3.) Second, physicians lacking formal training in occupational medicine may not be aware that diagnostic procedures of some efficacy in an individual clinical setting may be inappropriate in screening asymptomatic worker populations. Third, some screening is simply a "full employment program" for occupational physicians, a point of view expressed as far back as 1962 (a time of considerably less screening) by Dr. Thrift G. Hanks, then corporate director of health and safety for Boeing Company: "To be frank, if one were suddenly to remove physical examinations, a considerable number of physicians working in or for industry would have no reason for being. This, I believe, is why some industrial physicians are fearful of any argument against physical examinations. It attacks their security rather than their principles."[53] Finally, some procedures may be used for social and political reasons unrelated to medical concerns. Drug testing is perhaps the best example.[54]

Once all of the medical data are compiled, the occupational physician must decide whether the individual is medically qualified for employment. Perhaps not surprisingly, there is little information available on what specific conditions will automatically result in exclusion. Some employers have indicated that a positive drug test or HIV test will disqualify an applicant. For other conditions, the answer is not known. If, in testing for the presence of or propensity to contract nonoccupational illnesses, employers are acting as health insurers, perhaps data from health insurance is relevant. According to a recent study, commercial health insurers will deny coverage if the applicant has one of a variety of conditions, including diabetes, emphysema, and epilepsy.[55] Although employment discrimination on the basis of these and other health conditions may violate state and federal handicap discrimination laws (see Chapter 7), there is no requirement that applicants be informed of the basis for their not being hired. Thus, illegal discrimination could take place without the victim's awareness.

For medical conditions that do not result in an automatic exclusion (and this would probably include most medical conditions), how should the physician decide whether the individual is medically qualified? Pransky, Frumkin, and Himmelstein suggest that the two key factors are the certainty and the severity of the risk. They have illustrated these factors on the two-by-two table shown in Figure 1–1.

Few would question the recommended actions in Box 1 and Box 4. As to the more troublesome decisions in Box 2 and Box 3, it may be unrealistic and perhaps inappropriate to defer the decision-making to the applicant or employee. For example, a Box 2 case could involve an applicant whose allergic sensitivity made the individual quite likely to develop dermatitis from unpreventable workplace exposures. It is unlikely that many employers would permit an employee to decide to work under these conditions. A Box 3 case could involve an applicant for a bus driver job who had "substantially" controlled epilepsy. The degree of risk of the individual having a seizure would be a medical question, but even if the *individual* were willing to accept a "low" degree of risk, it would be irresponsible to permit an individual with more than a de minimis risk of a sudden, incapacitating illness to work in a job where there were direct, immediate, and severe public safety consequences. Pransky, Frumkin, and Himmelstein advance an important concept by suggesting greater worker autonomy in decisionmaking and by identifying certainty and severity of risk as important concerns. There are, however, several other relevant considerations, including public safety. For a further discussion, see Chapter 7.

Once a conclusion has been reached by the physician, two questions remain: What is management told? What is the applicant or employee told? The form in Figure 1–2 provides an answer to both questions. Management is told only the medical conclusions about employability without any specific medical facts. The applicant is told of both medical findings and the conclusion and also is asked to sign the report.

Figure 1–1

Certainty and Severity in Worker Risk Evaluation

		CERTAINTY OF ADVERSE OUTCOME	
		LOW	HIGH
SEVERITY OF ADVERSE OUTCOME	LOW	1 No disruptive intervention is justified	2 Provide information to worker and allow autonomous decision
	HIGH	3 Provide information to worker and allow autonomous decision	4 Worker exclusion, alternate placement, or job modification is necessary

Source: Pransky, Frumkin & Himmelstein, *Decision-Making in Worker Fitness and Risk Evaluation*, 3 Occup. Med.: State of the Art Revs. 179, 187 (1988). Reprinted by permission.

Withholding from management specific medical findings is in accord with Principle 7 of the AOMA Code of Ethics.

> "7. Physicians should treat as confidential whatever is learned about individuals served, releasing information only when required by law or by overriding public health considerations, or to other physicians at the request of the individual according to traditional medical ethical practice; and should recognize that employers are entitled to counsel about the medical fitness of individuals in relation to work, but are not entitled to diagnosis or details of a specific nature."[56]

Although "[f]ew contemporary occupational physicians would quarrel in principle"[57] with the policy of withholding specific medical information from management, it is not always adhered to in practice. One particular problem involves drug testing, where management often insists on the specific results of drug tests.[58]

Figure 1–2

Preplacement Evaluation Report Form

PREPLACEMENT EVALUATION REPORT FORM

Applicant Name _____ Date _____

Employer _____

Job Title _____

This individual is:

____ Medically qualified to perform the job described.

____ Medically qualified with the following restrictions and/or modifications:

_____

_____

_____

____ Not medically qualified.

____ Medical Hold pending further data.

The patient has been informed of any medical findings and my recommendations.

Signed _____ M.D.

_____ Applicant

Source: Pransky, Frumkin & Himmelstein, *Decision-Making in Worker Fitness and Risk Evaluation*, 3 Occup. Med.: State of the Art Revs. 179, 189 (1988). Reprinted by permission.

Perhaps the greatest threat to confidentiality of employee medical data is the increased use of preemployment and pretest waivers. Employees are often required to sign waivers authorizing physicians to disclose medical information to management. In essence, physicians are participating in a system in which employees are compelled to authorize the physicians to engage in otherwise unethical conduct. Although such waivers are legal, if this trend is not checked by legislation or self-regulation by occupational physicians, the lofty goals of Principle 7 will be rendered totally nugatory.

With regard to sharing medical findings and conclusions with the applicant or employee, there is less of a consensus, but some evidence suggests that the field has moved slowly toward embracing the concept of sharing the information.[59] Employees are more likely to receive examination reports than applicants. Massachusetts law provides that "[a]ny employer requiring a physical examination of an employee shall, upon request, cause said person to be furnished with a copy of the medical report following the said examination."[60] In addition, OSHA regulations provide that employees exposed to toxic substances have a right of access to their medical records.[61] There is no requirement that employees be informed of medical findings at the time the information is generated or recorded.

There is also a practical problem in sharing information with applicants and in obtaining their signatures. The physician may not reach a conclusion on employability until after laboratory and x-ray results are considered. By the time this occurs, it may no longer be possible to speak with the applicant or have the applicant sign the report. Interestingly, in other types of third-party medical examinations, such as insurance physicals and government benefits examinations, the physician is often expressly prohibited from disclosing any medical information to the individual being examined.[62]

Medical Records

More medical screening means more medical records and more medical records increase the chances of disclosure of sensitive information. In large companies that have their own medical departments, medical records usually are stored in the medical department and access is limited to medical personnel with a need to know. Even with such an arrangement, however, nonmedical personnel sometimes gain access to the records or are informed about specific medical facts in the records. At smaller companies, medical information obtained by contract physicians sometimes is maintained in personnel files where neither ethical canons nor legal strictures restrict access.

New computer technology, which facilitates the storage and transfer of medical data, also creates new threats to the confidentiality of medical information. Insurance companies long have shared health data on applicants through the Medical Information Bureau and large employers certainly have similar capabilities. New microchip technology also may make it possible to store an individual's entire medical history on a single, credit-card sized computer record. An employer could simply make submission of the record a condition of employment. The information, which then could be copied by the employer, would likely contain information of little relevance to employability and may well contain highly sensitive material.

Another significant threat to the confidentiality of medical records involves health insurance claims. To receive payment from an insurer, a health care provider must supply a diagnostic or procedure code number indicating the type of service performed. For a self-funded, self-administered health insurance plan, this information often goes directly to a personnel or benefits office, where it is stored in a file to which there is sometimes widespread access.

Employee medical records may contain information of a highly personal nature, such as reports of drug abuse, psychiatric conditions, reproductive health, and even HIV infection. Not surprisingly, the case law involving wrongful disclosure of medical records has tended to concern these types of medical conditions. For example, in *Levias v. United Airlines*,[63] a flight attendant's private physician, at her direction, supplied United's medical examiner with confidential information related to her gynecological condition. The medical examiner then disclosed this information to the flight attendant's male flight supervisor, who had no reason to know it, and gave a copy of the physician's report to the flight attendant's husband. A jury in Ohio awarded the flight attendant $34,000 in damages for invasion of privacy.[64]

Common law actions for invasion of privacy (as well as intentional infliction of emotional distress, defamation, negligence, and other torts) often do not work well in the workplace setting. For example, the lack of a physician-patient relationship may limit an employer-retained physician's duty to preserve confidentiality, and a limited privilege exists for employers to disclose certain employment records to others. Another obstacle to recovery is that the scope of publication must be broad enough to constitute "publicity."

In *Eddy v. Brown*,[65] Forrest Eddy, a worker at a Texaco refinery in Tulsa, brought an action for invasion of privacy after John Brown, his foreman, disclosed to coworkers that Eddy was undergoing psychiatric treatment. Although this disclosure led to such harassment and ridicule that Eddy quit his job, the Supreme Court of Oklahoma held that there could be no recovery for invasion of privacy because only a small group of workers was told of the treatment. In addition, a claim for intentional infliction of emotional distress was rejected because the conduct of Brown was considered insufficiently "extreme and outrageous."

The confidentiality of employee medical records is most likely to be protected by state statutes. Few laws, however, have so far been enacted. California's Confidentiality of Medical Information Act is perhaps the most sweeping law. It requires employers to take specific measures to protect the confidentiality of *all* employee medical records.[66] Other state laws are more limited in their applicability. For example, some recently enacted state drug testing laws provide for the confidentiality of drug testing records.[67] Nebraska's 1988 drug testing law, however, merely prohibits "public" disclosure of test results.[68]

2

Diagnostic Screening

Impairment, Disability, and Handicap

Diagnostic screening, the assessment of current health, involves the medical examination of applicants or employees to detect the presence of impairments. After this initial medical determination, nonmedical judgments can be made about an individual's employability or disability compensation.

The American Medical Association has provided useful definitions of "impairment" and "disability."

> "It is particularly important to understand the distinction between a patient's *medical impairment*, which is an alteration of health status assessed by medical means, and the patient's *disability*, which is an alteration of the patient's capacity to meet personal, social, or occupational demands, or to meet statutory or regulatory requirements, which is assessed by nonmedical means. In a particular case, the existence of permanent medical impairment does not automatically support the presumption that there is disability as well. Rather, disability results when medical impairment leads to the individual's inability to meet demands that pertain to nonmedical fields and activities."[1]

In other words, impairment refers to the individual's medical condition; disability refers to the administrative or legal conclusion of the effects of the impairment upon the individual. "Handicap" is a legislative classification (often protection from discrimination) based on the presence of certain impairments. Therefore, to be disabled, an individual must have an impairment; and to be handicapped (under many statutes), an individual must have an impairment, a history of impairment, or be perceived to have an impairment. An individual may be disabled but not handicapped (e.g., an alcoholic who is not in a recovery mode may be unable to work but excluded from coverage under a law protecting the handicapped); handicapped but not disabled (e.g., an orthopedically impaired individual with a sedentary job); or both disabled and handicapped (e.g., a stroke victim unable to work).

21

Occupational physicians are concerned not only with impairments, but with handicaps and disabilities as well. It may be necessary to decide what reasonable accommodations (e.g., wheelchair ramps) will permit an otherwise qualified individual with a handicap to perform the job. Physicians also may need to make disability assessments in determining an employee's eligibility for employer and government benefits, such as workers' compensation and disability insurance.

History, Physical, and Diagnostic Procedures

Medical screening of workers may involve the assessment of either asymptomatic or symptomatic individuals. The timing and purpose of the assessment, such as preemployment/preplacement or disability evaluation, will determine the physical conditions of the individuals being evaluated. With some allowances for the differing purposes of screening, most of the following discussion applies to all types of medical screening.

The first element of medical screening, the individual's health history, may be divided into the medical questionnaire, medical history, and occupational health history. Medical questionnaires remain in widespread use. Although they vary considerably, from short and general to long and detailed, they are considered an efficient and cost-effective way of generating information about possible health problems deserving further investigation. The main advantage of medical questionnaires—that they are completed by the worker without professional assistance—is also their main disadvantage. Applicants and employees may forget or have "selective" recall concerning their own medical histories, especially when not subject to further questioning.

Unlike the medical questionnaire, the medical history is taken by a physician, nurse, or other health professional. A medical history is important not only in assessing current impairments and employability, but also in proper job placement. The assessment includes efforts to identify illnesses that would be aggravated by workplace exposures. For example, "it might be desirable to place a worker with chronic perisistent hepatitis in an area without solvent exposure or to recommend the use of a respirator with even minor exposures to solvents."[2] The medical history should inquire about tobacco and alcohol use, allergies to medications, history of allergic contact dermatitis, or extrinsic asthma.[3] It is also important to note whether immunizations are up to date. For health care workers, this would also include vaccinations against rubella and hepatitis B.

The final part of the history, the occupational health history, has been called the "cornerstone of the occupational health examination."[4] A detailed occupational health history is certainly essential in evaluating a symptomatic patient in a clinical setting; it is also an important part of a preemployment or preplacement examination. Dr. Rose Goldman of Harvard Medical School has suggested that the initial occupational history for a new employee should consist of a job profile (including past jobs and exposures); a listing of symptoms, illnesses, or injuries related to past jobs; questions relevant to the requirements or potential hazards of the new job; and a listing of significant community and home exposures.[5] Figure 2–1 provides sample questions and areas of inquiry compiled by Dr. Goldman.

Dr. Goldman's short lists of questions illustrate the breadth of inquiry that may create some potential pitfalls for medical screening. Questions of doubtless relevance in a clinical assessment may have the potential for discrimination. For example, an individual with prior toxic exposures may be more of a risk (at least theoretically) than an individual without a record of such exposure, but rejecting people with prior exposures may have the effect of discriminating on the basis of age. It may be medically relevant how close to a factory an individual lives, whether there are environmental health problems in the community, and whether household members wear contaminated clothing into the home. Using this information in deciding employability, however, may have the effect of discriminating on the basis of socioeconomic class. These questions also show how hard it is to distinguish between "diagnostic" and "predictive" screening. (For a further discussion, see Chapter 3.)

Figure 2–2 is a medical history form used by a small, North-Central state manufacturer. The information solicited is not unusual in either breadth or depth. Yet it presents a significant potential for discrimination—through ignorance, negligence, or venial motive—by both medical and nonmedical personnel. For example, question 2(b) raises the issue of whether insurance risks are also employment risks and question 2(a) suggests that individuals denied employment by one employer may have difficulty with future prospective employers. Question 3 could be used as a basis for not hiring individuals who have filed workers' compensation claims. Ques-

Figure 2–1

Occupational History

Job Profile

A. Workplace name, location, products manufactured
B. Job title and description of operation
   1. Chemical (generic) or physical form of agents handled
   2. Operating and cleanup practices
   3. Protective equipment and clothing
   4. Ventilation or other engineering controls
   5. Eating or smoking at job site
C. Exposure monitoring information
D. Inclusion of part-time jobs and military service

Illnesses and Injuries Related to Past Jobs

A. Do you have any health problems, symptoms, or injuries associated with your most recent or past jobs?
B. Have you ever worked with any substance that caused you to break out in a rash?
C. Have you ever worked at a task that made you short of breath, cough, or wheeze?
D. Have you ever had to change jobs or work assignments because of a health problem or injury?
E. Have certain types of work caused you significant strain in your limbs (e.g., tendonitis) or back?

Home and Community Exposures

A. Do you live very close to a factory?
B. Do you know of any community environmental health problems, e.g., contaminated drinking water or chemical spills?
C. Do you have any hobbies that involve potentially hazardous exposures?
D. Do you use pesticides in the home or garden?
E. Do you have any conditions at home that you think might affect your health, e.g., use of aerosol sprays, chemicals, cleaning agents, recent reconstructions, painting?
F. Do any household members wear contaminated clothing into the home?

Source: Goldman, *General Occupational Health History and Examination*, 28 J. Occup. Med. 967, 969 (1986). Reprinted by permission.

Figure 2–2

Medical History Form

To be filled in by employer prior to medical examination:

Name _____   Soc. Sec. No. _____

Position for which examined _____   Date of birth _____

Name of Manager_____

Notify in case of emergency _____   Relationship _____

Address _____   Tele. No. _____

Name and address of personal physician _____

_____

_____

To be completed by applicant prior to examination by physician: (If possible, before date of exam)

Item	YES or NO or Specify	Comments by Applicant
1. Have you ever been hospitalized for any illness, injury or operation? (If so, describe and give names and addresses of physicians who cared for you.)		
2. Have you ever been: (If so, describe circumstances.) (a) refused employment because of your health? (b) refused or rated for life insurance?		
3. Have you ever filed for veterans' disability or workmen's compensation due to injury or disease? (If so, describe circumstances.)		
4. Have you ever had to take time off from work or have your work limited because of your health? (If so, describe.)		
5. Have you ever worked: (If so, describe.) (a) as a coal miner, quarryman, sandblaster, welder, or foundryman? (b) in a pottery factory, iron or steel mill, glass factory, cement, chemical, or paint manufacturing plant? (c) in a plant with asbestos, beryllium, lead, or plastics?		
Have any blood relatives ever had:		**Comments by Physician**
6. Turberculosis, asthma, hay fever, or hives, cancer?		
7. Diabetes, high blood pressure, mental illness?		
Have you ever had:		
8. Head injuries?		
9. Face, eye or ear injury resulting in loss of hearing, vision or visual difficulty?		
10. Spine, back, neck or chest injury, operation, pain, or disability?		
11. Any back examination, treatment, or adjustment by a physician osteopath, or chiropractor?		
12. Shoulder, elbow, arm, hand, or fingers—pain, injury, operation, or disability?		
13. Hip, knee, leg, or foot, or toes—pain, injury, operation, or disability?		
14. Fractures or disease of the bone?		
15. Varicose veins, vein ligations, phlebitis or thrombosis?		
16. Arthritis, rheumatism, neuritis, muscle weakness or multiple sclerosis?		
17. Hernia, rupture, tumors, growths, or cancer?		
18. Fainting, dizzy spells, fits, convulsions or epilepsy?		
19. Frequent or severe headaches, heat exhaustion or sunstroke?		
20. Mental disease, nervous breakdown or suffered from nerves?		
21. Heart trouble, rheumatic fever, or high blood pressure?		
22. Swelling of the hands, ankles or feet?		

Figure 2–2 continued

Have you ever had:	YES or NO or Specify	Comments by Physician
23. Lung trouble, chronic cough, or asthma?		
24. Hay fever, hives, or allergy to medicine, food, or injection?		
25. Skin rash or excessive oily or dry skin?		
26. Stomach trouble, ulcers, chronic indigestion or gall bladder trouble?		
27. Disease of the kidney, pancreas, spleen, or thyroid?		
28. Diabetes or sugar in the urine, venereal disease or bad blood?		
29. Bleeding disorder or needed a blood transfusion? Anemia?		
30. Any illness or injury not already mentioned?		
To be answered by female applicants only:		
31. Have you ever had painful or irregular menstruation?		
32. Last menstrual period — was it normal? Are you pregnant now?		
33. Have you ever been pregnant? Any miscarriages? Abortions?		
To be answered by male applicants only:		
34. Have you ever had testicle pains?		
35. Have you ever had prostate trouble?		

To be signed by the applicant at completion of above portion of the medical form:

> I have read the above and declare that I have had no injury, illness, or ailment other than as specifically noted; or any other ailment not included herein. I am not using drugs such as: marijuana, narcotics, barbiturates, amphetamines, L.S.D. or any other hallucinogen. Any falsification or misrepresentation will be sufficient grounds for my release from employment.

Signature

Note to examining physician: Please record pertinent information in appropriate space for all affirmative answers given by applicant. Space is provided below for additional notes if necessary. Please have applicant complete the following release.

To be signed by the applicant in the presence of the physician:

> I hereby authorize any physician, hospital, clinic, or medical institution to disclose to _____ or any of it's authorized agents, any information in his possession regarding my physical condition or past medical record.

Witness (Physician)	Signature	Date

Source: Bureau of National Affairs, Inc., *Recruiting and Selection Procedures*, PPF Survey No. 146 (May 1988), pp. 59–60.

tion 5 might work to deny employment to asymptomatic individuals with prior workplace exposures. Questions 6, 7, and 31–35 seek personal information of dubious relevance. Finally, the applicant is required to sign an unconditional release authorizing disclosure of all medical records.

With regard to the actual hands-on medical examination, Dr. Richard Schilling of the University of London, one of the world's leading authorities on occupational medicine, has questioned the value of many of the examinations as performed. He stated: "Many examinations are done as a perfunctory routine without any consideration of their value. . . . Routine examinations of large numbers of potentially healthy people may be boring to the examiner and may lower professional standards. They take up time that the health service staff could use more advantageously."[6]

As mentioned earlier, the specifics of the examination tend to vary by employer size and industry. Nevertheless, it is common for an examination to include a general evaluation and an evaluation of the following bodily parts or systems: skin and hair; eye, ear, nose, and throat; chest (pulmonary and cardiovascular); abdomen; genitourinary; musculoskeletal; neuropsychiatric; and hematologic.[7] Typically, any potential disease states or impairments suggested by the history or general examination are followed up by a more specific examination and other diagnostic procedures.

It should come as little surprise that laboratory and other diagnostic measures are the fastest growing areas of medical screening. After all, medical tests in all settings—the hospital, the doctor's office, in home, or the shopping mall—have become commonplace. Ours is a society with a blind faith in technology, especially medical technology. In 1987, medical testing cost as much as $27 billion in the United States[8] and there is increasing concern that medical tests are being overused. In the private practice of medicine, "defensive medicine" (trying to prevent claims of medical malpractice)[9] and increasing billing[10] are often accused of causing the growing use of tests, but there are many other reasons.[11] Dr. George D. Lundberg, editor of the *Journal of the American Medical Association*, compiled the list, in Figure 2–3, of reasons why physicians said they ordered medical tests.

Some medical tests of little efficacy have become entrenched. For example, until quite recently, it was standard procedure for all hospital patients to have a preadmission chest x-ray. A premarital Wasserman test used to be required in virtually every state. This proclivity for testing has led to patient demand for more tests, based on the cultivated but erroneous assumption that more procedures mean better medicine.

In the occupational setting, two leading explanations for overtesting are management pressure and habit. As with the *causes* of excessive testing, there are numerous *consequences* of too much testing. First is the overreliance on testing as a diagnostic tool.

Figure 2–3

Physician's Reasons for Testing

Confirmation of clinical opinion	Medicolegal need
Diagnosis	CYA (cover your ass)
Monitoring	Documentation
Screening	Personal profit
Prognosis	Hospital profit
Unavailability of prior result	Attempt to defraud
Previous abnormal result	Research
Question of accuracy of prior result	Curiosity
Patient-family pressure	Insecurity
Peer pressure	Frustration at nothing else to do
Pressure from recent articles	To buy time
Personal reassurance	"Fishing expedition"
Patient-family reassurance	To establish a baseline
Public relations	To complete a data base
Ease of performance with ready availability	Personal education
	To report to an attending physician
Hospital policy	Habit
Legal requirement	Others

Source: Lundberg, *Perservation of Laboratory Test Ordering: A Syndrome Affecting Clinicians*, 249 J.A.M.A. 639 (1983). Copyright 1983, American Medical Association. Reprinted by permission.

"Skills in history taking and physical examination . . . may suffer from overreliance on tests."[12] Tests can *aid* in a diagnosis, but they cannot *make* a diagnosis. In predicting whether an asymptomatic individual will become ill in the future, laboratory testing is even more problematic.

A second negative consequence of unnecessary testing is that it may produce inaccurate results. It is beyond question that "the more tests performed on a healthy subject the more likely is the discovery of an abnormal result."[13] This is because of the bio-statistical principles involved in screening groups with a low prevalence of the tested-for condition, a consideration further discussed in Chapter 3.

Many commonly used medical tests are simply not as predictive as widely believed. For example, the American College of

Obstetricians and Gynecologists estimates that the false negative rate on Pap smears (and thus failure to detect cervical cancer, which kills 7,000 women each year) at 20 to 40 percent.[14] Chlamydia tests have a 10 to 20 percent rate of false positives; mammography has a 10 to 20 percent rate of false negatives; and stress tolerance (treadmill) tests may have an 80 percent false positive rate and a 20 to 30 percent false negative rate.[15]

Even the most accurate tests are unreliable if they are performed by a substandard laboratory and there is considerable evidence that laboratory quality is not adequate. Between 4 and 6 billion tests are performed each year in over 100,000 laboratories.[16] According to the Centers for Disease Control, as many as one in seven test results are erroneous.[17] The errors are caused by, among other things, poor calibration of equipment, improper use of test chemicals, inadvertent switching of specimens, and technician error due to overwork or inadequate training.

The problems of technician fatigue are so great that researchers at Michigan State University have developed a computer program to convert normal graph lines on an analyzer into recognizable musical tunes. "A normal urine, for instance, might play 'America the Beautiful,' which is a tune everybody carries around in their head. . . . If the machine suddenly sounded a sour note, the technician would immediately know an abnormal urine had just been analyzed."[18]

Problems of inaccuracy also can be shown statistically. Each year about 100 million blood-cholesterol tests are performed to identify this important risk factor for heart disease. In 1985 the College of American Pathologists tested 5,000 laboratories, many of them hospital laboratories, to determine their proficiency in identifying a sample with a known cholesterol level of 262.6 milligrams per deciliter. The laboratories in the study reported levels ranging from 101 to 524 and almost 50 percent of the laboratories missed the result by more than five percent.[19]

Before 1988 federal regulations extended to only about 14,000 laboratories, principally through Medicare regulation or the regulation of laboratories sending specimens in interstate commerce.[20] The Clinical Laboratory Improvement Amendments of 1988[21] extends federal regulation to all clinical laboratories, including those operated by physicians in their offices, as well as those operated by health maintenance organizations (HMOs) and private companies.

It remains to be seen whether laboratory quality will improve as a result of the new regulation.

The final consequence or issue raised by overreliance on laboratory tests is relevance. In the nonoccupational setting, many laboratory tests ordered by physicians are inappropriate for diagnosis. For example, in one study of thyroid function tests ordered in hospitals, 37 percent of the test orders were judged inappropriate.[22] In the occupational setting, the question is even more fundamental: What is the appropriate scope of inquiry of an employer-retained physician? In the early part of this century, employment-based medical examinations served a public health function by providing medical examinations to many people who might otherwise never be seen by a physician. Today, it may be that a comprehensive history and physical examination, plus diagnostic procedures, have a salutary effect in the early diagnosis of illnesses and in proper job placement. It is also possible that these benefits do not justify their substantial costs in time, effort, expense, intrusion, and employee relations.

In the traditional practice of medicine, a physician who is entrusted with performing a comprehensive medical assessment also has a related set of professional (legal and ethical) duties. The examination must be voluntary; the patient must have a choice of physician; informed consent must be obtained before any procedure; medical information must be kept in the strictest confidence; the physician's loyalty must run to the patient; all relevant information, including test results, must be shared with the patient; and the patient must have autonomy in deciding how to act on the basis of the physician's medical advice. Few employers even attempt to comply with these duties.

Employers that are uncomfortable with these broad duties may want to opt for the less extensive role of only testing for a narrow range of job-related physical and mental abilities. With disclosure of the limited purpose of the examination, there would be no duty to make any of the further disclosures listed above. (This latter type of examination, however, would not aid in health risk screening.)

Employers cannot have it both ways. Increasingly, it appears that employers are likely to run into trouble (e.g., litigation, loss of trust) when they arrogate to themselves a system of comprehensive rights but only limited duties.

Psychological Screening

The psychological make-up of employees is an important part of both productivity (e.g., proper job placement and reducing absenteeism and turnover) and discipline at the workplace (e.g., preventing theft, violent crimes, and drug and alcohol abuse). Psychological screening provides a useful tool for determining the potential for these problems. Such screening also may be used in an attempt to avoid employing emotionally disturbed or violent employees, as well as the resulting harm and financial liability. For instance, in *Smith v. National Railroad Passenger Corp.*,[23] Charles Smith, a plant superintendent, reprimanded an employee, Joseph Leonetti, for having been in a restaurant eating breakfast when he was supposed to be at work. A few hours later, Leonetti entered Smith's office and fired two shotgun blasts at him, shattering his kneecap and adjoining bone. Smith sued Amtrak for negligence based on the failure to report or discipline Leonetti when he had previously displayed a propensity for violent behavior. The United States Court of Appeals for the Second Circuit affirmed a trial court jury's award of $3.5 million. Undoubtedly, a decision such as *Smith* gets the attention of management, which might fear a case brought on a theory of failing to engage in psychological screening rather than failing to discipline.

Concern for workers' compensation costs may be another factor encouraging psychological screening. According to the California Workers' Compensation Institute, claims for alleged stress-induced disease in California increased 430 percent from 1980 to 1986.[24] The increase may be attributable not only to more stress, but also to a growing employee perception of stress as work induced, to job dissatisfaction, and to attempts to obtain compensation.

There are also high costs associated with treating mental illness. Mental health benefits make up nearly 10 percent of health care costs and the figure would be higher without the benefit caps that are commonly imposed.[25] According to a study at Tenneco, Inc., only 2.8 percent of health claims were for mental health care, but they represented 8.1 percent of total health care dollars.[26] The average hospital stay for "other" illnesses was 6.1 days for employees, 6.2 days for spouses, and 4.4 days for dependents; the average hospital stay for mental health disorders was 20 days for employees, 15 days for spouses, and 43 days for dependents.[27] Consequently, psychological screening to control these costs is appealing to many managers for use in preemployment and preplacement settings.

Several types of psychological tests are used in the workplace, including general ability tests, vocational preference tests, and work simulation tests. The two most controversial types of tests in widespread use, however, are personality tests and honesty tests. These tests raise profound concerns about their accuracy, validity, intrusiveness, relevance, records generation, and stressfulness.

A. Personality Tests

"Personality" refers to the "unique synthesis of traits and functional characteristics defining an individual's lifestyle."[28] Personality testing, developed largely after World War II, is usually either objective or projective. Objective tests may be administered to a large group at the same time and are machine scored. Projective tests, such as the Rorschach Inkblot Test, are individually administered and require highly trained specialists to score and interpret the results. For cost and other considerations, objective tests are used almost exclusively in the workplace.

The best known objective personality test is the Minnesota Multiphasic Personality Inventory (MMPI). The MMPI was developed to assess and diagnose individuals who are mentally ill. It is a proven and respected tool for this purpose, but there is little evidence that the test has utility as a screening device for general populations, including job applicants taking it as a preemployment test.[29]

Despite the absence of any scientific basis, the MMPI has been used in the public and private sectors to screen applicants and employees. For example, in 1984 the Nuclear Regulatory Commission (NRC) proposed requiring psychological testing, including the MMPI, for all applicants for positions involving unescorted access to protected areas at nuclear power plants.[30] Although the proposed regulation was not adopted, in 1986 the NRC approved plans calling for the nuclear industry to adopt screening guidelines "voluntarily,"[31] and several utilities and other companies already have done so under pressure from the NRC.

Besides the lack of predictive value of the test, the MMPI's 566 questions have been challenged as being racially biased and as invading employee privacy by touching on a variety of sensitive and personal matters. The disclosure of even a single answer could lead to great embarassment to the individual. Figure 2–4 is a sample of questions from the MMPI.

Another surprisingly popular personality assessment technique is handwriting analysis ("graphology" or "graphoanalysis"). An estimated 2,000 to 2,500 U.S. employers use handwriting analysis to predict the personalities of individuals.[32] It is cheaper ($25 to $350) and simpler (12 to 14 lines of handwriting on unlined paper) than traditional psychological tests,[33] but its scientific validity is far from established. Many of the "handwriting consultants" to industry have no formal training or learned handwriting analysis through a correspondence course. Figure 2–5 gives some samples of handwriting analysis.

Honesty Tests

Although it is not a medical test (and perhaps not even a scientific test at all), the polygraph or "lie detector" test attempts to use biological data to draw behavioral inferences on which to base

---

Figure 2–4

Selected Questions From the Minnesota Multiphasic Personality Inventory

True or False

14. I have diarrhea once a month or more.
20. My sex life is satisfactory.
38. During one period when I was a youngster I engaged in petty thievery.
65. I loved my father.
69. I am very strongly attracted by members of my own sex.
133. I have never indulged in any unusual sex practices.
154. I have never had a fit or convulsion.
177. My mother was a good woman.
208. I like to flirt.
215. I have used alcohol extensively.
320. Many of my dreams are about sex matters.
432. I have strong political opinions.
488. I pray several times every week.

Source: Minnesota Multiphasic Personality Inventory (1943).

Figure 2–5

Handwriting Analysis Techniques

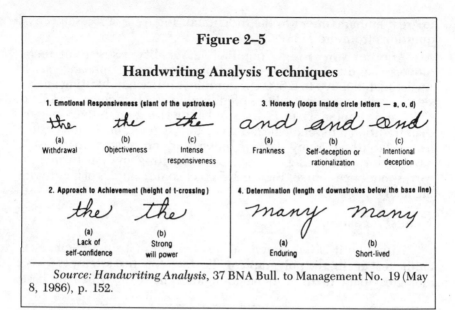

1. Emotional Responsiveness (slant of the upstrokes)	3. Honesty (loops inside circle letters — a, o, d)
(a) Withdrawal (b) Objectiveness (c) Intense responsiveness	(a) Frankness (b) Self-deception or rationalization (c) Intentional deception
2. Approach to Achievement (height of t-crossing)	4. Determination (length of downstrokes below the base line)
(a) Lack of self-confidence (b) Strong will power	(a) Enduring (b) Short-lived

Source: Handwriting Analysis, 37 BNA Bull. to Management No. 19 (May 8, 1986), p. 152.

employment decisions. More specifically, the theory underlying the polygraph is as follows: "lying leads to conscious conflict, which induces fear or anxiety, which in turn produces clearly measurable physiological change."[34]

Polygraphs usually measure three different types of physiological responses. The rate and depth of respiration is measured by pneumographs strapped around the chest and abdomen. Cardiovascular activity is measured by a blood pressure cuff (sphygmomanometer) placed around the bicep. Electrodermal response (galvanic skin response) is measured by electrodes attached to the fingertips.

In 1983 the Office of Technology Assessment (OTA) of the United States Congress undertook a detailed review of the scientific literature on the accuracy of polygraphs in various settings. OTA concluded that there are serious questions about the accuracy of polygraphs. "[T]here is very little research or scientific evidence to establish polygraph test validity in screening situations, whether they be preemployment, preclearance, periodic or aperiodic, random, or 'dragnet.'"[35] Overall, accuracy rates were estimated at from 50 percent to 90 percent.[36] When used as a preemployment screen, polygraphs may disqualify as many as 30 percent of applicants.[37] For a further discussion of test accuracy, see Chapter 3.

Based in part on the OTA study, Congress enacted the Employee Polygraph Protection Act[38] in 1988 to prohibit most uses of polygraphs in the private sector. Before enactment of the law, which took effect December 27, 1988, as many as two million polygraphs were performed in the private sector each year,[39] most frequently by banks, jewelers, retail stores, and fast food outlets.[40] Under the new law, roughly 85 percent of these polygraphs are prohibited. Preemployment polygraphs are illegal for most private sector employers, but polygraphs may be used to investigate cases of employee theft and sabotage if the employer has reasonable suspicion that the employee was involved. Security firms, drug companies, and federal, state, and local government employers are exempt from the ban.

Despite scientific evidence of the inaccuracy of polygraphs, numerous employers (especially the opponents of the federal law) have asserted that polygraphs are highly effective in screening out workers who steal and engage in other forms of misconduct. In fact, often the reason for the "effectiveness" of the polygraph is that many people who take polygraphs think the test is accurate and that it will detect lies. Therefore, they admit to various kinds of wrongdoing and are not hired or are fired as a result.[41] The polygraph is credited with ferreting out these people.

One consequence of the new federal polygraph law is that an equally suspect practice, "paper and pencil honesty testing," may increase. Before the federal law was passed, about half of the states prohibited or limited the use of polygraphs by employers. These legal constraints and the desire to find a less costly alternative to polygraphs led to the widespread use of objective, paper and pencil honesty tests.

There are several different companies in the honesty test business, each with its own test. The most important common element of the tests is the solicitation of "admissions," in which the test taker will be asked to admit any prior thefts or indiscretions. According to Dr. Philip Ash, research director for John E. Reid Associates, which markets honesty tests: "Incredible as it may seem, applicants in significant numbers do admit to practically every crime in the books."[42] People who do not admit to dishonesty may still be disqualified if they do not show sufficient "punitiveness" for those who are dishonest or if they have an "attitude toward theft" which indicates they seem to believe that theft is widespread. The tests "pass," as honest, people who report that they have never stolen and who believe that very few people steal, and that those who steal should be dealt with severely. The test traps the unwary and challenges the sophisticated (and not necessarily the honest) into a game of wits in trying to guess the answer the test makers think is the right one. There is very little scientific evidence to support the validity or accuracy of these tests.

In 1988 employers gave an estimated 3.5 million paper and pencil honesty tests.[43] These tests are not prohibited by current anti-polygraph laws.[44] Although taking these tests is less stressful and intrusive than taking a polygraph, the problem of inaccuracy may lead to legislative activity, especially if these tests continue to proliferate.

Mandatory Examinations

Generally speaking, there is no legal duty for employers to perform employee medical examinations or to engage in medical screening. Growing numbers of companies using medical screening have chosen to do so on their own. Medical screening by employers also is generally unregulated. Only an occasional state law, such as those in Oregon and West Virginia prohibiting employers from charging applicants or employees for mandatory medical examinations,[45] regulates medical examinations. Nevertheless, there are some governmentally mandated employee medical examinations. These medical examinations are for two main purposes: To protect the health and safety of the employee and to protect the health and safety of the public.

Perhaps the best example of medical examinations designed to protect the health of employees is OSHA-mandated examinations. These examinations, however, only pertain to employees with exposure to 24 specific toxic substances. In general, physicians must furnish employers with a copy of the physician's statement of suitability for employment in the regulated area; the employer must conduct periodic (usually annual) examinations; and in some instances, the employer must conduct examinations at termination of employment. The failure to conduct these required medical examinations may lead to the issuance of OSHA citations and the assessment of penalties. Table 2–1 contains a summary of the specific requirements.

Three of the most common questions regarding OSHA-mandated medical examinations are: (1) Is the medical examination

Table 2-1

Medical Requirements of OSHA Health Standards Regulating Toxic Substances

29 C.F.R.	Substance	Primary Health Risks	Required Medical Procedures
1910.1001	Asbestos	1. Asbestosis 2. Mesothelioma 3. Lung disorders	1. Pulmonary function tests 2. Chest x-rays
1910.1003 –.1016	13 car-cinogens[a]	1. Bladder cancer 2. Bronchogenic cancer 3. Lung cancer 4. Stomach cancer 5. Skin cancer 6. Liver cancer 7. Kidney cancer 8. Pulmonary edema 9. Central necrosis	1. Complete medical history, including genetic and environ-mental factors 2. Consideration of reduced immunological competence of employees, those undergoing treatment with steroids or cytotoxic agents, pregnant women and cigarette smokers
1910.1017	Vinyl chloride	1. Angiosarcoma 2. Lung cancer	1. Complete physical exam 2. Liver studies
1910.1018	Inorganic arsenic	1. Neuritis 2. Paralysis 2. Chest x-ray 3. Sputum cytology	1. Complete medical history and exam
1910.1025	Inorganic lead	1. Central nervous system disorders 2. Kidney damage	1. Complete medical history and exam 2. Detailed blood studies
1910.1028	Benzene	1. Leukemia 2. Blood disorders	1. Complete medical history and exam 2. Complete blood count
1910.1029	Coke oven emissions	1. Lung Cancer 2. Kidney cancer 3. Skin cancer	1. Complete medical history 2. Chest x-ray 3. Pulmonary function tests 4. Sputum cytology 5. Urine cytology
1910.1043	Cotton dust	1. Byssinosis	1. Complete medical history 2. Standardized respiratory questionnaire 3. Pulmonary function tests

Table 2–1   continued

29 C.F.R.	Substance	Primary Health Risks	Required Medical Procedures
1910.1044	DBCP[b]	1. Sterility	1. Complete medical and reproductive history 2. Examination of genitourinary tract 3. Serum specimen for radioimmunoassay
1910.1045	Acrylonitrile	1. Asphyxia 2. Weakness	1. Complete medical history and exam, with particular attention to peripheral and central nervous system, gastrointestinal system, skin, and thyroid 2. Chest x-ray 3. Fecal occult blood screening for all workers over 40 years of age
1910.1047	Ethylene oxide	1. Leukemia 2. Brain cancer 3. Stomach cancer 4. Central nervous system disorders 5. Reproductive harms	1. Complete medical history and exam 2. Complete blood count
1910.1048	Formaldehyde	1. Cancer 2. Respiratory disease	1. Medical disease questionnaire 2. Physical exam with emphasis on eyes, skin, and respiratory system 3. Pulmonary function tests

Source: Adapted from 29 C.F.R. §§1910.1001 to .1048 (1988).

[a]4-Nitrobiphenyl (§1910.1003); Alpha-Napthylamine (§1910.1004); Methyl chloromethyl ether (§1910.1006); 3,3'-Dichlorobenzidine (and its salts) (§1910.1007); bis-Chloromethyl ether (§1910.1008); Beta-Napthylamine (§1910.1009); Benzidine (§1910.1010); 4-Aminodiphenyl (§1910.1011); Ethyleneimine (§1910.1012); Beta-Propiolactone (§1910.1013); 2-Acetylaminofluorene (§1910.1014); 4-Dimethylaminoazobenzene (§1910.1015); N-Nitrosodimethylamine (§1910.1016).

[b]1,2-dibromo-3-chloropropane.

mandatory? (2) Who selects the physician? and (3) Who pays for the examination?[46]

First, section 6(b)(7) of the Occupational Safety and Health Act provides that medical examinations shall "be made available" to exposed employees. OSHA has interpreted this language to mean that the employer must offer the examination; however, the employee may refuse to take the examination. Nevertheless, OSHA does not protect a refusal to participate. Unless the issue is covered by the terms of a collective bargaining agreement, an employer may make cooperation with medical examinations a valid condition of employment.

Second, the Act does not specifically indicate whether the employer or employee has the right to select a physician to perform medical examinations. Early on, OSHA determined that the employer should have the option of choosing the physician and should have access to the results of the examination. This policy has been followed in all of the health standards.

Third, section 6(b)(7) of the Act makes it clear that medical examinations shall be made available "by the employer or at his cost." OSHA's health standards have included language indicating that all costs for medical examinations must be borne by the employer. The employer also may be required to compensate employees for time spent taking the examination (outside normal working hours) and for extra transportation expenses.[47]

Although physicians should be familiar with OSHA's medical examination provisions, these regulations are of limited value for the following four reasons: (1) the provisions only apply to specific occupational exposures and therefore are of limited scope; (2) the provisions list required procedures but often give little guidance as to the significance of specific clinical or laboratory findings; (3) the provisions do not indicate what procedures or tests may not be performed; and (4) with few exceptions, there is no mention about what personnel actions are required, permitted, or prohibited on the basis of test or examination results.

Another law requiring medical examinations to protect employee health is the Mine Safety and Health Act.[48] Section 203(a) of the Act[49] requires that all miners working in a coal mine be given a chest x-ray within six months after commencement of employment, a second x-ray three years later, and a third x-ray two years later if the second x-ray showed evidence of pneumoconiosis.

There are a number of federal laws mandating employee medical screening to protect the health and safety of the public. Two of the most important of these laws prescribe medical certification for over-the-road truckers and airline pilots.

The Department of Transportation's (DOT) Bureau of Motor Carrier Safety has issued detailed regulations for the physical examination of drivers operating motor vehicles in interstate commerce.[50] Successful completion of the examination is a prerequisite to driver certification. Physicians are provided with a form (Figure 2–6) and instructions about specific conditions to evaluate.[51]

Similar regulations have been promulgated by the Federal Aviation Administration (FAA) for airline flight crews.[52] Unlike the Motor Carrier examinations, which may be performed by any licensed physician, aviation medical examinations may be performed only by physicians designated by the FAA under the auspices of the Federal Air Surgeon.

The DOT and FAA examinations contemplate a role for the physician different from that in other examinations. Because of concern for public safety, detailed procedures and standards have been adopted that remove a great deal of the discretion from the physician. If the standards are excessively stringent and serve to disqualify individuals who would normally be considered fit, it is considered to be an acceptable price to pay for protecting the public.

A number of state laws also require preemployment medical examinations to protect public health and safety. Among the occupations for which a medical examination may be mandated are teachers,[53] school bus drivers,[54] frozen food processing employees,[55] and meat and poultry workers.[56] Police, firefighters, and transportation workers also may be subject to state-required examinations.

As in other types of medical screening, it is difficult to strike a proper balance between not unfairly restricting employment opportunities and protecting public health and safety. Legal challenges are inevitable, but sound medical and policy considerations should dictate the outcome of the legal proceedings rather than *vice versa*.

In *Davidson v. United States Department of Energy*,[57] security inspectors employed at the Oak Ridge, Tennessee, nuclear facilities operated by private contractors challenged Department of Energy regulations establishing minimum medical and physical fitness standards for security personnel. The regulations,[58] enacted in 1984 to deal with an increasing threat of terrorist activity, require that security inspectors be able to run certain distances within specified times as a prerequisite to carrying weapons. The plaintiffs claimed that the regulations had the effect of discriminating against female, older, and handicapped employees. The United States Court of Appeals for the Sixth Circuit, in affirming the district court's grant-

Figure 2–6

Department of Transportation Form
for Physical Examination of Interstate Drivers

EXAMINATION TO DETERMINE PHYSICAL
CONDITION OF DRIVERS

Driver's name ————□ New Certification
Address ——————□ Recertification
Social Security No. ————
Date of birth ———— Age ——

Yes	No	Health History
□	□	Head or spinal injuries.
□	□	Seizures, fits, convulsions, or fainting.
□	□	Extensive confinement by illness or injury.
□	□	Cardiovascular disease.
□	□	Tuberculosis.
□	□	Syphilis.
□	□	Gonorrhea.
□	□	Diabetes.
□	□	Gastrointestinal ulcer.
□	□	Nervous stomach.
□	□	Rheumatic fever.
□	□	Asthma.
□	□	Kidney disease.
□	□	Muscular disease.
□	□	Suffering from any other disease.
□	□	Permanent defect from illness, disease or injury.
□	□	Psychiatric disorder.
□	□	Any other nervous disorder.

If answer to any of the above is yes, explain:

————————————————————

————————————————————

PHYSICAL EXAMINATION

General appearance and development:
    Good —— Fair —— Poor ——
Vision: For distance:
    Right 20/ —— Left 20/ ——
    □ Without corrective lenses.
    □ With corrective lenses if worn.
    Evidence of disease or injury:
        Right —— Left ——
    Color Test ——————————— ————
    Horizontal field of vision:
        Right ——° Left ——°
Hearing:
    Right ear —— Left ear ——
    Disease or injury ——————— ————
Audiometric Test (complete only if audiometer is used to test hearing) decibel loss as
    500 Hz ——-, at 1,000 Hz ——, at 2,000 Hz
    ——

Figure 2–6 continued

Throat ————————————— ———
Thorax:
  Heart ————————— ————
If organic disease is present, is it fully comp-
    ensated? —————————
  Blood pressure:
    Systolic —— Diastolic ——
  Pulse: Before exercise —————
  Immediately after exercise ————
  Lungs ——————————
Abdomen:
  Scars —— Abnormal masses ——
    Tenderness ——
  Hernia: Yes —— No ——
  If so, where? ———————
    Is truss worn? ————————
Gastrointestinal:
  Ulceration or other disease:
    Yes —— No ——
Genito-Urinary:
  Scars ————————— ————
  Urethral discharge ————— ————
Reflexes:
  Romberg ————— —————
  Pupillary —— Light R —— L ——
  Accommodation Right —— Left ——
Knee Jerks:
  Right:
    Normal —— Increased —— Absent ——
  Left:
    Normal —— Increased —— Absent ——
  Remarks ————————— ————
Extremities:
  Upper ————————— —————
  Lower ————————— —————
  Spine ——————— —————
Laboratory and other Special Findings:
  Urine: Spec. Gr. —— Alb. ——
    Sugar ——
  Other laboratory data (Serology, etc.)
  ————————————————————
  Radiological data ————— ————
  Electrocardiograph ————— ————
General comments ————— —————

————————————————————
(Date of examination)

————————————————————
(Address of examining doctor)

————————————————————
(Name of examining doctor (Print))

————————————————————
(Signature of examining doctor)

Source: 49 C.F.R. §391.43 (1987).

ing of summary judgment for the Department of Energy, held that the physical fitness requirements were sufficiently correlated with essential emergency skills.

A physician who is too lenient in certifying the health of employees may risk personal liability in addition to creating dangers to innocent third parties. In *Wharton Transport Corp. v. Bridges*,[59] a truck driven by Martin Lawson, a Wharton employee, struck the rear of a car parked on the side of a road and occupied by the Rains family. The collision resulted in the death of one child, severe injuries to three other children, and minor injuries to the father. Lawson was not hurt. Wharton paid $426,314.25 to settle the case brought by the Rains family and then brought an indemnity action against Dr. James T. Bridges, the third-party physician it had retained to perform the DOT-mandated examination to determine whether Lawson was physically fit to drive a truck in interstate commerce. Wharton alleged that Dr. Bridges was negligent in certifying Lawson as physically fit when subsequent examination indicated that he had a variety of severe impairments as follows: (1) only five percent vision in his left eye and blurred vision in his right eye caused by chorioretinitis; (2) severe osteoarthritis in both legs causing a loss of flexion and range of motion; (3) chronic degenerative disc disease in his neck and lower back which impaired his ability to move his neck and head; and, (4) chronic fatigue, depression, and emotional exhaustion.

The Tennessee Supreme Court held that Dr. Bridges owed a duty to Wharton and that an action for idemnity would lie. It further held that a jury could find that the injuries sustained by the Rains family were reasonably foreseeable as a result of Dr. Bridges' negligence.

Medical screening and employee fitness standards also are being developed by state and local governments. These standards have been applied to police officers, firefighters, transit workers, and other job classifications. Perhaps the best known standards are those developed by the state of California and San Bernardino County.[60] Overall, it has been difficult and costly to develop job-related and nondiscriminatory medical criteria. National consensus standards development and data sharing would seem to be essential to avoid the needless duplication of these efforts.

3

Predictive Screening

Medical Screening and Occupational Illness

Predictive screening, the assessment of future health risk, is an attempt to calculate whether an asymptomatic or presymptomatic individual is at an increased risk of future impairment. As suggested in the last chapter, it is difficult from a medical standpoint to distinguish between the assessment of current and future health. From a legal standpoint, however, it may be important to draw these distinctions, because employer policies that screen out individuals currently capable of performing the job will be more difficult to defend from claims of discrimination.

Figure 3–1 indicates the various stages at which medical evaluation and medical screening may take place in the causal sequence of occupational disease. Although medical screening may take place at any point along the causal chain, there are three main types or stages of medical screening: preemployment/preplacement examinations, medical surveillance of exposed workers, and disability evaluations. In a general sense, the medical examinations in this sequence range from asymptomatic to presymptomatic to symptomatic. The key factor is that the endpoint for all the conditions discussed in this section is an *occupational* illness or injury.

In *Medical Screening of Workers*, I described in some detail how an increased risk of future occupational illness could be based on innate characteristics (age, race and ethnicity, familial health history); behavioral and environmental factors (geography, diet, tobacco, alcohol, medical drugs and radiation, recreation and hobbies, lifestyle, psychological factors); nonoccupational health factors (musculoskeletal, prior illness, clinical findings); and occupational health factors (prior exposures). I need not repeat that discussion. It bears noting, however, that new studies have continued to discover new associations between certain risk factors and future illness.

44

Figure 3-1
Medical Evaluation in the Causal Chain of Occupational Disease

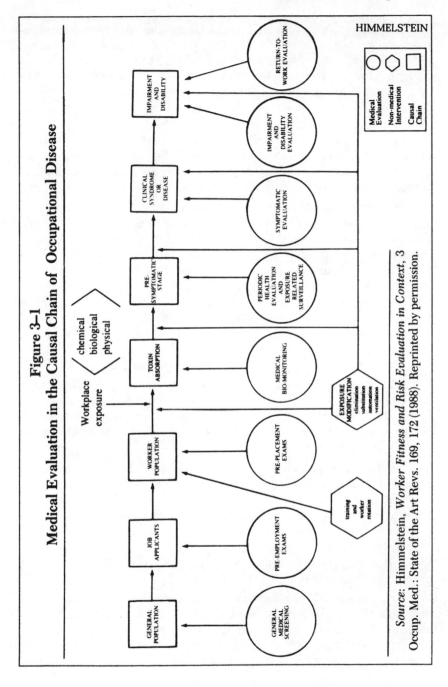

Source: Himmelstein, Worker Fitness and Risk Evaluation in Context, 3 Occup. Med.: State of the Art Revs. 169, 172 (1988). Reprinted by permission.

A few examples help to illustrate the different types of predictive risk factors that continue to be discovered. First, already recognized cause-effect relationships may be found to exist at lower levels than previously documented. For example, asbestos is known to cause, among other diseases, mesothelioma, a cancer of the pleura, peritoneum, or pericardium. New data suggest that individuals exposed to even small quantities of asbestos may develop mesothelioma.[1] Thus, an individual with a prior nonoccupational exposure to asbestos (such as could occur in hobbies like pottery and automotive brake repair) might be at increased risk of this fatal, usually occupational neoplasm.

A second kind of new study is one that marshalls new data to describe and document a poorly characterized, but known, illness. For example, a 1988 study documented the etiology of a form of hypersensitivity pneumonitis, "humidifier fever," caused by contamination in heating, cooling, and humidifying systems.[2] Immunologic screening for sensitization already is the most common form of hazard-specific medical screening. For instance, 97.4 percent of workers in large plants who were exposed to the sensitizing liquid toluene diisocyanate (TDI), were subject to preplacement and periodic examinations.[3] Consequently, new documentation of hypersensitivity reactions could lead to more screening.

Third, new evidence of additional adverse health effects of a known hazard may be developed. For instance, recent studies have found that cigarette smoking will increase the risk for a variety of occupational illnesses including bladder cancer,[4] polymer-fume fever,[5] and even noise-induced hearing loss.[6]

Finally, new risk factors may be established for both cause and effect. A study of the risk factors for occupational hand injury identified cardiovascular disease (consistent with automobile crash studies, but for reasons not entirely clear), being less than 25 years of age (older workers were less prone to these injuries), and sleeping nine or more hours per night (long sleepers are more likely to be anxious or depressed).[7] Interestingly, the study also found that fewer accidents occurred on Mondays.

The traditional function of medical screening is to aid in selection and placement. Even if new attention is given to medical screening for nonoccupational illness, predictive screening for occupational illness will continue to be an important and growing role of occupational health professionals. In focusing increased attention on personal risk factors for occupational illness,[8] privacy concerns also will need to be considered.

Reproductive Hazards

From the mid-1970s to the mid-1980s there was growing public concern about reproductive hazards in the workplace and the measures that some employers were using in attempting to restrict exposure to these hazards. Although public interest in the issue seems to have diminished (replaced, perhaps, by concern over AIDS and drugs), the underlying issues remain unresolved. Simply stated, the problem is how to protect the reproductive health of male and female workers and the health of their offspring without engaging in discriminatory employment practices. Complicating the problem are the limitations of economic and technological feasibility in hazard reduction and the relative dearth of scientific data on the effects of workplace hazards on reproduction.

The starting point for any discussion of reproductive hazards is the realization that the human reproductive process is fragile. It is highly sensitive and, unfortunately, often works imperfectly. An estimated 10 percent of couples attempting to parent children are infertile.[9] For every 3,000,000 births per year in the United States there are 450,000 to 600,000 spontaneous abortions and 33,000 fetuses die in utero.[10] Of live births, about 10 percent are premature,[11] approximately seven percent have a low birth weight,[12] and another three to seven percent have congenital anomalies.[13] The cause of the anomaly is unknown for 65 to 70 percent of the cases.[14] About 30,000 babies per year die during the neonatal period and at least 15,000 die in the first year.[15]

Although conclusive epidemiological evidence exists for relatively few environmental factors as the causes of congenital anomalies,[16] animal studies, in vitro studies, and case reports clearly suggest that exposure to numerous occupational and other hazards can result in a variety of negative reproductive effects. Among these effects are altered fertility, chromosomal abnormalities, spontaneous abortions, congenital malformations, behavioral disorders, and malignancies.[17] Some of the numerous substances and agents commonly in use in industry known to cause negative reproductive effects are arsenic, benzene, cadmium, formaldehyde, lead, mercury, radiation, and vinyl chloride.[18] Table 3–1 lists some of the numerous agents and substances under review for their possible reproductive effects.

Despite this lengthy list of possible harmful substances and agents, it represents only a small fraction of the potential hazards. There are over 63,000 chemicals listed in the Toxic Substances Control Act inventory and no publicly available toxicity information exists for more than 70 percent of the chemicals.[19] OSHA has promulgated permanent health standards for only three substances (DBCP, lead, ethylene oxide) that include specific provisions for the protection of reproductive health. OSHA's inactivity in regulating reproductive hazards in the workplace can be traced to a lack of research, both by the scientific community generally[20] and by OSHA and NIOSH.

Dr. Peter F. Infante, Director of OSHA's Office of Standards Review, has observed that regulation of reproductive hazards is made more difficult because there are comparatively fewer studies on reproductive effects of substances found in the occupational setting than there are on other effects, such as carcinogenicity. "We're no better off today in terms of studying reproductive hazards than we were in the 1950s. However, in terms of regulating hazards, we're worse off because we've done little or nothing to contain substances shown to be teratogenic to humans exposed in the occupational setting."[21] Only recently, have EPA and NIOSH devoted more resources to the study of reproductive and developmental toxicology.

While much is not known about reproductive hazards, much information already has been discovered.[22] As illustrated in Table 3–2, toxic substances may cause a wide range of reproductive effects.

Table 3–3 indicates some developmental effects in children based on parental exposure to reproductive hazards.

Two main problems complicate the control of reproductive hazards. First, with regard to at least some agents, the developing embryo and fetus may suffer severe effects at exposure levels that have no effect on the mother (or father).[23] These levels may be so low as to render their elimination technologically and economically infeasible. Second, the nature and severity of developmental defects depends on the degree of exposure and the time of exposure. Significantly, the greatest risks appear to be during the early stages of pregnancy.

Table 3-1

Agents and Substances Under Review for Reproductive Health Effects

Metals:
  Lead
  Boron
  Manganese
  Mercury
  Cadmium
  Arsenic
  Antimony
Chemicals:
  Agricultural chemicals:
    Carbaryl
    Dibromochloropropane (DBCP)
    DDT
    Kepone (Chlordecone)
    2,4,5-T, Dioxin (TCDD), and
      Agent Orange
    2,4-D
  Polyhalogenated biphenyls:
    Polybrominated biphenyls
      (PBB)
    Polychlorinated biphenyls
      (PCB)
  Organic solvents:
    Carbon disulfide
    Styrene
    Benzene
    Carbon tetrachloride
    Trichlorethylene
  Anesthetic agents:
    Epichlorohydrin
    Ethylene dibromide (EDB)
    Ethylene oxide (ETO)
    Formaldehyde
  Rubber manufacturing:
    1,3-Butadiene
    Chloroprene
    Ethylene thiourea

Vinyl halides:
  Vinyl chloride
Hormones
Undefined industrial exposures:
  Agricultural work
  Laboratory work
  Oil, chemical, and atomic work
  Pulp and paper work
  Textile work
Physical factors:
  Ionizing radiation:
    X-rays
    Gamma rays
  Nonionizing radiation:
    Ultraviolet radiation
    Visible light
    Infrared radiation
    Radiofrequency/microwave
    Laser
    Ultrasound
    Video display terminals
    Magnetic field
  Hyperbaric/hypobaric
    environments
  Hot environments
  Cold environments
  Noise
  Vibration

Stress

Biological agents:
  Rubella
  Cytomegalovirus
  Hepatitis B
  Other infectious agents
  Recombinant DNA

Source: Office of Technology Assessment, U.S. Congress, Reproductive Health Hazards in the Workplace 7 (1985).

Table 3–2

Some Examples of Reproductive Toxic Effects

Compound	Effects
Benzene	Menstrual disorders
Styrene	Menstrual disorders
Chlordecone (Kepone)	Decreased sperm count and motility, abnormal morphology
Chloroprene	Decreased libido, impotence, decreased sperm count, motility, abnormal morphology. Increased spontaneous abortion in wives of exposed male workers
DBCP	Testicular atrophy, decreased sperm count, decreased fertility
Arsenic	Low birth weight, spontaneous abortions
Carbon monoxide	Fetotoxic, low birth weight, fetal brain damage
PCB	Low birth weight, high postnatal mortality, skin discoloration, menstrual disorders
Lead	Wide spectrum: both sexes
EDB	Reduced fertility in men
Carbon disulfide	Sperm abnormalities, spontaneous abortions: women workers

Source: Adapted from Office of Technology Assessment, U.S. Congress, Reproductive Health Hazards in the Workplace 169 (1985).

"In the first three weeks of embryonic life, the most probable effect of significant exposure is severe damage and death of the embryo; organogenesis has not yet begun. The period from four to nine weeks is the time where classic birth defects can be induced. . . . Exposures after nine weeks gestation may cause postnatal functional abnormalities."[24]

Table 3–4 identifies the time periods when major organ systems are most sensitive to toxins.

As Table 3–4 suggests, exposures causing birth defects often occur so early during gestation that the mother is unaware that she is pregnant. Most women do not learn of their pregnancy until four to

Table 3–3

Some Reported Developmental Effects of Exposure to Reproductive Hazards

Agent	Reported Site
Anesthetic gases	Hemangiomas, hernias, skin, heart
Smelter emissions (lead and/or arsenic)	Multiple malformations
Polybrominated biphenyls	Skin discoloration, enlarged fontanelles
Alcohol	Facial, central nervous system
Vinyl chloride	Neural tube
Warfarin	Nose, bones (case reports only)
Diphenylhydantoin	Cleft lip, cleft palate, other craniofacial, mental deficiency
Aminopterin	Multiple malformations
Busulfan	Eye, cleft palate (1 report)
Methotrexate	Skull, ribs, toes (2 reports)
Methylmercury	Central nervous system

Source: Adapted from Office of Technology Assessment, U.S. Congress, Reproductive Health Hazards in the Workplace 170 (1985).

six weeks after conception, although early pregnancy test kits are now in increased use.

Based on the problems of low dose and early harm, many employers have adopted the much-debated policy of refusing to employ any fertile women in jobs where there is exposure to possible teratogenic agents. Because of the ubiquitous nature of many of these substances, as many as 20 million jobs may be affected.[25] (Nearly 30 percent of the nation's work force is made up of women of childbearing age.)[26] Some of the companies known to have exclusionary policies are Allied Chemical, American Cyanamid, B.F. Goodrich, Dow Chemical, DuPont, Firestone, General Motors, Goodyear, Gulf Oil, Johnson Controls, Monsanto, Olin, St. Joe's Minerals, and Sun Oil.

From a policy standpoint, there are at least two main problems with female exclusionary policies—they are underinclusive and

Table 3-4

Periods of Sensitivity for Major Organ Systems

Embryonic Period*									Fetal Period*	
Organ	3	4	5	6	7	8	9	16	20–36	38
CNS	XXXXXXXXXXX ---									
Heart		XXXXXXXXXX ---------------------								
Upper Limbs		XXXXXXXXXXXXXXXXX -----------								
Eyes		XXXXXXXXXXXXXXX --								
Lower Limbs		XXXXXXXXXXXXXXXXXXX ---------								
Teeth					XXXXXXXX --					
Palate					XXXXXXXXX ----------					
External Genitalia						XXXXXXXX --				
Ear		XXXXXXXXXXXXXXXXXXXXXXXX -------------------								

*Period is in weeks
XXXXX = highly sensitive period
--------- = less sensitive period

Source: Welch, *Decisionmaking About Reproductive Hazards*, 1 Seminars in Occup. Med. 97, 99 (1986). Copyright 1986, Thieme Medical Publishers, Inc. Reprinted by permission.

they are overinclusive. They are underinclusive because they focus solely on women and consequently only on post-conception, teratogenic workplace hazards. (Teratogens are substances absorbed by the mother which cross the placental barrier and act on the dividing cells of the growing embryo or fetus and cause structural or functional defects.) A comprehensive reproductive hazards policy also needs to consider preconception exposure of the mother *and father* to mutagens.[27]

Many substances that are teratogens are also mutagens (substances which damage the germ cells of males and females, resulting in mutations).[28] Mutagenic damage to a woman is irreversible because all of the oocytes are present in the ovaries at birth and are subject to harm from cumulative exposure. Mutagenic damage to a man may be reversible. If only the sperm is damaged, the constant production of new sperm means that the defective sperm will be replaced within 74 days. If the germinal epithelium is damaged, however, all new sperm produced will be genetically defective.[29]

The essence of the underinclusiveness argument is that female-only policies ignore the dangers to the offspring of male employees. Table 3–5 lists some of the agents with suspected effects on male reproduction. For some of these agents, such as ionizing radiation, the hazards to men are greater than the hazards to women.[30]

The overinclusiveness claim is based on the fact that female exclusionary policies usually apply to all fertile women, regardless of the woman's use of contraception, the fertility of the woman's partner, the woman's sexual orientation or activity, or the woman's reproductive plans. According to one estimate, of women at risk for unintended pregnancy, 93 percent of currently married and 80 percent of currently unmarried women use contraception.[31] It is not known what percentage of women (presumably higher) would use contraception if they were informed that they were working with substances suspected of being teratogenic.

Legal challenges to exclusionary policies have, implicitly or explicitly, relied on the underinclusiveness/overinclusiveness arguments. In *Wright v. Olin Corp.*,[32] a group of female employees argued that Olin's "fetal vulnerability policy" constituted sex discrimination in violation of Title VII of the Civil Rights Act of 1964. Pursuant to the policy, fertile women were excluded from jobs with

---

Table 3–5

Occupational Agents with Suspected Effects on Male Reproduction

Heat	Chlordecone
Ionizing radiation	Oral contraceptives
Mumps virus	Carbon disulfide
Lead	Ethylene dibromide
Manganese	Ethylene glycol ethers
Dibromochloropropane	Vinyl chloride

Source: Paul, *Reproductive Fitness and Risk*, 3 Occup. Med.: State of the Art Revs. 323, 329 (1988). Reprinted by permission.

exposure to toluene, carbon disulfide, and lead. The United States Court of Appeals for the Fourth Circuit held that the health of the fetus was a legitmate concern of the employer and would support a "business necessity" defense to a female exclusionary program, but only if the employer could prove, among other things, that there are no similar risks to the unborn children of male workers. [33]

California[34] and Connecticut[35] have enacted laws prohibiting employers from requiring sterilization as a condition of employment. In 1988 the Equal Employment Opportunity Commission (EEOC) issued new guidelines for determining whether an employer's fetal protection policy violates Title VII. [36] Under the guidelines, EEOC will consider whether a substantial risk of harm to employees' offspring exists through exposure to a reproductive or fetal hazard in the workplace, whether the harm takes place through the exposure of employees of one sex but not the other, and whether the employer's policy effectively eliminates the risk of fetal or reproductive harm.

Another line of cases has involved the removal of pregnant employees, especially x-ray technicians. The courts have applied a similar approach to that used in the fetal protection cases. [37] Because of the uncertainty of the scientific evidence, the allocation of the burden of proof is crucial. An employer will have an extremely difficult time proving the negative proposition that a one-sex policy is not underinclusive as a matter of science. In other words, the employer may be able to prove that there are risks to women workers, but not that there are no similar risks to men workers.

The concept of overinclusiveness, although frequently raised, has been applied in only one case. In *Steele v. B.F. Goodrich Chemical Co.*, [38] the Illinois Human Rights Commission held that Goodrich's exclusionary policy constituted sex discrimination as applied to Mrs. Steele, because of her age (48), her professed desire not to have children, and the availability of birth control. The Commission concluded that, as to Mrs. Steele, the Goodrich policy was "overkill."[39] Although it is a simple case decided largely on the facts, *Steele* is noteworthy because it values worker autonomy in an employment system that has been structured on paternalism since the early 1900s, when workers' compensation abrogated the assumption of risk defense.

Companies, unions, health professionals, and the government continue to wrestle with the problem of reproductive health. [40] New industries (e.g., semiconductor) and new work practices (e.g., video display terminals) raise new questions about reproductive health hazards from occupational exposures.[41] But reproductive problems from nonoccupational exposures is also of growing concern to employers. Reproductive harms require health care expenditures for men and women workers. In addition, since 1983 over 150 companies, including Pillsbury, Eastern Airlines, and Quaker Oats, have adopted prenatal health programs.[42] Problem pregnancies and deliveries are very expensive. Moreover, because many employer-provided health insurance programs cover dependents, each child born with a birth defect represents a tremendous additional expense. While much attention has been focused on the possibility of lawsuits and adverse publicity for occupation-related birth defects, the largest expense, health care costs, is the same regardless of the cause of the birth defect. As with other health conditions, the costs associated with occupational and nonoccupational reproductive injuries are often closely related.

Medical Screening and Nonoccupational Illness

It is often difficult to distinguish between occupational and nonoccupational illnesses. For example, exposure to benzene causes leukemia, but only some individuals exposed to benzene will get leukemia and only a small percentage of leukemias are attributable to benzene exposure. It is virtually impossible to determine whether any single case of leukemia is an occupational or nonoccupational illness. Fortunately, medico-legal causation, a key aspect of workers' compensation and personal injury cases, is one issue that need not be addressed in this book.[43] Predictive screening to contain health care costs is concerned with nonoccupational as well as occupational illness.

There is little doubt that employer interest in predictive screening for nonoccupational illness will continue to grow. Risk reduction of current employees via health promotion and wellness programs already is well established. (See Chapter 10 under the heading of Health Promotion and Wellness Programs). It is only logical that a company spending thousands of dollars encouraging employees to, among other things, exercise regularly, stop smoking, and lose weight, might prefer to hire someone in the first place who has a healthy life style.

Because medical screening is used for selection purposes, it is important to focus on the predictive value of the screening criteria. Some predictive screening measures correlate closely with future illness. A genetic test, for example, may indicate that a currently healthy individual is virtually certain to develop a late-onset genetic disease. An individual with a positive HIV test is now considered likely to develop an AIDS-related illness, including possibly a clinical case of AIDS over a period of five to ten years. Other possible screening criteria or procedures only establish an increased risk. An elevated serum cholesterol level is a risk factor for heart disease, but it lacks the predictive power of a genetic or HIV test.

One way of illustrating some concepts of risk is to look at cancer. Table 3–6 is based on an admittedly imprecise ranking system developed by Dr. Bruce Ames and his associates.

Ames' purpose in compiling the data from which Table 3–6 is drawn is to influence regulatory priorities. "It is important not to divert society's attention away from the few really serious hazards, such as tobacco or saturated fat (for heart disease), by the pursuit of hundreds of minor or nonexistent hazards."[44] This view has been applauded by industry, which has argued that many carcinogenic chemicals pose much less of a risk than naturally occurring substances. But Ames also has his share of critics, who assert that his ranking system may be off by a thousandfold,[45] that he is trivializing cancer risks,[46] and that he is overlooking the noncancerous health effects of many substances.[47]

Even with these caveats, Table 3–6 is helpful in illustrating the concepts of absolute and relative risk. Cooked bacon is carcinogenic; three times as carcinogenic as tap water. But the chances of getting cancer from eating bacon in a year are only one in a million and someone eating 15 slices of bacon a day is likely to have other more immediate health concerns besides the risk of cancer. Thus, the absolute and relative risk of any hazard must be considered.

With these principles in mind, it is appropriate to contemplate a few diverse, recent studies of nonoccupational cancer risk. Indoor radon exposure may be causing 5,000 to 20,000 cancer deaths each year.[48] As much as 10 to 15 percent of childhood cancer may result from residential exposure to electromagnetic fields caused by power lines and electrical appliances.[49] Alcohol has been linked with several malignancies, including breast cancer[50] and ovarian cancer.[51] Dietary fat intake is a risk factor for prostate cancer,[52] colo-rectal cancer,[53] and cancer of the lower urinary tract.[54] One study of adult

Table 3–6

Ranking of Possible Carcinogenic Hazards

Relative Ranking	Source	Daily Amount	Carcinogen	Risk of Cancer/yr.
1	Tap water	1 qt.	chloroform	3 in 10 million
3	Cooked bacon	15 slices	dimethylnitro-samine	—
8	Swimming pool	1 hr.	chloroform	—
30	Peanut butter	1 sandwich	aflatoxin	—
60	Diet cola	12 oz.	saccharin	—
67	Background radiation	at sea level	radiation	1 in 50,000
70	Brown mustard	5 g.	allyl isothio-cyanate	—
100	Raw mushroom	one	hydrazines	—
100	Dried basil	¾ tsp.	estragole	—
600	Indoor air	14 hrs.	formaldehyde	—
2100	Mobile home air	14 hrs.	formaldehyde	—
2800	Beer	12 oz.	ethyl alcohol	—
5800	Formaldehyde	6.1 mg.	formaldehyde	—
12,000	Cigarettes	1 pack	tobacco smoke	1 in 300 (all diseases)
140,000	Ethylene dibromide	150 mg.	ethylene dibromide	—

Source: Based on Ames, Magaw & Gold, *Ranking Possible Carcinogenic Hazards*, 236 Science 271, 273 (1987); Tierney, *Not to Worry*, Hippocrates, Jan./Feb. 1988, at 29, 31. The information about brown mustard, mobile homes, and ethylene dibromide appeared only in *Science*; the other information appeard in both *Science* and *Hippocrates*. The *Science* article is copyright 1987 by the American Association for the Advancement of Science. Excerpted by permission.

men in Iowa and Minnesota even found a two-fold risk of leukemia and non-Hodgkin's lymphoma among men who had dyed their hair.[55]

Is it too far-fetched to think that an employer would base hiring decisons on any of these studies? Would a health insurer be interested in this information? New methods of early cancer detection are being developed all the time. For example, the quantitative fluorescence image analysis is a new urine test for the early detection of bladder cancer. Suppose new technologies were developed to measure antibodies produced by the body when it begins to fight off cancer cells. Would the detection of these antibodies (or elevated levels of oncogenes) justify screening out job applicants? Should these tests be given more weight than mere associational findings? Should it depend on the basis of the risk?

A number of vocations (and avocations) have been associated (at least in a preliminary way) with a heightened risk of cancer and other illnesses. Artistic painters may be at risk for bladder cancer,[56] printers are at risk of malignant melanoma,[57] amateur radio operators have been shown to have a significant excess mortality due to acute myeloid leukemia and multiple myeloma,[58] and photographers with long-term exposure to sulfuric and acetic acid fixers may develop acute respiratory disease.[59] Is employment screening based on controllable (and behavioral) factors, such as prior exposures, an acceptable basis for screening?

Whites are ten times as likely as blacks (1 in 100 versus 1 in 1,000) to get malignant melanoma.[60] People with freckles, light colored hair, blue or gray eyes, and birth marks such as moles are also much more susceptible to skin cancer.[61] Yet, even these arguably stronger associations and higher relative risks are unlikely to persuade any employer to engage in screening based on skin tone—regardless of the illegality of such a practice. Skin color would simply be an inappropriate basis for medical screening. But would other bases be acceptable?

There are a variety of risk factors for nonoccupational illness. Drawing distinctions among possible screening criteria based on epidemiological, economic, political, ethical, and legal concerns is a difficult task. The number of questions greatly exceeds the number of answers, but the questions must be asked.

Cigarette Smoking

The treatment of cigarette smokers (and other tobacco users) by employers provides a good example of decisionmaking in employment based on concerns over nonoccupational illness. The logical starting point, assessing the health consequences of smoking, is an area of little debate. According to the Surgeon General, cigarette smoking is "clearly the largest single preventable cause of illness and premature death in the United States."[62] It is associated with heart and blood vessel diseases; chronic bronchitis and emphysema; cancers of the lung, larynx, pharynx, lip, oral cavity, nasal sinus, kidneys, esophagus, pancreas, and bladder; and with other ailments ranging from minor respiratory infections to stomach ulcers.[63] Some evidence suggests that smokers also have an increased risk of dying of pneumonia and influenza.[64] The estimated 314,000[65] to 390,000[66] premature deaths annually in the United States attributed to smoking is greater than the number of people who die each year from the following causes combined: AIDS, cocaine, heroin, alcohol, fire, automobile accidents, homicide, and suicide.[67]

Smokers suffer 10 times the risk of nonsmokers of developing lung diseases,[68] three times the risk of developing coronary heart disease,[69] and two times the risk of fatal coronary disease.[70] Smoking is linked annually to 88 percent of the deaths due to chronic lung disease, 13 percent of the deaths due to cardiovascular disease, and 32 percent of all cancer deaths.[71] Smoking-related deaths resulting from these three diseases alone account for 16 percent of all deaths in the United States annually.[72]

In addition to the general health risks to the smoker, certain sectors of the population face heightened risks. Smoking during pregnancy increases the risks of complications of pregnancy, low birth weight, and retardation of fetal growth.[73] Tobacco smoke interacts with occupational exposures to toxic substances, such as asbestos, multiplying the smoking employees' risks of developing chronic bronchitis, emphysema, diminished lung function, and bronchogenic carcinoma.[74]

Not all smokers face identical risks. The age at which a person began smoking, the total number of years of smoking, the number of cigarettes smoked per day, the degree of inhalation, as well as genetic and other factors affect an individual smoker's risk of smoking-related disease or death.[75] Although cigarette smoking has been the most carefully studied, cigar and pipe smoking, as well as tobacco chewing and snuff, present serious health risks.[76]

Recently, much attention has focused on the hazards to non-smokers of "passive inhalation" of environmental tobacco smoke. Indeed, much of the regulation of cigarette smoking in public places is designed to protect the health and comfort of nonsmokers. There is legitimate cause for concern. Tobacco smoke contains between 3,000 and 4,000 chemicals, more than 20 of which have been shown to cause cancer or benign tumors.[77] Undiluted sidestream smoke, the primary source of environmental tobacco smoke, contains higher concentrations of some of these toxic compounds than the mainstream smoke which the smoker inhales.[78] Because the smoke is diluted in the atmosphere, however, the passive smoker's actual "dose" is less than a smoker's exposure.[79] Thus, nonsmokers' health risks per person are smaller than the risks faced by smokers. Nevertheless, the number of individuals receiving passive exposure is larger than the number of smokers; therefore, more persons may be harmed through passive smoking.[80]

Many of the health effects of active smoking have been evaluated for nonsmokers exposed to environmental tobacco smoke. The most common effects associated with exposure to secondary smoke are eye, nose, and throat irritation.[81] For some persons, eye tearing can be so intense it is incapacitating.[82] In one study, 69 percent of the nonsmoking subjects suffered eye irritation and 31 percent reported headaches. The sensitivity increased for individuals with allergies.[83] Additionally, environmental tobacco smoke triggers immunological responses in some individuals, though the components of smoke eliciting these responses are unknown.[84]

Despite a wealth of data about the health effects of smoking to both smokers and passive inhalers, smoking in the workplace was largely unregulated until the 1980s. In less than a decade, however, over a dozen states and scores of municipalities have passed laws regulating smoking in the workplace.[85] By 1987, 75 percent of American companies either had a smoking policy or were considering adopting one.[86] As indicated in Table 3–7, the existence of a state or local law is one of the three main reasons why employers have adopted a policy on smoking.

As might be expected, the actual smoking policies adopted by employers vary widely.[87] A majority of the policies ban smoking in hallways, meeting rooms, restrooms, and customer and visitor

Table 3-7

Employer Reasons for Adopting a Smoking Policy

Reasons	Percent
Concern for employees' health/comfort	71
Complaints from employees	54
State or local law	39
Order by top executive	17
Insurance cost concerns	12
Absenteeism concerns	10
Productivity concerns	8
Other	10

Source: American Society for Personnel Administration/Bureau of National Affairs Survey (1987), cited in Bureau of National Affairs, *Where There's Smoke: Problems and Policies Concerning Smoking in the Workplace* 19 (2d ed. 1987).

areas; limit smoking in cafeterias to designated areas; and permit smoking in private offices and company vehicles.[88]

Restricting smoking in the workplace may protect the health and comfort of nonsmoking co workers and customers. It may even improve productivity and reduce fires and accidents. But employees who smoke, even if only off work, represent an increased cost for employers. According to Marvin M. Kristein, Professor of Economics at City University of New York, smokers use $500 to $600 more medical care each year than nonsmokers and they are absent from work more often than nonsmokers.[89] In addition, family members of a smoker are more likely to get heart disease, lung disease, lung cancer, and other illnesses.[90] Only with a work force of nonsmokers can these latter costs be eliminated.

In the last few years some public and private employers have begun to refuse to employ individuals who smoke off the job. Although the current number of employers with this policy appears to be small, the potential exists for a rapid growth in their number. According to one report, about 40 major employers currently hire only nonsmokers.[91] Other employers give a preference to nonsmokers. Many of the employers are hospitals and other health care providers, municipal police and fire departments, and insurance companies.[92]

There are four main reasons why employers have adopted policies of refusing to employ smokers: synergism with workplace exposures, "heart and lung" statutes, effectuating workplace smoking restrictions, and reducing health costs.

A number of studies have demonstrated the synergistic effect of cigarette smoking and occupational exposure to various substances. The best documented of these effects is with asbestos. Table 3–8 shows that smoking increased the death rate from lung cancer for both "blue collar" and asbestos workers by ten-fold. Asbestos workers had a five-fold higher death rate from lung cancer than other "blue collar" workers. Thus, smoking asbestos workers had a death rate 50 times higher than nonsmoking "blue collar" workers.

In addition to the synergistic effects of smoking and asbestos, gold mine, and certain rubber industry exposures, there may be additive effects from smoking and exposures to chlorine, cotton dust, coal dust, and other substances.[93] With the exception of miners (who never have been permitted to smoke on the job for safety reasons), there are few studies of workers who smoke only off work. Nevertheless, even off-work smoking is likely to produce the synergistic or additive health effects demonstrated with workplace smoking.

Table 3-8

Asbestos and Cigarette Smoking: Death Rate From Lung Cancer

Worker Group	No Smoking	Smoking
"Blue-collar" working men	11.3	122.6
Asbestos workers	58.4	601.6

Source: I. Selikoff, Disability Compensation for Asbestos-Related Disease in the United States 333, 335 (1982)(report to U.S. Department of Labor).

Note: Figures are per 100,000 man-years, standardized for age.

The foregoing suggests that industries in which employees work with substances shown to have a synergistic or additive effect with smoking may well be among the first to attempt to prohibit off-work smoking. A reduction in employee illness could mean substantial savings on workers' compensation; health, disability, and life insurance; personal injury litigation; and lost productivity. The Manville Corporation, with 8,000 employees, hires only non-smokers.[94] In 1987 the USG Acoustical Products Company (formerly United States Gypsum), which makes glass wool and mineral wool, ordered its 1,500 employees to stop smoking on and off the job after studies showed that the risk of lung disease from glass and mineral wool exposures was increased by smoking.[95]

Management's interest in off-work regulation is apparently not shared by workers, regardless of whether they smoke. According to a recent survey of workers in high risk industries, 82.0 percent supported restrictions on smoking in the workplace, but only 39.5 percent said that companies or unions should be concerned about smoking off the job.[96]

The second reason for refusing to employ smokers relates to workers' compensation law. Over half the states have enacted provisions in their workers' compensation laws creating an irrebuttable presumption that any cardiovascular or respiratory impairment suffered by a firefighter is work related.[97] These "heart and lung" statutes were enacted to provide a fringe benefit for incapacitated firefighters and to eliminate the difficult problems of proving the work-relatedness of an impairment where the individual was exposed to a variety of gases, vapors, and smoke.

Benefits mandated by heart and lung presumptions can be expensive and some state and local governments blame much of the expense on cigarette smoking. Because these laws make any impairment of the heart or lungs presumptively compensable as occupationally induced, smoking by employees can be extremely expensive to fire departments. In 1988 Massachusetts enacted a law that prohibits newly hired police officers and firefighters from smoking on or off the job.[98] Other states may follow suit.

Another reason for not employing individuals who smoke off the job is that it makes it easier to enforce bans on smoking *on* the job. Over 150 companies, including Boeing, Campbell Soup, and Adolph Coors, are entirely smoke free or limit smoking to certain lounges or cafeteria areas. Numerous other companies, including IBM, AT&T, and Honeywell, provide extensive smoke-free areas, including work stations.[99] According to its medical director, Dr. W. Edwin Magee, Ralston Purina banned all smoking at its corporate offices in St. Louis because: "We just finally decided that there was no way to separate smokers and nonsmokers."[100] For some companies, employing only nonsmokers might be the next logical step, especially if enforcing no-smoking rules becomes difficult.[101]

Finally, there is the issue of employee health costs. According to the health insurance industry, rates for both individual and group health insurance are six to 10 percent lower for nonsmokers[102] and reductions may be as high as 22 percent.[103] According to one estimate, health care cost savings per nonsmoking employee ranged from $75 to $150 annually.[104] In addition to these substantial savings, an employer with a work force of only nonsmokers would save considerable amounts on sick leave, absenteeism, turnover, and similar costs.[105] This additional savings is estimated to be $40-80 per worker annually.[106]

The legal issues raised by employer refusals to employ smokers are quite complicated[107] and need not be discussed at this point. The employment relations implications are enough to establish considerable doubt about the desirability of such policies. A crucial question that comes to mind concerning no-smoking policies is the following: How is an employer going to be able to verify whether employees are complying with their pledges to refuse to smoke off the job as well as on the job. There are a variety of possibilities, but the following three methods already have been used.

First, employers can rely on reports of employees being observed smoking. In *Grusendorf v. City of Oklahoma City*,[108] Greg Grusendorf was hired as a firefighter trainee by the city. He was required to sign an agreement not to smoke on or off duty during his first year of employment.[109] Grusendorf had quit smoking, in order to improve his physical condition, about three months before being hired. After two months of work, during unpaid lunch time, another city employee observed Grusendorf taking three puffs of a cigarette. When the incident was reported to the fire department, Grusendorf admitted the observed conduct and was discharged. The United States Court of Appeals for the Tenth Circuit upheld the discharge and ruled that Grusendorf had failed to prove that the city's policy was irrational.

Although in *Grusendorf* the observation was the result of happenstance, more elaborate systems for reporting off-work activities are not without precedent. For example, some companies have established "hotlines" to permit employees to report anonymously any drug use by coworkers.[110] Even if such a system were legal and effective in reducing drug abuse (or cigarette smoking), it is highly unlikely that the employee relations disruptions and other costs would justify its use.

A second way of checking on whether employees are genuine nonsmokers is to give them a polygraph. The Non-Smokers Inn, a 135-room motel in Dallas, hires only nonsmokers and gives applicants a polygraph to verify that they do not smoke.[111] It is not clear what the Inn will do now that the use of polygraphs violates federal law.

Third, because cigarette smoking causes detectable physiological changes, urine or blood tests could be used to detect the biochemical changes in body fluids caused by smoking.[112] Already there are reports of such testing[113] and it would be easy to test for smoking when other preemployment or periodic urine or blood tests were being performed. The proliferation of drug testing in recent years, however, has raised a storm of controversy. If courts and commentators have been reluctant to accept a public safety justification for random drug urinalysis, it is hard to imagine their approval of urinalysis to detect off-work cigarette smoking, where the risks are largely personal to the smoker and the harms are not immediate.

Cigarette smoking and other forms of tobacco use in the United States cause the deaths of about 1,000 people every day and cost the economy about $178 million daily. Serious and far-reaching measures are needed. Smoking should be discouraged, smoking cessation programs should be encouraged, and smoking in public places should be restricted. But refusing to employ smokers goes too far. It is especially inappropriate when viewed in the context of predictive screening for nonoccupational illness that, increasingly, equates employability with health insurance risks.

The Limits of Predictive Screening

Conclusions about the desirability of employee medical tests and other screening criteria, from legal, ethical, economic, and policy standpoints, depend to a great extent on the accuracy of the screening device. As discussed in Chapter 2, History, Physical, and Diagnostic Procedures, both laypersons and professionals often give much more credence to test results than they deserve. Moreover, the various medical screening tests vary widely in their accuracy, both in theory and in practice.

The starting point for analyzing the accuracy of a test is its sensitivity and specificity. The sensitivity of a test is a measure of the test's ability to correctly identify persons with the tested-for condition. It is the percent of persons with the condition who have a positive test, or:

$$\frac{\text{true positives}}{\text{true positives} + \text{false negatives}} \times 100\%$$

Therefore, if 100 persons have a condition and the test is able to identify 90 of them, the test would be 90% sensitive.

The specificity of a test is a measure of the test's ability to correctly identify persons free of a condition. It is the percent of persons free of the condition who have a negative test, or:

$$\frac{\text{true negatives}}{\text{true negatives} + \text{false positives}} \times 100\%$$

Therefore, if 100 persons are free of a condition and the test is able to identify 90 of them, the test would be 90% specific.

The predictive value (positive) of a test is the value of a positive test result in predicting the presence of the condition. It is the percent of those persons with a positive test who really have or will develop the condition, or:

$$\frac{\text{true positives}}{\text{true positives} + \text{false positives}} \times 100\%$$

In other words, when a test is positive, the predictive value represents the likelihood that the condition is actually present or will develop within a specified time interval.

One also needs to keep in mind the question to be answered by the test. A blood cholesterol test may have a high predictive value (positive) in correctly identifying individuals with elevated levels of serum cholesterol. It is quite another matter, however, to calculate whether an elevated cholesterol level predicts future heart disease.

Chapter 6 at the heading Drug Testing Technology contains a discussion of current drug testing technology. One of the most widely used screening tests is the EMIT (enzyme multiplied immunoassay technique) test, developed and marketed by the Syva Company. According to independent studies,[114] the EMIT test has a sensitivity of about 99% and a specificity of about 90%.[115] The predictive value (positive) of the test, however, varies greatly depending on the prevalence of drug usage in the tested population. Tables illustrate 3–9 and 3–10 illustrate how important prevalence is to the predictive value of a test.

Table 3–9 assumes a 50 percent prevalence—perhaps individuals in a drug treatment program or, if in a workplace setting, individuals selected for testing based upon reasonable suspicion. The test correctly identifies 4,950 of the 5,000 true positives, with 50 false negatives. It correctly identifies 4,500 of the 5,000 true negatives, with 500 false positives. Therefore, of the 5,450 positives, 4,950 are true positives. The predictive value (positive) of the test is 4,950/5,450 or 90.8 percent.

Table 3–10 assumes a 5 percent prevalence—a reasonable estimate of the prevalence of recent users of any particular illicit drug among job applicants.[116] The test correctly identifies 495 of the 500 true positives, with 5 false negatives. It correctly identifies 8,550 of the 9,500 true negatives, with 950 false positives. Therefore, of the 1,445 positives, only 495 are true positives and 950 are false positives. The predictive value (positive) of the test is 495/1445 or 34.3 percent. According to Table 3–10, two out of three positives identified by the test will be false positives. Although confirmatory testing will increase the specificity and predictive value (positive) of the test, many companies do not want to pay for the more expensive confirmatory tests, especially for applicants.

Table 3-9

Predictive Value of EMIT Test With 99% Sensitivity, 90% Specificity, 50% Prevalence, and 10,000 Subjects

Subjects	Test Results	
5,000 +	True Positives 4,950	False Negatives 50
5,000 −	False Positives 500	True Negatives 4,500

Table 3-10

Predictive Value of EMIT Test With 99% Sensitivity, 90% Specificity, 5% Prevalence, and 10,000 Subjects

Subjects	Test Results	
500 +	True Positives 495	False Negatives 5
9,500 −	False Positives 950	True Negatives 8,550

The infamous polygraph provides another good example of how statistics can be used to point out the shortcomings of a test. Analog (simulation) and field studies of polygraph "accuracy" have a range of 50 percent to 90 percent.[117] Table 3–11 assumes a sensitivity of 80 percent and a specificity of 80 percent. Assume that 1,000 applicants for jobs as janitors in day care centers are asked if they have ever molested a child. Further assume that one percent of the applicants *have* molested children. (In polygraphs, this is referred to as the base rate of guilt.)[118]

Of the 206 individuals with a positive test only eight would be true child molesters. The predictive value (positive) of the test is

---

Table 3-11

Predictive Value of Polygraph With 80% Sensitivity, 80% Specificity, 1% Prevalence, and 1,000 Subjects

Subjects	Test Results	
10 +	True Positives 8	False Negatives 2
990 −	False Positives 198	True Negatives 792

3.88 percent. While the predictive value (negative) is 792/794 or 99.7 percent, the predictive value (negative) of using nothing is 99.0 percent. Note also, that if the question is changed to: "Are you an agent of a foreign government?" (assumed base rate of guilt of 1 in 1,000), the predictive value (positive) falls to 0.4 percent.

Polygraphs are inadmissible in criminal cases because they are thought to be inaccurate, but they have been used extensively in other (including preemployment) settings. Ironically, it is in the criminal area that the polygraph is most predicitve. Through the use of detective work, the number of suspects is narrowed and therefore the base rate of guilt (or prevalence) increases and, with it, the predictive value (positive) of the test.[119]

These same principles apply to more established methods of medical screening. "Indiscriminate use of laboratory tests on subjects selected at random is doomed to failure if the prevalence of the disease is low."[120] Medical detective work— the history and physical examination—*first* should identify individuals for whom testing, such as chest or back x-rays, are indicated. For example, American Occupational Medical Association guidelines recommend that preplacement chest x-rays should be taken *selectively* based on the individual's occupational and medical history, clinical examination, and proposed work assignment.[121] The nonselective use of medical tests and procedures compromises their predictive ability (by increasing the number of false positives), is a waste of resources, and in the case of x-rays, needlessly exposes individuals to risks.[122]

4

Genetic Testing

Biochemical Genetics: 1963–1983

Since at least 1917, scientists have speculated that genetic factors may predispose workers to occupational disease.[1] In 1938 the geneticist J.B.S. Haldane first suggested the possibility of genetic screening of workers as a way of preventing occupational illness.

> "The majority of potters do not die of bronchitis. It is quite possible that if we really understood the causation of this disease, we should find that only a fraction of potters are of a constitution which renders them liable to it. If so, we could eliminate potters' bronchitis by rejecting entrants into the pottery industry who are congenitally disposed to it."[2]

Even if there had been an interest in genetic screening of the kind suggested by Haldane, scientists lacked the technical means to do so. During the next 25 years most of the emphasis on genetic variability in relation to environmental exposures was confined to pharmacogenetics, the effect of individuals' genetic make-ups on their responses to pharmaceuticals.[3]

In 1963 Dr. Herbert E. Stokinger, then chief toxicologist with the Public Health Service and executive secretary of the American Conference of Governmental Industrial Hygienists (ACGIH), and John T. Mountain published the first of several articles advocating the use of genetic screening to identify individuals who were "hypersusceptible" to occupational chemicals.[4] Three specific tests were proposed to reduce worker exposures to hemolytic chemicals: glucose-6-phosphate dehydrogenase (G-6-PD) testing, glutathione (GSH) instability testing, and methemoglobin reduction testing. Ten years later, Dr. Stokinger and L.D. Scheel published a "consensus report," which they claimed represented national and international opinion on the subject.[5] They complained that despite the scientific evidence only three

U.S. chemical companies used the tests and only one used them for screening purposes.[6] The "unbelievably bad response" was blamed on the "ultra-conservative American physician" who ignored the scientific evidence to avoid any confrontation with labor unions.[7] On the subject of employment discrimination the authors stated that "the tests do not deny employment; they merely orient job placement to the advantage of both the employer and the employed."[8] Employers were encouraged to screen for even more genetic traits: alpha$_1$ antitrypsin deficiency, G-6-PD deficiency, carbon disulfide sensitivity, reagenic antibodies to allergenic chemicals, and sickle cell trait.

In 1978 an article in the *Journal of Occupational Medicine* by Dr. Charles Reinhardt indicated that Du Pont had conducted sickle cell testing of black employees.[9] In February 1980, Richard Severo published a series of four articles in the *New York Times*,[10] which moved the issue of genetic testing in employment from the pages of obscure professional journals to front page news. It was not known, however, the extent to which genetic testing actually was being used in industry.

The almost-immediate public clamor surrounding genetic testing led to a series of congressional hearings in 1981 and 1982 before the Subcommittee on Investigations and Oversight of the House Committee on Science and Technology, chaired by then-Representative Albert Gore, Jr.[11] The Office of Technology Assessment (OTA) also was asked to conduct a detailed study of genetic testing. As a part of its study, in 1982 OTA conducted an anonymous survey of the "Fortune 500" companies, the 50 largest private utilities, and 11 major labor unions.[12] Of the 366 (65.2 percent) organizations responding, six (1.6 percent) were currently using biochemical or cytogenetic tests, 17 (4.6 percent) had used the tests in the past 12 years, and 59 (16.1 percent) said they would consider using the tests in the next five years. Of the specific tests performed, sickle cell testing was the most prevalent, followed by G-6-PD, alpha$_1$ antitrypsin deficiency, unspecified immune system markers, and cytogenetic testing for chromosomal aberrations.

In April 1983, OTA issued its final report, *The Role of Genetic Testing in the Prevention of Occupational Disease*, which concluded: "None of the genetic tests evaluated by OTA meets established scientific criteria for routine use in an occupational setting. However, there is enough suggestive evidence to merit further research."[13] There was insufficient evidence that bio-chemical genetic traits, such as sickle cell trait or G-6-PD defi-ciency, would predispose an individual to occupational disease when exposed to certain hazardous environments.[14] Moreover, serious legal and ethical concerns were raised because each of the various biochemical genetic traits or conditions (and the tests used to identify them) tended to have a disparate effect along racial or ethnic lines. Genetic monitoring of previously exposed workers to detect chromosomal changes induced by workplace exposures, a lesser focus of the study, was thought to hold prom-ise as a diagnostic tool, but the technology was still viewed as being in its infancy.

Inadequate scientific data and overwhelmingly adverse pub-licity are the two main reasons why most observers concluded that genetic testing in the workplace had virtually stopped by the mid-1980s.[15] Certainly, any companies still performing genetic tests were not about to admit it by name. A 1987–88 survey of 245 personnel and industrial relations executives found that only three companies admitted using genetic screening.[16] The survey did not ask what screening was performed or why.

Recombinant DNA Technology: 1983–1993

The ink had hardly dried on the OTA report when, in the fall of 1983, Dr. James Gusella and his colleagues at Massachusetts General Hospital announced a major breakthrough in the fast-moving field of molecular genetics.[17] Using recombinant DNA technology, they had identified a genetic marker closely identi-fied with Huntington's disease. Although this was not the first time a genetic disease marker had been discovered, Huntington's disease was a unique case. An autosomal dominant disease, any affected individual's or carrier's offspring would have a 50 percent chance of inheriting a variant dominant allele. In such an event, the individual would eventually develop Huntington's disease, an incurable neurological disease. Because the disease does not man-ifest itself until the late 30s or early 40s, previously, there was no way to know whether the individual had inherited the gene for Huntington's. After this discovery, using familial linkage studies, a prediction could be made with at least 95 percent accuracy about whether the individual was a carrier who would develop the disease.

Another breakthrough occurred in 1983 when Dr. Michael Brown and Dr. Joseph Goldstein, geneticists at the University of Texas Health Science Center in Dallas, identified several mutations in a gene involved in the premature onset of atherosclerosis. About one in 500 individuals carries the mutant gene, which prevents the efficient removal of low-density lipoproteins. Such people are prone to heart attacks in their 30s. Brown and Goldstein won the Nobel Prize in medicine for this discovery.

After 1983 all the assumptions about the workplace application of genetic testing had changed. We had entered a decade of recombinant DNA technology development. Important biochemical genetic research continues, such as that involving pharmacogenetic polymorphisms associated with an increased risk of cancer. Nevertheless, after 1983 the main focus of research was no longer testing for the biochemical manifestations of genetic diseases (e.g., enzyme deficiencies, variant proteins, cellular surface antigens), but probing the DNA itself. In other words, as related to the workplace, the emphasis was quickly shifting from genetic susceptibility to occupational illness to genetic predetermination or predisposition to nonoccupational illness.

Before recombinant DNA technology was developed there were two types of genetic tests available.[18] The first test examined the structure or activity of the defective gene protein. This approach has been used in the testing of, for example, sickle cell anemia, the thalassemias, and Tay Sachs disease. The second method measured the concentration of low molecular weight compounds to identify individuals who have abnormal concentrations of these compounds due to a defective gene. This method has been used to screen for phenylketonuria (PKU) in the newborn by measuring the concentration of phenylalanine in the blood. These techniques are only useful if the defect is present in accessible tissues such as blood or urine. If gene expression cannot be demonstrated in accessible tissues the tests cannot be used to predict a genetic disorder in asymptomatic individuals.

Recombinant technologies do not rely on gene expression because the tests detect alterations in nucleotide sequences in the DNA itself. Each individual's nucleated cells contain a full complement of DNA and this information is identical in all of the individual's somatic cells, as long as no somatic cell mutations have occurred. Therefore, DNA tests can be performed on any nucleated cell in any tissue. For example, it is possible to obtain and test white blood cells or the cells of the villi of the chorionic membrane surrounding the fetus as soon as the ninth week of pregnancy.

Eventually, direct gene probes will be able to focus directly on the specific gene. More commonly, however, linkage studies generally have been developed first. To perform linkage studies, both affected and unaffected members in families in which the disease has occurred must be studied. These studies examine segments of the genome where normal variations (polymorphisms) in the nucleotide base sequences exist. These sequences are examined until one segment is found in affected members which has an allele of the DNA variant linked to the disease or defect in question. Those family members that do not have the disease have a different allele in this segment. This segment is said to be the linkage between the locus where the disease-causing allele is located and the polymorphism. It serves as a marker for the disease locus and can be used for other families having a disease which results from a mutation at the same gene locus. Once the defect is localized to a region near a marker, the gene responsible for the disease can be identified.

Over 1,000 such markers now exist, in the form of biochemical signposts called restriction fragment length polymorphisms (RFLPs), and more are being identified each week. Each RFLP defines a specific site on the human genome where a variation in the DNA sequence occurs. If the RFLP happens to be situated close to a disease-causing gene, the inheritance of the RFLP can help predict passage of the gene from parent to child.

Recombinant DNA technology already has been applied to a variety of genetic diseases, including Huntington's disease,[19] Alzheimer's disease,[20] retinoblastoma,[21] hypercholesterolemia,[22] adult polycystic kidney disease,[23] hemophilia A,[24] Duchenne muscular dystrophy,[25] cystic fibrosis,[26] neurofibromatosis,[27] and manic depression.[28] DNA probes now can be used to screen for 30 genetic diseases during the first trimester of pregnancy.[29] Table 4–1 lists some of the currently available genetic tests.

With these important discoveries, many scientists are eager to embark on an even more ambitious project—mapping and sequencing the entire genome. The project could cost as much as $3 billion and would be extremely intricate. The human genome

Table 4–1

Some Available Genetic Tests by Type of Test, 1988

Test type	Disease
Linkage RFLP tests:	Becker's muscular dystrophy
	Carbamyl phosphate synthetase deficiency
	Chronic granulomatous disease
	Cystic fibrosis
	Fragile X syndrome
	Hemophilia A and B
	Huntington's disease
	Myotonic dystrophy
	Neurofibromatosis
	Polycystic kidney disease (adult)
Direct tests:	Alpha$_1$ antitrypsin deficiency
	Duchenne muscular dystrophy
	Growth hormone deficiency
	Lesch-Nyhan disease
	Ornithine transcarbamylase (OTC) deficiency
	Retinoblastoma
	Sickle cell anemia
	Thalassemia (some forms)
Tests for very tightly linked polymorphisms:	Hemoglobinopathies
	Phenylketonuria (PKU)
	Thalassemias

Source: Office of Technology Assessment, U.S. Congress, Medical Testing and Health Insurance 138 (1988).

consists of more than 3 billion nucleotides. If it were an encyclopedia, the entire sequence would take up more than 500 volumes, with each volume 1,000 pages in length and each page having 1,000 words of the six-letter DNA language.[30] In 1987 the first genetic linkage map spanning the entire human genome was completed.[31] Its markers, about 9 million base pairs apart, provide a rough frame on which the "cosmid" map can be constructed, which will have a resolution of about 50,000 base pairs.[32]

The effort, expense, and effect on other research of a gene sequencing project has caused much debate in the scientific community.[33] Dr. James D. Watson, who along with Dr. Francis H.C. Crick discovered the chemical structure of DNA in 1953, is convinced of the merits of the project. "It has got to go ahead, it is so obvious. The only question now is the rate and under whose auspices."[34] In September 1988, Dr. Watson was appointed to direct the human genome project of the National Institutes of Health.

Applied Genetics: 1993 and Beyond

Undoubtedly, much good will result from emerging discoveries in genetics. Reproductive planning, disease prevention, and gene therapy to treat previously untreatable diseases are all possible. To see the possible benefits of genetic testing, one need only look at the success of phenylketonuria (PKU) screening of newborns. Mass screening is feasible, despite an incidence of only one in 11,500, because of the discovery by Guthrie in 1961 of a bacterial growth inhibition assay for measuring blood phenylalinine. A low phenylalanine diet begun in the first few weeks of life can prevent mental retardation in affected children.[35] PKU screening is now legally mandated in every state.

According to a 1988 survey of biotechnology firms involved in developing future genetic tests, by the early 1990s genetic testing is expected to double.[36] With about 4,000 known genetic diseases, there is a tremendous potential for genetic testing. Table 4–2 provides an indication of that potential.

Preconception, prenatal, neonatal, and carrier screening all raise extraordinarily complicated issues of medicine, ethics, law, economics, religion, and social policy. To take just one example, women who decide to have prenatal genetic screening, which reveals a genetic disease, will often choose to have an abortion. Termination rates for muscular dystrophy, cystic fibrosis, and alpha and beta thalassemia are nearly 100 percent; they are 60 percent for hemophilia; and 50 percent for sickle cell anemia.[37] What if the disease is a late-onset disease, such as Huntington's disease, or the condition is not fatal, such as Down's syndrome, or the test only reveals a "predisposition" to cancer or heart disease? According to Barbara Katz Rothman, author of The Tentative Pregnancy, this puts a "terrible burden" on women. "You are asking them to evaluate what kind of life is worth living."[38]

Table 4-2

Genetic Tests Available and Total Americans Affected

Genetic Condition	Total Cases
Currently Available	
Adult polycystic kidney disease	500,000
Fragile X syndrome	100,000
Sickle cell anemia	65,000
Duchenne muscular dystrophy	32,000
Cystic fibrosis	30,000
Huntington's disease	25,000
Hemophilia	20,000
Phenylketonuria	16,000
Retinoblastoma	10,000
Potential Future Tests	
Hypertension	58 million
Dyslexia	15 million
Atherosclerosis	6.7 million
Cancer	5 million
Manic-depressive illness	2 million
Schizophrenia	1.5 million
Type 1 diabetes	1 million
Familial Alzheimer's	250,000
Multiple sclerosis	250,000
Myotonic muscular dystrophy	100,000

Source: Med. World News, Apr. 11, 1988, at 58. Reprinted by permission.

As if these questions were not difficult enough, it is inevitable that there will be time lags between initial discoveries in genetics and more usable or meaningful information. For instance, genetic testing through linkage studies will often precede the availability of a direct gene probe. Do family members have a duty to participate in linkage studies? Is there a duty to inform family members of test results? Another time lag problem arises because testing will be available long before a cure or treatment. According to Dr. Kurt Hirschhorn of Mount Sinai Medical Center: "If you're going to screen, it must be for a condition you can do something about."[39] But even if mass screening may be inappropriate, many individuals will want to know their fate. Will adequate counseling be available? What are the social implications of having this information? How will the confidentiality of this information be maintained?

Nobel Laureate Walter Gilbert has called the human genome the "Rosetta stone of biological information."[40] With medical science on the verge of deciphering the genetic code, profoundly difficult questions arise concerning the use of the information. Resolution of these questions will be inextricably intertwined with society's emerging ethic on access to health care, discrimination, and allocation of resources and opportunities.

An article appearing in the *Journal of the American Medical Association* a century ago recognized that information about an individual's genetic predisposition to disease would have great practical value. The article noted that "in each individual there are certain constitutional peculiarities, congenital and not acquired, which govern not only the course and termination of disease, but likewise the susceptibility to its invasion. . . . [This information would be] of no small importance to life insurance companies."[41]

With regard to life insurance, even if insurers were denied access to previously run genetic tests, they would likely want to perform the testing themselves. Insurers argue that they need to know any risk information possessed by the insured because their entire industry is based on risk assessment. If life expectancy based on genetic factors could not be determined, then life insurers would not necessarily be concerned. They could rely on standard mortality tables. But, when such information is available, insurers must assume that applicants have this information and thus the insurance company would need it too. This illustrates the principle of "adverse selection" or "anti-selection," in which those who know that they are at greatest risk are likely to seek the most insurance. Without equal access to medical information, insurers could not engage in the necessary risk underwiting and would either lose substantial amounts of money or would raise the premiums of all policyholders so that low-risk policyholders subsidize the rates of those at high risk.

Insurance is risk sharing against unknown contingencies. If individual life expectancy can be estimated by using genetic tests, there will be far fewer unknown contingencies. Eventually, life insurance may be primarily for accidents and diseases with little genetic component.

The issues in health insurance are different. Life insurance is not a necessity; health insurance is. Access to quality health care depends on access to health insurance. Genetic testing to exclude individuals from health insurance (more likely for individual health insurance), will have major social consequences. According to Dr. Le Roy Walters of Georgetown University's Kennedy Institute of Ethics: "To have insurance companies free to screen would seem to me to sentence people who couldn't do anything about their genes to facing potentially very large costs. The development of these new diagnostic techniques may bring to a point questions of what approach we as a society want to take to people born with a genetic disease."[42] Issues concerning insurance are further explored in Chapter 10.

With respect to genetic testing by employers, if the cost is low, the accuracy is high, and the testing can be done quickly and easily, it must be assumed that many employers would have an interest. After all, genetic screening is the ultimate predictive screening technique and, as discussed earlier, employers have shown a substantial interest in other, less promising screening methods. Moreover, future developments in genetics may relate to areas already of interest to employers, such as a genetic predisposition to alcoholism, tobacco-induced lung cancer, or mental illness.

Current employment laws are inadequate to deal with the myriad new issues that are certain to be raised by genetic testing. Four states have laws prohibiting discrimination based on genetic traits. Florida,[43] Louisiana,[44] and North Carolina[45] prohibit discrimination based on sickle cell trait. These laws were passed in the early 1970s when sickle cell testing was being widely encouraged and were an attempt to prevent any resulting discrimination. New Jersey's law,[46] passed in 1981, prohibits discrimination in employment based on all of the following genetic traits: sickle cell, hemoglobin C, thalassemia, Tay Sachs, or cystic fibrosis.

Other, more general, employment discrimination laws may not extend to discrimination based on genetic factors. It is clear that an individual with a genetic disease would be considered "handicapped" under federal and state handicap discrimination laws, but it is not clear whether an individual with a specific ge-

notype would be considered "handicapped." (For a further discussion, see Chapter 7.) Title VII of the Civil Rights Act of
1964,[47] which prohibits discrimination based on race, color,
religion, sex, and national origin, affords protection against discriminatory use of biochemical genetic tests because of the disparate impact of many of the tests.[48] The relevance of Title VII
would depend on showing a similar disparate impact of a particular gene probe.

Legal regulation of genetic testing by employers will depend
on what public policies are ultimately developed on genetic testing generally. The public debate is destined to be a lively one.
According to Dr. Arthur Caplan of the University of Minnesota,
when genetic tests are available for susceptibility to heart disease,
depression, or alcoholism, "drug testing is going to look like
happy holiday."[49]

In a sense, genetic screening will require society to make a
judgment about how it wants to treat individuals who are currently asymptomatic but who are likely to become ill at some
point in the future. Ironically, we will need to make decisions
about this issue before the perfection of genetic technology. The
impetus will be AIDS. Dr. Nancy Wexler, president of the
Hereditary Diseases Foundation, has observed: "In a bizarre way,
AIDS may be setting a precedent for genetic diseases."[50]

5

AIDS

need for info

Background

The epidemic of acquired immune deficiency syndrome (AIDS) is the most dramatic, pervasive, and tragic medical event in recent history. AIDS has caused a reassessment of our society's approaches to public health strategy, health care resource allocation, medical research, and sexual behavior. It has affected virtually all of our institutions and our culture. Sadly, those effects will continue to be felt for the foreseeable future.

The first cases of AIDS were identified in 1981,[1] but after 10 years there will have been at least 270,000 cases of AIDS in the United States, causing more than 179,000 deaths.[2] There are currently one to two million people in the United States infected with the human immunodeficiency virus (HIV) associated with AIDS and most of these people will probably die of AIDS-related causes. Indeed, the "null hypothesis" postulates that all who have HIV will eventually succomb to AIDS.

Three distinct conditions after infection with HIV are the seropositive state, AIDS-related complex (ARC), and clinical or "full blown" AIDS.[3] In the seropositive state, blood tests reveal the presence of antibodies to HIV, indicating infection with that virus. Most people become seropositive within two or three months of infection. As many as 10 million people world-wide are estimated to be seropositive. Although a seropositive person does not show symptoms of ARC or AIDS and may not develop such symptoms for many years, he or she does carry the virus and can transmit it to others.

A person who is seropositive may develop ARC or AIDS. ARC causes moderate damage to the immune system and is characterized by nonspecific symptoms of illness. Under the Centers for Disease Control (CDC) definition for ARC, at least two of the following clinical signs lasting three or more months must be present: fever,

81

weight loss, lymphadenopathy, diarrhea, fatigue, and night sweats. There must be two laboratory findings: a low number of T-helper cells and a low ratio of T-helper to T-suppressor cells. Additionally, there must be at least one of the following: low white blood cell count, low red blood cell count, low platelet count, and elevated levels of serum globulins.

Clinical AIDS represents a major collapse of the immune system, which allows opportunistic infections and Kaposi's sarcoma (a rare dermal malignancy) to invade the body. About half of all patients die from *pneumocystis carinii* pneumonia, which is extremely rare in persons whose immune systems are working properly.[4] The incubation period for the disease—the time between the initial infection by the virus and the onset of AIDS—has so far been reported to be up to seven years, with the average being four and a half years. AIDS is fatal, on average, two years after diagnosis.

The virus spreads from infected persons either by anal or vaginal intercourse or by the introduction of infected blood (or blood products) through the skin and into the bloodstream, which may occur in intravenous (IV) drug use, blood transfusion, or treatment of hemophilia. In addition, it can spread from an infected mother to her infant during pregnancy or at the time of birth. Studies show no evidence that the infection is transmitted by so-called casual contact—that is, contact that can be even quite close between persons in the course of daily activities. Thus, there is no evidence that the virus is transmitted in the air, by sneezing, by shaking hands, by sharing a drinking glass, by insect bites, or by living in the same household with an AIDS sufferer or an HIV-infected person.[5]

Because HIV is transmitted almost exclusively in certain narrow circumstances, the CDC has been able to classify almost all people with AIDS into six groups: (1) sexually active homosexual and bisexual men (74 percent); (2) heterosexual intravenous drug abusers who share injection needles (17 percent); (3) heterosexuals who have intercourse with people who are seropositive or at high risk (four percent); (4) hemophiliacs who have received contaminated blood-clotting factor products (one percent); (5) other people who have received transfusions of contaminated blood (two percent); and (6) newborn infants of infected mothers (one percent).[6]

Although new anti-viral medications have prolonged the survival of people with AIDS, neither a cure nor a vaccine is likely in the near future. Education programs and safe practices to prevent new cases of HIV infection offer the only realistic approach to control the spread of the epidemic.[7] The scientific development with the greatest effect on prevention remains the discovery of a method of screening blood for HIV, which has been used to prevent the spread of infection through transfused blood and blood products.[8]

In March 1985, after several months of testing, the Food and Drug Administration (FDA) approved the first of the blood tests for commercial use. Although the approved tests differ slightly, all use the Enzyme-Linked Immunosorbent Assay (ELISA) technique to detect antibodies to HIV.[9] The test measures the presence of antibodies stimulated by the AIDS virus. The ELISA test is relatively inexpensive, costing between two and three dollars a test.[10] To be accurate, however, an ELISA test with a positive result should be repeated and then confirmed by another test procedure. The most commonly used confirmation test, the Western Blot, is much more expensive (about $100), difficult, and time-consuming to perform.[11] The Western Blot identifies proteins of a specific molecular weight and therefore helps to eliminate false positives.[12]

It is important to note what the HIV antibody test does and does not measure. First, the test does not identify individuals with AIDS. As mentioned earlier, the CDC defines AIDS by its clinical symptoms. While a positive antibody test may help support a diagnosis, the test is not a primary diagnostic tool.[13] Further, a positive test does not necessarily mean that a person will get AIDS in the future.

Second, the test does not identify individuals with ARC, whose definition is also based on clinical features and by laboratory abnormalities indicative of immunodeficiency. The test does not necessarily predict ARC, either.

Third, the test does not identify all blood containing the AIDS virus. Since it was designed to detect only nonneutralizing antibodies stimulated by the virus, the test would not identify an individual as positive during the period of time between exposure to the virus and seroconversion—the development of antibodies— which usually takes from six to eight weeks, but may take a year or more.[14] It also would not identify as positive individuals whose immune systems were so severely damaged by the virus that they were not producing antibodies.[15]

New, improved HIV tests are being developed. The polymerase chain reaction (PCR) test, for example, is believed to be faster and more accurate than other tests because it measures the

HIV's genetic material in DNA molecules, rather than measuring antibodies. With PCR, it is possible to detect the virus while it is still dormant. Better test techniques are important from a medical standpoint, but one essential legal and policy issue is largely unaffected by an advance in test technology—how to deal with asymptomatic seropositive individuals.

AIDS and the Workplace

Any discussion of AIDS would be incomplete without mentioning the psychological effects of the epidemic. AIDS has a stigma shared by few other diseases in modern times.[16] The fact that AIDS is fatal, it is sexually transmitted, and, in the United States, it is concentrated in homosexual and bisexual men and intravenous drug users—unpopular groups—no doubt contributes to the stigma. The result has been irrational ignorance, fear, and discrimination. Tables 5–1 and 5–2, based on some recent polls, demonstrate the continuing public fears of and misconceptions about AIDS.

Table 5–1

Public Views on Transmissibility of AIDS

"It is likely that someone would contract AIDS from . . ."

Conduct	Percent
Kissing with saliva exchange	69
Shared utensils	47
Eating at a restaurant where the cook had AIDS	36
Mosquitos and insects	35
Public toilets	31
Blood donation	26
Working near a person with AIDS	18

Source: Public Health Service (Nov. 1987); Centers for Disease Control (Jan. 1988).

Table 5–2

Fears Concerning Contact With Employees Known to Have AIDS

	Yes(%)	No(%)
Would you be concerned about using the same bathroom?	66	34
Would you be concerned about eating in the same cafeteria?	40	60
Would you be willing to share tools or equipment with the individual?	63	37
Would you favor making special work arrangements for the individual if his or her health deteriorated?	75	25
Do you believe the reported evidence that AIDS can only be transmitted by sexual contact or blood contamination?	65	35

Source: D. Herold, Employees' Reactions to AIDS in the Workplace 5–7 (Center for Work Performance Problems, Feb. 1988). Reprinted by permission.

Not surprisingly, polls of employees reveal similar fears about working with someone with AIDS. These fears persist despite the fact that since the 1985 publication of its *Guidelines on AIDS in the Workplace*,[17] the CDC has continued to emphasize that HIV cannot be spread by casual contact in the workplace and that HIV testing is not recommended for health care, personal service, food service, and other workers.

More surprising are the views on AIDS of top executives of some of the nations' largest corporations. While several thoughtful and well-conceived programs have been adopted at companies of all sizes, Table 5–3 indicates that even by 1988 many of our leading executives had given little thought to AIDS or they favored irrational or illegal practices.

Although Congress has shown concern about AIDS, particularly in funding research and health care, most of the legislative activity regarding AIDS has taken place at the state level. In 1987 alone, more than 550 bills were introduced in state legislatures and

Table 5–3

AIDS Policies of Corporate CEOs

Answer	Percent
1. Does your company have an AIDS policy?	
Yes, written	10
Yes, unwritten	8
Developing one	11
No	71
2. Should the company have an active AIDS education program?	
Yes	41
No	15
Neutral	38
3. What is the company policy with regard to HIV testing?	
Test job applicants	2
Would not hire HIV positives	39
Not sure whether HIV positives would be hired	38
Test current employees	1
Favor testing current employees in the future	8

Source: Allstate Insurance Co./Fortune Magazine (Jan. 1988). Reprinted by permission.

more than 90 of them were enacted, addressing various AIDS-related issues such as antibody testing, blood banks, confidentiality, housing, informed consent, insurance, marriage, prisons, and reporting.[18]

The states also have taken the lead in prohibiting AIDS-based discrimination in employment. At least nine states (California,[19] Delaware,[20] Florida,[21] Iowa,[22] Massachusetts,[23] Rhode Island,[24] Vermont,[25] Washington,[26] Wisconsin[27]) have enacted laws prohibiting HIV testing or other forms of discrimination in employment based on AIDS or HIV infection. Texas[28] prohibits employers from performing or using HIV tests unless the employer can prove that being uninfected is a bona fide occupational qualification (BFOQ), which would be extremely difficult to prove. A number of cities, including Austin,[29] Los Angeles,[30] Philadelphia,[31] and San Francisco[32] also have ordinances prohibiting discrimination in employment based on AIDS.

Besides these specific laws, federal and state laws prohibiting discrimination in employment on the basis of handicap have been held to prohibit discrimination based on AIDS. (Federal and state handicap discrimination laws are discussed in greater detail in Chapter 7.) In *School Board v. Arline*,[33] Gene Arline, an elementary school teacher in Nassau County, Florida, was discharged after a third relapse of tuberculosis. The school board based its decision on fear that students or co-employees might contract the disease. Arline sued under section 504 of the federal Rehabilitation Act of 1973, alleging that the school board had engaged in unlawful handicap discrimination. The United States district court ruled in favor of the school board; United States Court of Appeals for the the the Eleventh Circuit reversed.[34]

When the Supreme Court agreed to hear the *Arline* case, many observers believed that, in addressing the issue of whether the Rehabilitation Act applied to contagious diseases, the Supreme Court would decide whether AIDS is a "handicap" under federal law. The Court, however, expressly declined to address the issue of AIDS,[35] but the analysis in its opinion would unmistakenly apply to cases involving AIDS.[36]

The Court held, based on the Act's legislative history and statutory intent, that contagious illnesses are handicaps covered under section 504.

> "By amending the definition of 'handicapped individual' to include not only those who are actually physically impaired, but also those who are regarded as impaired and who, as a result, are substantially limited in a major life activity, Congress acknowledged that society's accumulated myths and fears about disability and disease are as handicapping as are the physical limitations that flow from actual impairment. Few aspects of a handicap give rise to the same level of public fear and misapprehension as contagiousness. Even those who suffer or have recovered from such noninfectious diseases as epilepsy or cancer have faced discrimination based on the irrational fear that they might be contagious. The Act is carefully structured to replace such reflexive reactions to actual or perceived handicaps with actions based on reasoned and medically sound judgments. . . ."[37]

The Court went on to point out, however, that only individuals who are both handicapped and otherwise qualified are eligible for relief. The case was remanded for a determination of whether reasonable accommodation will eliminate the risk of contagion.[38]

The Court specifically adopted the four factors suggested in the American Medical Association's *amicus curiae* brief to determine whether a person handicapped with a contagious disease is otherwise qualified: (1) the nature of the risk (how the disease is transmitted); (2) the duration of the risk (how long is the carrier infectious); (3) the severity of the risk (what is the potential harm to third parties); and (4) the probabilities the disease will be transmitted and will cause varying degrees of harm.[39]

On remand, the United States District Court for the Middle District of Florida held that Arline was otherwise qualified and posed no threat of communicating tuberculosis to her students. She was on medication, her medical tests indicated only one colony surrounded by negative cultures, none of her family tested positive, and she had limited exposure to students. The court ordered the school board to reinstate Arline or give her the amount of her salary until she reaches retirement age— $768,724.[40]

Post-*Arline* cases have applied these factors to hold as unlawful under the Rehabilitation Act discrimination on the basis of AIDS. For example, in *Chalk v. United States District Court*,[41] Vincent Chalk, a teacher of hearing-impaired students in Orange County, California, was barred from the classroom and reassigned to administrative duties after he was hospitalized with *pneumocystis carinii* pneumonia and diagnosed as having AIDS. The United States Court of Appeals for the Ninth Circuit reversed a district court's denial of an injunction ordering reinstatement. It held that there was no showing of a risk of harm to the students and that possible fear and apprehension among parents and students was an inadequate justification for his reassignment.[42]

In 1988 Congress passed the Civil Rights Restoration Act over the veto of President Reagan.[43] One provision of that law, section 9, amends the Rehabilitation Act to clarify the coverage of individuals with contagious diseases.

"(C) For the purpose of sections 503 and 504, as such sections relate to employment, such term does not include an individual who has a currently contagious disease or infection and who, by reason of such disease or infection, would constitute a direct threat to the health or safety of other individuals or who, by reason of the currently contagious disease or infection, is unable to perform the duties of the job."[44]

Based on this amendment, an individual with a contagious disease is covered by sections 503 and 504 so long as the individual does not pose a direct threat to the health or safety of others and is able to perform the duties of the job. Furthermore, the legislative history of this provision, sponsored by Senators Tom Harkin of Iowa and Gordon Humphrey of New Hampshire, makes it clear that the amendment "does nothing to change the current laws regarding reasonable accommodation."[45]

At the state level, virtually every state to consider the issue has held that AIDS and AIDS-related conditions are handicaps.[46] Only in a state such as Tennessee, which statutorily excludes all infectious, contagious, or "similarly transmittable" diseases or conditions from the definition of "handicap,"[47] would AIDS not be a protected handicap. While the federal cases are the trend-setters, most of the AIDS cases are adjudicated or resolved under state or local handicap or AIDS laws. The number of these cases continues to grow. National figures are unavailable, but in 1987, New York City's Human Rights Commission handled 600 cases of AIDS discrimination in employment and public accommodations.[48] Over 90 percent of the cases were resolved in favor of the complainant.[49]

A particularly difficult problem involves the treatment of employees who are frightened about contracting AIDS in the workplace. In the vast majority of workplace settings, these fears are completely unfounded and usually can be dissipated with an educational program. The issue is more difficult in the health care and laboratory settings where there are slight but legitimate risks. It would appear that compliance with CDC infection-control measures would be a prerequisite to any employer discipline for refusing to perform work.

In *Stepp v. Review Board*,[50] Dorothy Stepp, a laboratory technician in Indianapolis, refused to work on specimens which contained AIDS precautionary labels. The laboratory had complied with CDC guidelines and she was provided with protective gloves, aprons, masks, and other equipment. Thus, her refusal was not based on concern for her personal safety. Stepp refused to perform the tests because, according to Stepp, "AIDS is God's plague on man and performing the tests would go against God's will."[51] The Indiana Court of Appeals held that Stepp was discharged for just cause and therefore was not entitled to unemployment compensation.

AIDS and Cost Containment

Early on in the AIDS epidemic it became apparent that, in addition to the human toll, AIDS was going to exact substantial costs from our economy. The first study of the cost of AIDS over a patient's lifetime was $147,000 per case.[52] This estimate, based on the first 10,000 cases, was heavily weighted with high-cost cases from New York City and other cases requiring inpatient care and was widely viewed as being too high. Subsequent estimates, based on more outpatient treatment, community support programs, and hospice care, generally ranged between $23,000[53] and $55,000.[54] These estimates, however, are probably too low, especially in light of increased survival rates and the use of new, expensive drugs such as AZT, which can cost as much as $8,000 per year per patient.[55] Current thinking, which certainly could change, suggests total lifetime costs of $80,000 per patient.[56]

The question with AIDS-related health care costs is not whether our society will pay for this health care. Of course it will. We would never deny medical treatment to thousands of sick and dying people. The question is not even who will pay the bills. If it is through employer-provided health benefits, the costs will be passed along to consumers. If it is through private health insurance, the costs will be passed along to policyholders. If it is through the government, the costs will be passed along to taxpayers. Inasmuch as consumers, policyholders, and taxpayers tend to be the same people, the real question is *how* will the bills be paid. This, in turn, depends on broad policy decisions related to Medicare, Medicaid, access to health care, and other matters not specifically related to AIDS.

In the workplace setting, AIDS policies seem to be at odds with widespread corporate attempts to contain health care costs. Indeed, there is a growing tension between handicap discrimination laws (and AIDS discrimination laws), which require employers to disregard future health risks in deciding employability, and the traditional underwriting function of an insurer, which employers have increasingly assumed.[57] For example, assuming that 50 percent of HIV positive individuals will develop AIDS within five to ten years and that each case of AIDS costs $80,000, each HIV positive person hired represents an average cost of $40,000. According to one estimate, by 1991 the present value of expected costs borne by employers for AIDS in that year will be about $11.3 billion in 1986 dollars.[58] In view of these costs, is it reasonable to believe that only a few rogue employers would choose to engage in HIV testing when at least 90 percent of commercial insurers, Blue Cross/Blue Shield plans, and health maintenance organizations (HMOs) screen individual applicants for HIV infection?[59]

In terms of its relationship to employer health care expenses, HIV testing is no different from genetic testing, early cancer screening, or other forms of predictive medical screening for a serious and costly illness. AIDS has forced us to ask ourselves many questions—most before we were ready—and one of those questions involves the efficacy and desirability of predictive medical screening as a means of health care cost containment. The policies developed for HIV testing could serve as the model for decisionmaking about other forms of predictive medical screening.

Employer Policies

Employers do not have the luxury of awaiting the final outcome of a prolonged debate over national policy on AIDS, health care, and employment. They need to act immediately to implement policies that are sound from both a legal and business standpoint. They also need policies that are sufficiently flexible to apply to a broad spectrum of medical and legal issues associated with AIDS.

Perhaps the easiest way of analyzing the legal issues of AIDS and employment is to work backwards from the most seriously ill people with clinical AIDS to the people who are asymptomatic but HIV positive. People with AIDS vary widely in their ability to work. As with other disabling conditions, whether a person with AIDS is able to continue work will depend on the nature of the job and an individualized determination of fitness. The employer, however, also may be required to make reasonable accommodations, such as adopting more flexible scheduling or leave policies, that will permit the employee to work while undergoing treatment.

Because AIDS is not transmitted in the workplace setting, fears or preferences of co-workers or customers will not justify discrimination in hiring, firing, promotions, assignments, or other terms and conditions of employment. Co-worker and customer preference have been argued unsuccessfully in race, sex, and other employment discrimination cases, and these arguments are unlikely to succeed in AIDS and other handicap discrimination cases. Essentially, employers will be responsible for educating co-workers about AIDS rather than discriminating against employees with AIDS or HIV infection.

Another commonly asserted reason for refusing to employ people with AIDS is concern that workplace exposures (e.g., heat, cold, infections) could be hazardous to the employee with AIDS. This is a legitimate concern, and it should be a part of the persons' individualized determination of fitness. Nevertheless, employer actions must be based on sound medical evidence and not assumptions, stereotypes, or speculation.

In short, people with AIDS must be treated in the same way as other workers with a serious and life-threatening illness. If they miss excessive amounts of work time or are unable to perform the job safely and efficiently, they need not be retained. Otherwise, any adverse personnel action will violate AIDS discrimination or handicap discrimination laws.

The same principles applicable to AIDS also apply to ARC. With regard to asymptomatic seropositives, it is clear that these individuals are not prevented from safely and efficiently performing job-related activities, and therefore it would be illegal to discriminate against them. Accordingly, the serological status of an individual is irrelevant to a medical determination of fitness.

Because an individual's HIV status is information that cannot be used in deciding employability, it becomes clear that this is information that no reasonable employer would want to know. Even if legally obtained (such as where HIV testing is offered to current employees on a voluntary basis), this information is probably the most sensitive information that would ever appear in an employee's medical file. If this information were inadvertently, negligently, or intentionally disclosed to any party, the employer might be exposed to enormous potential liability for negligence, defamation, invasion of privacy, negligent or intentional infliction of emotional distress, or other torts. Testing also raises numerous other legal problems, such as the duty to provide counseling or to notify spouses or other sexual partners.

There is simply no good reason for an employer to perform HIV testing.[60] The AOMA Guidelines on AIDS in the workplace provide, in part: "The AOMA supports voluntary testing of high risk groups including intravenous drug abusers, homosexuals, bisexuals, and their contacts."[61] Although this recommendation is consistent with CDC policy, there is no compelling reason for employers to become involved in the testing. It is unfortunate that AOMA did not support off-site testing. Such a policy would be in the interest of employers, employees, and public health. Testing is widely available at little or no cost and even can be done anonymously in many places. To the extent that employers obtain HIV test results, they must be kept with the utmost confidence.

A number of carefully considered AIDS policies have been developed by employer, employee, and community groups. Those policies emphasizing education and compassion have been very successful in allaying the fears of co-workers and maintaining good employee relations. The Citizens Commission on AIDS for New York City and Northern New Jersey has developed the following 10 principles for a policy on AIDS in the workplace:

1. People with AIDS or HIV (Human Immunodeficiency Virus) infection are entitled to the same rights and opportunities as people with other serious or life-threatening illnesses.

2. Employment policies must, at a minimum, comply with federal, state, and local laws and regulations.

3. Employment policies should be based on the scientific and epidemiological evidence that people with AIDS or HIV infection do not pose a risk of transmission of the virus to coworkers through ordinary workplace contact.

4. The highest levels of management and union leadership should unequivocally endorse nondiscriminatory employment policies and educational programs about AIDS.

5. Employers and unions should communicate their support of these policies to workers in simple, clear, and unambiguous terms.

6. Employers should provide employees with sensitive, accurate, and up-to-date education about risk reduction in their personal lives.

7. Employers have a duty to protect the confidentiality of employees' medical information.

8. To prevent work disruption and rejection by coworkers of an employee with AIDS or HIV infection, employers and unions should undertake education for all employees before such an incident occurs and as needed thereafter.

9. Employers should not require HIV screening as part of general pre-employment or workplace physical examinations.

10. In those special occupational settings where there may be a potential risk of exposure to HIV (for example, in health care, where workers may be exposed to blood or blood products), employers should provide specific, ongoing education and training, as well as the necessary equipment, to reinforce appropriate infection control procedures and ensure that they are implemented.[62]

These principles already have been endorsed and adopted by a number of leading companies, including IBM, AT&T, Johnson & Johnson, Prudential Insurance, and Xerox. Moreover, the broader principle of nondiscrimination based on AIDS has been advocated by every serious group to consider the issue, including the Presidential Commission on the Human Immunodeficiency Virus Epidemic,[63] the National Academy of Sciences,[64] and the American Medical Association.[65] Nondiscrimination is not just a matter of civil rights, it is a matter of public health. According to Admiral James Watkins, chairman of the Presidential Commission on AIDS: "People simply will not come forward to be tested, or will not supply names of sexual contacts for notification, if they feel they will lose their jobs and homes."[66]

6

Drug Testing

Drugs and the Workplace

Drug abuse is one of America's most widespread, serious, tragic, and seemingly intractable social problems.[1] According to the National Institute on Drug Abuse (NIDA), over 70 million Americans have experimented with illegal drugs and 23 million Americans are currently using some type of illegal substance.[2] Over 22 million Americans have experimented with cocaine and 10 million are cocaine dependent.[3] In the last 10 years there has been a 200-percent increase in cocaine-related deaths and a 500-percent increase in admissions to drug abuse treatment programs.[4]

The abuse of legal drugs, especially alcohol, also is a source for great concern. Over 100 million Americans use alcohol,[5] and there may be as many as 18 million adult alcoholics in the United States.[6] Alcohol is involved in nearly half of all automobile accidents and homicides, one-fourth of all suicides, and four-fifths of all family court cases.[7]

Although the greatly increased attention given to drug abuse by politicians and the media imply the problem is worsening,[8] recent studies suggest that drug abuse may have stabilized or decreased for most substances. Table 6–1 is based on the annual survey of high school seniors.

Although every study of drug use raises some methodological concerns,[9] the results in Table 6–1 are revealing. First, the use of marijuana, hallucinogens, and cocaine has declined 28.5 percent, 35.4 percent, and 14.2 percent, respectively, from 1979 levels. Some experts consider marijuana use the best predictor of the future use of other drugs.[10] Second, alcohol consumption rates are fairly constant over the entire period and seem largely unaffected by changing patterns of illicit drug use. Moreover, alcohol consumption rates declined only modestly when the legal age for drinking was raised to 21, which took place in many states from 1985 to 1987.

Table 6–1

**Percent of High School Seniors Who Said They Used Drugs
Within the Preceding 12 Months, 1975 to 1987**

Drug	% of Drug Users by Class Year						
	1975	1977	1979	1981	1983	1985	1987
Marijuana/hashish	40.0	47.6	50.8	46.1	42.3	40.6	36.3
Hallucinogens	11.2	8.8	9.9	9.0	7.3	6.3	6.4
Cocaine	5.6	7.2	12.0	12.4	11.4	13.1	10.3
Heroin	1.0	0.8	0.5	0.5	0.6	0.6	0.5
Alcohol	84.8	87.0	88.1	87.0	87.3	85.6	85.7

Source: Institute for Social Research, University of Michigan (1988). Reprinted by permission.

(Measures of heavy drinking also showed modest declines during this period.) Third, something not reflected in the table, is the changing pattern of drug use. More educated and affluent people have shown a significant decline in drug use, while less educated and poor people have had no decline.[11] This is especially true with crack, the smokable and highly addictive form of cocaine, which has become entrenched in inner-city areas.[12]

Two other categories of drugs are essential to note. First, "designer drugs" are synthetically produced narcotics that may be hundreds or thousands of times stronger than plant-based narcotics.[13] These drugs are easily formulated, often impossible to detect or identify, and legal until specifically criminalized. In 1982 more than six million Americans used synthetic drugs such as methamphetamine and phencyclidine (PCP).[14] The latest designer drug of abuse is "ecstacy," a hallucinogenic stimulant, which is a combination of a synthetic mescaline and an amphetamine. Ecstacy and other potent designer drugs have caused hundreds of deaths and thousands of hospitalizations.

Second, prescription and over-the-counter medications are widely abused. Americans are the most over-medicated people in history. In terms of numbers alone, this may be our number one drug abuse problem. Analgesics, barbiturates, benzodiazepines, antihistamines, and other common medications are often misused, frequently resulting in serious illness or injury.[15]

Drug abuse exacts a heavy toll from our society—from the health care system, from the criminal justice system, and from drug abusers and their families. Drug abuse is also very costly to employers. According to one estimate, 90 percent of drug and alcohol abusers work[16] and a significant number of employees use drugs on the job. The national cocaine helpline, a telephone treatment and referral service, averages 1,000 calls a day, with the "average" caller being white, male, 30 years old, and employed. Fifty percent of the callers report using cocaine daily.[17]

Different occupations often tend to have a particular type of drug problem. For instance, marijuana use on the job is most prevalent in the entertainment/recreation industry (17 percent), construction industry (13 percent), personal services (11 percent), and manufacturing of durable goods (10 percent).[18] On the other hand, alcohol abuse is most prevalent among "blue collar" workers. Undoubtedly, age, education, income, and other characteristics of the work force are responsible for these trends.

Regardless of the drug involved, it is clear that employee drug abuse is a legitimate concern. Moreover, despite contradictory studies, many employers believe that the problem is worsening[19] and that the costs to employers are increasing. The costs of employee drug abuse borne by employers can be divided into six categories: (1) lost productivity; (2) accidents and injuries; (3) insurance; (4) theft and other crimes; (5) employee relations; and (6) legal liability.

Lost Productivity

Several studies have attempted to measure whether the use of drugs by employees adversely affects their performance on the job. Using verbal, written, physiological, and physical testing, the studies concluded that drug abusers were functioning at only 50 to 67 percent capacity.[20] Specifically, drug abusers demonstrated poor work quality, failure to follow up or complete assignments, inadequate preparation, impaired memory, lethargy, reduced coordination, carelessness, mistakes, and slowdowns.[21]

A second measure of lost productivity attributed to drug abuse is absenteeism. Drug-abusing employees have a higher rate of absenteeism, with estimates ranging from 2.5 to 16 times higher than employees who do not use drugs.[22] Thus, employers are faced with increased costs for additional sick leave and medical insurance.

Finally, drug abusers have a higher turnover rate. According to one study, illicit drug users (particularly marijuana users who also use alcohol or other drugs) had average termination dates 10 months earlier for males and 16 months earlier for females.[23]

Estimates of the total financial impact of lost productivity from drugs borne by American business vary widely. The most frequently cited estimates are those of the Research Triangle Institute, which estimates that lost productivity totals $99 billion annually, with two-thirds of that amount attributable to alcohol.[24]

Accidents and Injuries

In 1984 American business lost an estimated $81 billion due to accidents, and many people believe that drug abuse is responsible for a significant share of the losses.[25] In the last 10 years there have been a number of highly publicized accidents where employee drug abuse was a factor, including 37 deaths in the railroad industry.[26] Overall, it has been reported that drug users have three to four times as many accidents as nonusers.[27]

There has been little scientific study, however, of the relationship between drugs and accidents. In a study by the National Institute for Occupational Safety and Health (NIOSH), out of 2,979 workplace injuries in the chemical industry in 1984 and 1985, drugs were a primary factor in only two injuries and a partial factor in only six more.[28] Similarly, a study by the Mine Safety and Health Administration (MSHA) found only 10 accidents in four years involved drugs.[29]

Despite any doubts raised by these contradictory studies, there is a perception that many workplace accidents are caused by drugs, and there is certainly the potential for drug-related accidents. Thus, many policies appear to be based on the assumption of a causal relationship between drugs and accidents.

Insurance

Drug and alcohol abuse may increase insurance costs by as much as $50 billion annually.[30] Employers that provide employees with insurance coverage as a part of the employee benefits package pay a substantial part of these increased costs. For example, employees with drug problems are more likely to use medical insurance and file workers' compensation claims.[31]

Theft and Other Crimes

A common concern about the employment of people who use drugs is whether, to support their drug habit, they are likely to steal from their employer, embezzle money, sell company products or trade secrets without authorization, steal from coworkers or customers, and sell drugs on company premises. Although these concerns have not been proven empirically, there is anecdotal evidence, and many employer policies appear to be based on the assumption that these concerns are valid.

Employee Relations

Another cost associated with drug abuse that is difficult to quantify is the negative impact of drugs on employee relations. Lost productivity, safety risks, and "work shifting" (nonusers being forced to do more than their share of work) can lower employee morale. Employees who use drugs also may try to sell drugs to coworkers or to spread the use of drugs to coworkers. Consequently, management must resolve intra-employee frictions and disputes. Meanwhile, management energies also must be committed to drug detection, crime prevention, drug education, quality control, accident prevention, and rehabilitation—all without invading employee privacy or undermining labor-management relations.

Legal Liability

Employer policies dealing with drugs in the workplace also must consider the issue of legal liability. Every injured person, damaged piece of property, defective product, breached contract, or other wrongful act attributable to employee drug usage has the potential for substantial employer liability. For example, several cases have held companies liable when alcohol-intoxicated employees injured other motorists while driving home after a company Christmas party or after being discovered intoxicated at work and ordered home by the company.[32]

These same principles are likely to be applied in drug cases. For example, in *Chesterman v. Barman*,[33] after an evening meeting with potential customers, the president of a one-man construction company took a "chocolate mescaline" pill in order to stem a feeling of depression and provide him with energy to continue work. The pill caused him to hallucinate and he broke into a nearby house and sexually assaulted the occupant. The Supreme Court of Oregon held that the actions could be imputed to the corporation because the man took the drug in order to perform work for the corporation.

On the other hand, overzealous efforts to combat drug abuse in the workplace also have the potential for liability. Heedless drug testing and dissemination of results may lead to liability for invasion of privacy, defamation, and other torts. This type of litigation is discussed in Chapter 9 under the section on Dignitary Torts. Thus, employers must navigate a careful course between insouciance and overreaction to the threat of drugs in the workplace.

Drug Testing in the Public and Private Sectors

There is little debate over the fact that drug abuse in the workplace is a serious problem and that measures should be taken to reduce, if not eliminate, the use of drugs by American workers. There is considerable debate, however, about the most appropriate means of achieving that end. Specifically, it is not clear whether mandatory urine testing is effective in reducing the workplace effects of drug use[34] and, even if it is, whether the benefits of reducing drug use outweigh the expense, intrusiveness, legal challenges, and employee relations costs that often accompany urine testing.

There is an unmistakable political component to drug testing in both the public and private sectors. With a media-conscious "war on drugs," much drug testing has been initiated by government entities and private companies because the failure to do so might be perceived as condoning drug use. This sentiment was aptly expressed by President Reagan. "I have heard critics say employers have no business looking for drug abuse in the workplace, but when you pin the critics down, too often they seem to be among the handful who still believe that drug abuse is a victimless crime."[35] This statement, of course, miscasts the issue as simply that a person either supports drug testing or drug taking. President Reagan, it may be recalled, had his own much-publicized drug test in 1986 and, in fact, the test was moved up two days so that he would not get a false positive result from the anesthesia he was to receive for a scheduled urological examination.[36]

Widespread drug testing actually began in the military in 1981. By 1985 over three million drug tests were performed annually[37] at a cost of over one-half billion dollars.[38] The Department of Defense credits its drug testing program for a decline in drug usage in the military.

In July 1983, President Reagan established the President's Commission on Organized Crime. In its March 1986 report on drug abuse, the Commission recommended drug testing for public and private sector employers.

> "The President should direct the heads of all Federal agencies to formulate immediately clear policy statements, with implementing guidelines, including suitable drug testing programs, expressing the utter unacceptability of drug abuse by Federal employees. State and local governments and leaders in the private sector should support unequivocally a similar policy that any and all use of drugs is unacceptable. Government contracts should not be awarded to companies that fail to implement drug programs, including suitable drug testing."[39]

On September 15, 1986, President Reagan issued Executive Order 12,564,[40] which requires the head of each Executive agency to establish a program to test for illegal drug use by employees in sensitive positions. "Sensitive positions" is defined as those handling classified information; those serving as Presidential appointees; those in positions related to national security; those serving as law enforcement officers; those charged with the protection of life, property, and public health and safety; and those in jobs requiring a high degree of trust and confidence. This extremely broad definition authorized the testing of 1.1 million of the nation's 2.1 million federal employees.[41]

The Executive Order specifically authorizes testing under four circumstances: (1) where there is reasonable suspicion of illegal drug use; (2) in conjunction with the investigation of an accident; (3) as a part of an employee's counseling or rehabilitation for drug use through an employee assistance program (EAP); and (4) to screen any job applicant for illegal drug use. The Order mandates confirmatory testing and allows the employee to provide a urine specimen in private unless there is reason to believe adulteration will occur.

The Executive Order also prescribes the action agencies must take when an employee's test is positive. Employees will be referred to an EAP and refusal to participate in the EAP will result in dismissal. Employees in sensitive positions are removed from duty pending successful completion of rehabilitation through the EAP. Agencies must initiate disciplinary action against any employee found to use illegal drugs unless the employee satisfies three criteria: (1) the employee must voluntarily identify himself or herself as a drug user before being identified through other means; (2) the employee must seek EAP rehabilitation; and (3) the employee must refrain from illegal drug use in the future. The employee must be dismissed if he or she is found continuing to use illegal drugs after initial identification.

Although the Executive Order was controversial, Congress passed an appropriations bill in 1987[42] that permitted implementation of the Order for the federal employees subject to drug testing.[43] Meanwhile, the federal government has moved swiftly to mandate the testing of workers in federal employment (e.g., Executive Office of the President, Department of Justice, Federal Aviation Administration, Department of Defense) as well as federally regulated employment (e.g., merchant marines, railroads, airlines, pipelines). By 1988, 42 federal agencies had begun drug testing. The federal government also has mandated the testing of millions of private sector employees in the transportation industry and those employed by government contractors. In addition, numerous municipal and state employees, including police, firefighters, transit workers, and school employees have been required to undergo drug testing.

The Department of Health and Human Services (HHS) is charged with promulgating scientific and technical guidelines for the federal drug testing program. The guidelines, issued in August 1987,[44] detail the scientific and technical requirements, including collection of specimens, laboratory analysis, and transmittal and interpretation of test results. The guidelines require testing for marijuana and cocaine and permit testing for any drug listed in Schedule I or II of the Controlled Substances Act.[45] The guidelines also include specific information on other drugs "most likely to be included in agency drug testing programs"—opiates, amphetamines, and PCP. Significantly, the guidelines contain no specific mention of testing for alcohol or other legal drugs of abuse. This fact tends to refute official claims that the testing program is an attempt to assure safety and productivity rather than a law enforcement measure.

The specimen collection procedures detailed in the guidelines have generated considerable controversy. The employee may urinate in privacy "unless there is reason to believe that a particular individual may alter or substitute the specimen to be provided." "To ensure that unadulterated specimens are obtained," the guidelines also detail the "minimum precautions" to be taken in the collection of urine specimens: (1) toilet bluing agents must be placed in the toilet bowl (presumably to prevent dilution of the sample); (2) there is to be no other source of water available in the area where the sample is given; (3) the person must present photo identification upon arrival; (4) the person must remove any unnecessary outer garments that could conceal items used to adulterate the sample; (5) the person must wash his or her hands upon arrival but may not wash again until after the sample collection has been completed; (6) immediately after collection the sample must be inspected for color and signs of contaminants and, within four minutes of urination, its temperature must be measured; and (7) if the temperature of the specimen gives rise to reasonable suspicion of adulteration or if other cause for suspicion is established, a second specimen must be obtained under direct observation.

The guidelines provide procedures to verify the chain of custody and also detail the required analytical procedures. The initial screen must be an immunoassay with confirmation using gas chromatography/mass spectrometry (GC/MS). The guidelines also set forth the necessary quality assurance measures, including laboratory proficiency testing.

Although drug testing began in the private sector, it was not until public employers began testing that private sector drug testing became so widespread. As Professor Elinor P. Schroeder of the University of Kansas has observed, "the federal government's enthusiastic propaganda campaign undoubtedly has encouraged the adoption of drug screening programs by some employers who otherwise might not have done so . . . [although] even without Presidential support, . . . drug testing probably would still have been popular among employers."[46] For the most part, it is the large companies that have embraced drug testing. Among *Fortune* 500 corporations, only 10 percent performed urinalysis in 1982; by 1985 the figure had reached 25 percent, and by 1988 nearly 50 percent of the largest corporations performed drug testing.[47]

As the size of the company declines, so too does the prevalence of drug testing. In a 1987 survey of companies with more than 500 employees, 17 percent of the companies tested current workers for drugs and 23 percent tested applicants.[48] Smaller companies reported less testing. Transportation and manufacturing companies were most likely to test, electronics/communications and insurance/finance companies were least likely to test.

The specifics of drug testing also vary by size of the company, geography, industry, and other factors. Larger companies are more likely to use confirmatory testing and to refer those testing positive to an EAP; smaller companies are more likely to use only screening tests and to respond to a positive test with summary dismissal.[49] In a 1988 study of small businesses south of metropolitan Boston, over 50 percent of companies using preplacement screening did not hire applicants on the basis of a single, unconfirmed screening test and nearly 30 percent of the companies did not inform the applicant of the results.[50]

According to another study, almost all of the companies (94.5 percent) using urinalysis test job applicants, and nearly three-fourths of the companies (73 percent) test current employees on a "for cause" basis.[51] Only 14 percent conducted random tests and those companies tended to be smaller, with a significant number of them testing people in jobs of a "sensitive or high risk nature." The most widely cited reason for testing (37 percent) was health and safety. Other reasons for testing were the identification of a work-place substance abuse problem (21 percent), the awareness of drugs as a national problem (11 percent), and the high-risk nature of the job (9 percent).

It is also valuable to consider why the companies without drug testing programs have declined to engage in testing. According to the American Management Association, the most common reasons for not performing drug testing are as follows: moral issues or privacy (68 percent); inaccuracy of tests (63 percent); negative impact on morale (53 percent); tests show use, not abuse (43 percent); employee opposition (16 percent); and union opposition (7 percent).[52] Interestingly, fear of litigation was not mentioned, but it certainly may be an increasingly significant consideration.

Drug Testing Technology

Current drug testing methods were developed in the late 1960s and early 1970s as a way of monitoring heroin use among people at drug treatment centers.[53] Since 1972, when the Syva Corporation first marketed its EMIT test, drug testing has become increasingly sophisticated (e.g., using recombinant DNA techniques to amplify trace chemicals in urine), automated, and competitive. Drug testing is now estimated to be a one billion dollar a year industry.[54]

All drug tests analyze a body specimen for the presence of drugs or their by-products, metabolites. The most commonly used specimen for workplace testing is urine,[55] although blood, breath, saliva, hair, and other specimens have been used in settings other than the workplace.[56] Blood testing by employers is mostly limited to retrospective testing after the occurrence of an accident.[57]

Scientifically valid drug testing is a two-step process.[58] In the initial step, a "screening" test eliminates from further testing those specimens with negative results, indicating either the absence of targeted substances or the presence of levels below a designated threshold or "cut-off" point. A result which reveals substance levels at or above the cut-off is considered positive. All positive specimens are then retested using a "confirmatory" test. According to the Toxicology Section of the American Academy of Forensic Sciences, the confirmatory test must be "based upon different chemical or physical principles than the initial analysis method(s)."[59] Confirmatory testing is essential to establish both the identity and quantity of the substances in the specimen.

There are three main types of initial screening tests: color or spot tests,[60] thin layer chromatography,[61] and immunoassays. The most widely used are the immunoassays, which are of three types, enzyme, radio, and fluorescence. All of these latter tests are based on immunological principles. A known quantity of the tested-for drug is bound to an enzyme or radioactive iodine and is added to the urine. If the urine contains the drug, the added, "labeled" drug competes with the drug in the specimen and cannot bind to the antibodies. As a result, the enzyme or radioactive iodine remains active. By measuring enzyme activity or radioactivity, the presence and amount of the drug can be determined.

The most commonly used immunoassay is the enzyme multiplied immunoassay technique or EMIT. An advantage of EMIT is that it tests for a broad spectrum of drugs and their metabolites, including opiates, barbiturates, amphetamines, cocaine and its metabolite, benzodiazepines, methaqualone, methadone, phencyclidine, and cannabinoids. It is also fast and cheap. A single test may cost about five dollars. In addition, portable kits starting at $300 are sold for on-site use by individuals with minimal training.

The radioimmunoassay (RIA)[62] can measure only one drug at a time but has broad-spectrum detection capabilities similar to EMIT. RIA is more expensive than EMIT, requires a more highly trained technician, and produces radioactive waste. It is used mostly by the military. The fluorescence polarization immunoassay (FPIA) is a relatively new technique and, as yet, not widely used.[63]

The most widely used confirmatory test is gas chromatography/ mass spectrometry (GC/MS). In GC the sample is pretreated to extract drugs from the urine. The drugs are converted to a gaseous form and transported through a long glass column of helium gas. By application of varying temperatures to the column the compounds are separated according to their unique properties, such as molecular weight and rate of reaction. These particular properties are used to identify the compound. Although GC can be used alone, the superior method combines it with a mass spectrometer (MS), which breaks down the compound molecules into electrically charged ion fragments. Each drug or metabolite produces a unique fragment pattern, which can be detected by comparison with known fragment patterns. GC/MS requires expensive equipment ($50,000 to $200,000) and highly trained technicians to prepare the sample and interpret test results. The process is also time-consuming because only one sample and one drug per sample may be tested at a time. High performance liquid chromatography (HPLC) is also used as a confirmatory test,[64] but GC/MS has become the standard confirmatory test.

The pricing structures for drug tests vary widely. Some laboratories charge customers a flat fee per specimen tested; others divide the fee so that those samples requiring a confirmatory test incur an additional charge.[65] Other factors affecting price are the type of analysis used, the number of specimens tested, and the types of drugs tested for. In general, laboratory charges for single-procedure methods range from $5 to $20; GC/MS confirmation costs from $30 to $100.[66]

It is essential to understand that a positive result on a drug test does not indicate impairment of the subject.[67] Drug metabolites detected in urine are the inert, inactive by-products of drugs and cannot be used to determine impairment. Although a blood test can reveal the presence of drugs in the blood in their active state, there is no known correlation, with the exception of ethanol, between the detection of metabolites in urine and blood concentrations.[68] Moreover, there is no agreement among experts on what level of drug indicates impairment.[69]

Many variables influence how a drug will affect an individual user, including the type of drug, dose, time lapse from administration, duration of effect and use, and interactions with other drugs. The individual's age, weight, sex, general health state, emotional state, and drug tolerance also are important factors.[70] Consequently, the wide individual variations make generalizing extremely speculative. According to one expert: "Testing does only one thing. It detects what is being tested. It does not tell us anything about the recency of use. It does not tell us anything about how the person was exposed to the drug. It doesn't even tell us whether it affected performance."[71]

A final factor that complicates interpretation of a positive result is the often-considerable duration of detectability of drugs in urine. As indicated in Table 6–2, drug metabolites can be detected in urine from one day to several weeks following exposure. The usual effects of most drugs, however, persist for only a few hours after use. Therefore, drugs are detectable long after their effects have subsided, and any correlations between a positive test and impairment are impossible.

The predictive value (positive) of the EMIT test has been calculated in Tables 3–9 and 3–10 in Chapter 3. With a prevalence of five percent, the predictive value (positive) is only 34.3 percent. In other words, two out of three positives identified by the test will be false positives. Thus, confirmatory tests are essential. Due to the much higher costs of confirmatory tests, however, even some of the large companies do not use confirmatory tests on applicant drug screens.

Because drug tests detect metabolites of drugs rather than the drugs themselves, commonly used screening tests sometimes incorrectly identify as metabolites of illicit drugs the metabolites of other substances or normal human enzymes such as lysozyme and malate dehydrogenase.[72] Table 6–3 indicates some of the substances for which this effect, cross-reactivity, has been documented.

Theoretically, confirmatory testing will eliminate the problem of cross-reactivity. For example, eating poppy seeds may result in a positive test for opiates, but the GC/MS will spot that a key metabolite of heroin (6-0-acetylmorphine) is not present.[73] The problem of cross-reactivity demands not only confirmatory testing, but also

Table 6–2

Detectability of Selected Drugs in Urine

Drugs	Approximate Duration of Detectability
Amphetamines	2 days
Barbiturates	1–7 days
Benzodiazepines	3 days
Cocaine metabolites	2–3 days
Methadone	3 days
Codeine	2 days
PCP	8 days
Cannabinoids	
single use	3 days
moderate smoker (4 times/week)	5 days
heavy smoker (daily)	10 days
chronic heavy smoker	21 days

Source: Council on Scientific Affairs, American Medical Association, *Scientific Issues in Drug Testing*, 257 J.A.M.A. 3110, 3112 (1987). Copyright 1987, American Medical Association. Reprinted by permission.

necessitates using pretest questionnaires inquiring about medications and other cross-reactants, and giving individuals an opportunity to explain a positive result.

A related concern is that a drug test will be positive because of "passive inhalation." There is disputed evidence about whether a marijuana test using a cutoff of 20 nanograms (billionths of a gram) per milliliter of urine will test positive if the subject was exposed to the marijuana smoke of other people.[74] Using a higher cutoff, however, such as 100 nanograms per milliliter of urine, will eliminate this problem.[75]

Table 6–3

Some Commonly Available Substances That Cross-React With Widely Tested-For Drugs

Type of Drug	Cross-Reactants
Amphetamines	over-the-counter cold medications (decongestants) over-the-counter and prescription dietary aids asthma medications anti-inflammatory agents
Barbiturates	anti-inflammatory agents phenobarbital (used to treat epilepsy)
Cocaine	herbal teas (made from coca leaves)
Marijuana (cannabinoids)	nonsteroidal anti-inflammatory agents ibuprofen (Advil, Motrin, Nuprin)
Morphine, opiates	codeine prescription analgesics and antitussives poppy seeds over-the-counter cough remedies
Phencyclidine (PCP)	prescription cough medicines Valium

Source: Rothstein, *Drug Testing in the Workplace: The Challenge to Employment Relations and Employment Law*, 63 Chi.-Kent L. Rev. 683, 698 (1987), and authorities cited therein. Reprinted by permission.

The accuracy of drug tests also may be affected by several other factors. Alteration of the specimen, such as by substitution or dilution,[76] improper calibration of equipment or cleaning of equipment (the so-called "carry-over effect"), mislabeling, contamination, or technician error all may undermine test accuracy. Indeed, even the best methodologies will yield valid results only to the extent that the testing laboratory adheres to rigid standards of quality control. Laboratory proficiency criteria, however, have been extremely inadequate.[77]

Legal Challenges

As a result of the workplace drug testing controversy, lawyers are often asked whether drug testing is legal. It is a question that is impossible to answer in the abstract. Indeed, soliciting the most basic information needed to give a reasonable answer to the question is practically a short course in employment law. The lawfulness of drug testing depends on the answers to, at least, the following questions: Is the employer public or private? If private, is the testing government-mandated? Did the testing occur in a state with a drug testing law? Is the employer covered under the federal Rehabilitation Act or state handicap discrimination law? Are the employees unionized? If so, does the collective bargaining agreement cover drug testing? Was the testing conducted in an invasive manner, were the results publicized, or was there any other conduct on the part of the employer or other parties that would be actionable in contract or tort? (Issues related to collective bargaining and civil litigation involving drug testing are discussed in Chapters 8 and 9 respectively.)

Constitutional Law

A number of constitutional arguments have been raised to challenge the legality of employee drug testing. Because the federal Constitution only applies to governmental actions, federal constitutional protections are limited to public employees and private employees where drug testing is mandated by federal, state, or local governments.

The most frequently raised argument is that drug testing constitutes an unreasonable search and seizure in violation of the fourth amendment, which provides: "The right of the people to be secure in their persons, houses, papers, and effects, against unreasonable searches and seizures, shall not be violated. . . ." In *Schmerber v. California*,[78] the Supreme Court held that taking a blood sample from a criminal defendant to determine whether he was intoxicated was a search within the meaning of the fourth amendment. Lower court decisions after *Schmerber* have recognized that requiring a urine sample is far less intrusive than extracting blood but have nonetheless concluded that a mandatory urine screen also is a search for purposes of the fourth amendment.[79] The limited nature of the intrusion, however, may be important in determining the validity of the search.

The fourth amendment does not bar all searches, only unreasonable ones. Therefore, it must be determined whether the drug test is unreasonable. This in turn often depends on the nature of the search: who is searched, when the search is made, how it is made, and what is done with the results. Courts balance the degree of intrusion of the search on the person's fourth amendment right of privacy against the need for the search to promote some legitimate governmental interest.[80]

One essential factor affecting the constitutionality of a search is whether the individual has a reasonable expectation of privacy relative to the circumstances of the search. Government employees have a reasonable expectation of privacy at work and "do not surrender their fourth amendment rights merely because they go to work for the government."[81] Yet, government employers maintain rights in conducting warrantless searches "for the proprietary purpose of preventing future damage to the agency's ability to discharge effectively its statutory responsibilities."[82]

A related but distinct constitutional protection has been established to protect the "right of privacy." Although this right is not explicit in the Constitution, the Supreme Court has found that it includes the individual's interest in avoiding disclosure of personal matters and independence in making certain kinds of important decisions, such as those involving marriage, procreation, and family relationships.[83] This privacy interest, however, is not absolute and must be balanced against legitimate governmental interests in disclosure. In the context of drug testing, the courts have been reluctant to apply privacy principles distinct from those recognized under the fourth amendment.[84]

Another constitutional argument often raised in drug testing cases is procedural due process. The argument has been used to challenge both test procedures and employee termination procedures. As to the former, it has been held that termination of employment on the basis of an unconfirmed EMIT test violated due process[85] and that it violated due process when voluntarily submitted urine samples were destroyed before they could be sent out for independent testing.[86] Even the addition of confirmatory testing may not satisfy due process concerns about the proper handling of the specimen and cleaning and calibration of test equipment. As to the latter, employee termination procedures, the termination of an individual's employment must be preceded by notice and opportunity for a hearing appropriate to the nature of the case, although a full, predischarge hearing is not required.[87]

Several other federal constitutional theories have been advanced to challenge drug testing. It has been asserted that drug testing violates the first amendment freedom of religion, fifth amendment ban on self-incrimination, ninth amendment protection of liberty, and fourteenth amendment substantive due process and equal protection. None of these theories have met with much success.

Federal constitutional arguments have been used to attack a wide range of government and government-mandated drug testing. The cases have involved various employees, such as police officers,[88] firefighters,[89] prison guards,[90] Army employees,[91] nuclear power plant employees,[92] transit employees,[93] school bus attendants,[94] school teachers,[95] and jockeys.[96] The results also have varied widely. In 1989 the Supreme Court upheld the drug testing of employees of the U.S. Customs Service[97] and railroad employees.[98] The narrow opinions relied on the drug interdiction and public safety roles of the two classes of employees. Additional cases will be needed to clarify the constitutionality of drug testing.

State constitutional law also may be relevant to drug testing in one of two ways. First, the drug testing of government employees may violate a state constitution that prohibits unreasonable searches and seizures. Second, unlike the United States Constitution, there is no governmental action requirement under certain state constitutions. In several states,[99] the state constitution contains a protection for the right of privacy that may be violated by the mandatory drug testing of private sector employees. For example, the California State Constitution has been used to challenge preemployment drug testing by Matthew Bender & Company, a publisher of law books.[100]

State Drug Testing Laws

The political significance of drug testing has not been lost on state and local politicians. During the 1986 gubernatorial campaign, Kansas Governor Mike Hayden campaigned for a drug-free state government from the top down.[101] In 1988 he signed legislation authorizing the drug testing of all state employees in safety-sensitive positions, including the governor, lieutenant governor, appointed heads of state agencies, and governor's staff.[102] Tennessee also enacted legislation in 1988 to authorize the drug testing of the state's Department of Corrections employees.[103]

Utah's Drug and Alcohol Testing Act[104] encourages drug testing in the private sector. The Utah law permits drug testing as a condition of hiring or continued employment so long as employers and managers also submit to testing periodically. In encouraging drug testing, the statute requires that employers performing drug testing have a written testing policy and that confirmatory tests be used. If an employer satisfies these requirements, the law immunizes the employer from liability for defamation or other torts based on the drug testing. It also prohibits any action based on the failure to conduct a drug test.

The other states to enact drug testing legislation, Connecticut,[105] Iowa,[106] Minnesota,[107] Montana,[108] Nebraska,[109] Rhode Island,[110] and Vermont[111] all restrict drug testing. The laws are similar in the following respects: (1) all of the laws seek to limit drug testing but do not prohibit testing completely; (2) all of the laws permit the preemployment testing of applicants and some permit the periodic testing of employees if advance notice is given; (3) exceptions are often made for public safety officers and employees in safety-sensitive jobs; (4) "for cause" testing is generally allowed if there is "probable cause," "reasonable cause," or "reasonable suspicion" that an employee is impaired; (5) most of the laws require that the sample collection be performed in private; (6) all of the laws require confirmatory testing; and (7) most of the laws specifically require drug testing records to be kept confidential.

The most important local drug testing law yet enacted is San Francisco's ordinance,[112] which applies to any person working in San Francisco except uniformed police, firefighters, police dispatchers, and emergency vehicle operators. The ordinance prohibits employee drug testing unless "the employer has reasonable grounds to believe that an employee's faculties are impaired on the job; and . . . the employee is in a position where such impairment presents a clear and present danger to the physical safety of the employee, another employee or to a member of the public."

Rehabilitation Act and State Handicap Discrimination Laws

The Rehabilitation Act of 1973,[113] the primary federal law prohibiting employment discrimination against individuals with handicaps (discussed in detail in Chapter 7) was amended in 1978 to clarify the Act's coverage of alcoholics and drug abusers. The 1978 amendment specifically provides that the denial of employment opportunities on the basis of alcohol or drug use is justified only under limited circumstances. "[The term handicapped individual] does not include any individual who is an alcoholic or drug abuser whose current use of alcohol or drug abuse . . . would constitute a direct threat to property or the safety of others."[114]

There is little legislative history surrounding the 1978 amendment. The amendment was sponsored by conservative members of Congress to correct a perceived flaw in the Act, whereby affirmative action plans seemingly would mandate the hiring of "active" alcoholics and drug abusers, resulting in a threat to public safety.[115] Viewed as a narrow, clarifying exception (and the provision is written in the negative), it merely excludes *some* alcoholics and drug abusers—those not currently capable of performing the job. Other alcoholics and drug abusers (those not posing a direct threat) would be covered if they met the statutory definition of "handicapped individual": "any person who (i) has a physical or mental impairment which substantially limits one or more of such person's major life activities, (ii) has a record of such an impairment, or (iii) is regarded as having such an impairment."[116]

In *School Board v. Arline,*[117] the Supreme Court noted that Congress did not intend to ban completely the hiring of alcoholics or drug abusers.

> "Congress recognized that employers and other grantees might have legitimate reasons not to extend jobs or benefits to drug addicts and alcoholics, but also understood the danger of improper discrimination against such individuals if they were categorically excluded from coverage under the Act. Congress therefore rejected the original House proposal to exclude addicts and alcoholics from the definition of handicapped individual, and instead adopted the Senate proposal excluding only those alcoholics and drug abusers "whose current use of alcohol or drugs prevents such individual from performing the duties of the job in question or whose employment . . . would constitute a direct threat to property or the safety of others."[118]

There are three categories of drug users to consider for possible coverage under the Rehabilitation Act: (1) former drug abusers and current drug abusers (such as those on methadone maintenance) who are currently able to perform the job safely and efficiently; (2) current drug abusers whose current use constitutes a direct threat to property or the safety of others; and (3) current or former casual drug users (such as an occasional marijuana user). (This categorization does not contain a separate category for individuals with a record of impairment or regarded as having an impairment.)

The first category is the easiest. The language of the amendment and its legislative history make it clear that former drug abusers and current abusers able to perform the job may not be discriminated against.[119] For example, in *Wallace v. Veterans Administration*,[120] a registered nurse who was a recovering drug addict was held to be "handicapped" under the language of the 1978 amendment.

An example of a case from the second category, current drug abusers, is *Heron v. McGuire*.[121] A police officer was dismissed because of his addiction to heroin. The United States Court of Appeals for the Second Circuit held that the dismissal did not violate section 504 of the Rehabilitation Act. The court reasoned that because Heron's heroin addiction made him unfit for duty, the plaintiff was not a "handicapped individual" under the Act. It was therefore unnecessary to reach the issue of whether the plaintiff was "otherwise qualified."

In terms of the size of the employment pool, the third category, current or former casual drug users, is the most important. It is also the most difficult conceptually. For example, in *McCleod v. City of Detroit*,[122] firefighter applicants were rejected from employment on the basis of positive tests for marijuana. They brought an action under section 504 claiming discrimination on the basis of handicap. The action was dismissed on the ground that the plaintiffs were not "handicapped individuals" within the meaning of the Rehabilitation Act. The court reasoned that, under the Act's definitional provisions, section 706(7)(B), the plaintiffs must show that the impairment "substantially limits one or more of such person's major life activities." The regulations under the Rehabilitation Act interpret "major life activities" to include such activities as "caring for one's self, performing manual tasks, walking, seeing, hearing, speaking, breathing, learning and working."[123] Nevertheless, simply because the defendant refused to hire an individual on the basis of an impairment does not mean there has been a substantial limitation of the individual's ability to work. An impairment "substantially limits" working only if the individual would be disqualified from all or a significant number of similar jobs.

A similar result was reached in *Burka v. New York City Transit Authority*,[124] involving a challenge to the drug testing policy of the city transit authority. The court adopted a narrow view of the coverage of alcoholics and drug abusers under the 1978 amendment. The court held "that section 504 protects only those otherwise qualified drug abusers who have been or are being rehabilitated. It does not protect the illegal narcotics abuser who has not sought or is not seeking treatment for his or her condition."[125]

The court's reasoning in *Burka* raises the question of whether it is logical to extend the protections of the Rehabilitation Act to former (and some current) drug addicts, but to deny coverage to occasional drug users or those regarded as occasional drug users. The answer is that the Rehabilitation Act was not intended to prohibit all unfairness in employment or even all unfairness in employment related to physical or medical conditions. It was designed to prevent discrimination against the *severely* handicapped.[126] Although alcoholics are specifically covered by the Rehabilitation Act, it is unlikely that Congress also sought to cover every casual drinker, even though it may be more logical for an employer to want to discharge an alcoholic instead of a casual drinker.

The distinction between drug users and drug addicts raises a fundamental policy question. How should employers, the law, and the rehabilitation community deal with casual, "recreational" drug users. Many employers treat all users of illegal drugs as if they were drug addicts by referring them to an employee assistance program for rehabilitation. In many instances, this approach is inappropriate and a waste of money. It is like referring every drinker—social drinker as well as alcoholic—to Alcoholics Anonymous. (Of course, it may be necessary to have a rehabilitation professional assess the extent of the individual's drug usage and dependence inasmuch as "denial" often accompanies addiction.) It is certainly desirable and appropriate for employers to refer drug addicts to rehabilitation. For casual drug users whose drug use affects their job performance, employers would be justified in taking disciplinary measures. For casual drug users whose drug use does not affect their job performance, it is not clear whether any employer intervention is warranted.

Finally, with regard to state handicap laws, all 50 states and the District of Columbia have laws prohibiting discrimination in employment on the basis of handicap. Some of the laws specifically include alcoholics and drug abusers; others specifically exclude them from coverage. Some other states have resolved the issue through case law.[126] Many of the cases have involved the nature of the employer's duty of reasonable accommodation.

Developing a Sound Policy

Although the legal parameters of drug testing are still evolving, it is likely that employers will be legally permitted to require more employee drug testing than they need or ought perform. Consequently, before embarking on a drug testing program, managers should undertake a detailed and thoughtful consideration of whether there is a workplace drug abuse problem, whether drug testing is essential to combat the problem, whether the benefits of drug testing outweigh the costs to employers and employees, and whether drug testing can be undertaken in a way that will ensure accuracy, fairness, and privacy.

While some people have recommended unrestricted drug testing or no drug testing at all, there is a growing consensus—from the AFL-CIO[128] to the AMA[129] that limited drug testing is permissible. For example, the AMA's Council on Scientific Affairs recommended:

> "That the AMA take the position that urine drug and alcohol testing of employees should be limited to: (a) preemployment examinations of those persons whose jobs affect the health and safety of others, (b) situations in which there is reasonable suspicion that an employee's job performance is impaired by drug and alcohol use, and (c) monitoring as part of a comprehensive program of treatment and rehabilitation of alcohol and drug abuse or dependence."[130]

Placing careful controls on drug testing is an attempt to accommodate the legitimate concerns about test accuracy and privacy with legitimate concerns about public health and safety. It is even more difficult to move beyond generalities to concrete guidelines on workplace drug testing. A legal, ethical, and effective drug testing program should satisfy each of the following requirements.

Reasonable suspicion exists to believe that there is at least some class-wide problem of drug abuse among the relevant group of employees.

Drug testing is an extreme measure and it should not be undertaken lightly. The only compelling reason to test is to protect employee and public safety. Although drug testing should not be started only *after* a tragic accident, there are sound reasons why it should not be initiated unless there is at least some evidence of a drug abuse problem in the locality, in a particular profession or job classification, or at a particular place of employment. This information may come in many forms, such as drug-related arrests of employees, direct observation of drug use, discovery of drugs or paraphernalia in the workplace, drug-related accidents, reliable reports by employees and supervisors, and published studies.

Of the first 5,300 people tested by the U.S. Customs Service, only six had a positive result. [131] Of the first 8,064 workers tested by the Department of Transportation, only 61 tested positive and four people were discharged. [132] It is hard to imagine that in the private sector, in the absence of any evidence of a need to test, such a low yield could justify the expense and intrusiveness of testing. Nevertheless, the federal government seems undeterred and has continued to support even wider testing. In an era of budget cutting, it is surprising that the costs of drug testing are rarely discussed. Testing every federal employee once a year would cost $300 million annually and testing all workers in both the public and private sectors would cost $8 to $10 billion annually. [133]

There are no feasible alternatives to detecting impairment, including supervision and simulation.

The primary concern underlying drug testing is that drug-impaired employees will be impaired on the job. Drug testing, however, does not measure impairment. It measures prior exposure, which is used as a surrogate for impairment based on one of the two following theories. First, employees who use drugs off the job are more likely to use drugs on the job or to report to work under the influence of drugs. [134] Second, prior drug use may impede performance even though no impairment is noticeable. If impairment or the effects of impairment are detectable, then there is no need for drug testing. One way to detect impairment is through regular, close supervision. Supervision would not necessarily detect *drug* impairment, but it would detect reduced efficiency. From an employer's perspective it should not matter whether the reduced efficiency is caused by drugs, lack of sleep, personal problems, or other factors. Only the treatment of the problem will be affected. Another way to monitor impairment is for the employee to demonstrate fitness via simulation.

The drug testing program is limited to workers who, if working while impaired, would pose a substantial danger to themselves, other persons, or property.

Among the numerous asserted justifications for employee drug testing are the following: (1) drug use is illegal and therefore employers have a responsibility to discover employees who may be breaking the law; (2) drug abusing employees often need substantial sums of money to buy drugs and these employees are likely to steal from their employer or to accept bribes on the job; (3) employees using drugs are likely to have a reduction in their productivity; (4) maintaining a drug-free workplace is essential to an employer's public image; and (5) drug testing is essential to protect safety and health.

First, as to illegality, it is clear that employers are not concerned about illegality per se. If they were concerned simply about lawbreaking, measures other than drug testing are likely to be much more effective in detecting wrongdoing. For example, an employee (and management) federal income tax return screening every April 15th would undoubtedly be quite revealing. At the same time that the Reagan Administration was proclaiming "zero tolerance" for lawbreaking drug users,[135] former Attorney General Edwin Meese was "forgetting" to pay his income tax for 15 months.[136] Of course, it is the responsibility of the Internal Revenue Service and not employers to detect tax irregularities. Similarly, it is the responsibility of law enforcement agencies and not employers to prevent illegal drug use.

Second, as to theft and bribery, the sudden need for more money to support a drug habit is only one reason why an employee might become dishonest. To be thorough, employers would need to know if an employee were gambling, suffering losses in the stock market, or even having an extra-marital affair. Preemployment background and reference checks and post-hiring supervision and auditing are much more effective in preventing theft and bribery than urinalysis.

Third, productivity is a legitimate concern of an employer. Productivity, however, is directly measurable and is done so on a continual basis by employers. A decline in productivity is an endpoint and it is irrelevant whether the decline is caused by boredom, personal problems, or drug abuse.

"If daily dope smoking is making someone lethargic, fire him for lethargy. If coke has a worker alternating between intense but shabby work, mindless chattiness, and sloughs of despond, fire him on all three grounds. As for PCP, . . . [w]hy waste money on lab work when you can just be on the lookout for workers who ask the Xerox machine out to lunch?"[137]

Fourth, from a legal and policy standpoint, public image is a deeply troubling rationale for employment policies. Historically, many forms of employment discrimination have been defended on grounds such as "customer preference." The law has correctly rejected such asserted defenses. Public image, a valid justification according to the ill-advised AOMA guidelines on drug testing,[138] is not only so vague as to justify nearly any action, but it is a two-edged sword. Drug abuse in the United States is so widespread, the fact that an employer has, among its employees, one or more individuals with a substance abuse problem is unlikely to generate public disdain. The way in which the employer deals with the problem, however, may directly affect its public image. Indiscriminate drug testing without regard for employee rights can influence the way in which the employer is regarded by current employees, potential employees, customers, and shareholders.

Fifth, safety is the only justifiable reason for employee drug testing. It is true that current drug tests do not measure impairment and only measure prior exposure. Nevertheless, there is ample evidence that individuals who use drugs often take them at work or report to work impaired. For employees in safety-sensitive positions, prudence demands that public safety considerations outweigh even the legitimate concerns of employees. For employees not in safety-sensitive positions, such as retail or clerical workers, there is no justification for drug testing. Reasonable supervision will ensure that satisfactory performance is not impeded for any reason, including drugs.

If safety is the only compelling reason for drug testing, the nature of this exception needs to be further defined. The danger posed by an impaired worker must be *substantial*. This is based on the severity of the consequences, the likelihood of danger, and the immediacy of the harm. To justify drug testing, the risk of harm from an impaired worker also must be otherwise unpreventable (as by supervision, quality control, and work review) and the consequences irreparable. Nuclear power, chemical plant, and transportation workers are the best examples. Even as to these employees, however, the other elements still need to be satisfied.

Testing not based on individualized, reasonable suspicion is limited to preemployment and periodic testing.

Preemployment and periodic testing (especially as part of a preemployment or annual medical examination) are the least objectionable forms of testing. They permit the discovery of individuals who have a substance abuse problem within the context of a medical examination. There is no stigma attached to supplying a urine sample in this context. The medical setting also helps to encourage truthful disclosure by a substance-abusing employee, protects confidentiality, and facilitates treatment.

The other acceptable time for testing is when there is reasonable suspicion of impairment. This is a closer case. If an employee in a safety-sensitive job is observed to be drowsy, dizzy, disoriented, or otherwise is suspected of being impaired, the employee should not be permitted to continue work and should be referred to a physician. Thus, the need for a drug test under these circumstances may be questioned because the behavior establishing reasonable cause also demands action immediately and cannot await the results of a drug test. The other point raised by reasonable cause testing is that clear guidelines must be established for determining reasonable cause. Without such guidelines there is a danger of arbitrariness in selecting the employees for testing.

Despite the drawbacks of reasonable cause testing, employers should be provided with some basis for a periodic or unprogrammed testing, because recreational as well as compulsive drug users may be able to forego the use of drugs for a short period of time each year to test negatively. In those job categories where drug testing is acceptable, it ought to be effective. Reasonable cause testing, including post-accident testing, should be permissible.

Some people have suggested that the *only* permissible drug testing is for reasonable cause. For employees working alone (such as truck drivers), it is hard to imagine that there ever would be reasonable cause until after a tragic accident occurred. Thus, reasonable cause testing should not be the only basis for drug testing. Periodic, scheduled (e.g., annual) testing would be otherwise reasonable. Other forms of testing, however, such as random testing and surprise, mass testing have been justifiably rejected by several courts as being overly intrusive and oppressive.

State of the art screening and confirmatory test procedures are performed by trained professionals, off-site, under laboratory conditions.

Employers that use "do-it-yourself" drug testing kits and unconfirmed screening tests are engaged in a false economy or worse. Unless the best technology is used, drug test results are unreliable and more likely to be challenged successfully in court. Even the best analytical techniques are only as good as the people performing the tests. Careful laboratory selection and ongoing quality review are essential.

Specimen collection is not observed.

With the growth of employee drug testing there have been numerous reports of employees attempting to substitute "clean urine" or otherwise tampering with specimens. Some employers, in response, have taken to observing employees in the act of urination. For many employees, this aspect of drug testing is the most objectionable, degrading, and insensitive element. It is highly unlikely that the benefits of observation (preventing tampering by a few individuals whose drug problems were not otherwise detectable) outweigh the human relations, employment relations, and public relations costs of observation.

Testing is performed for the presence of prescription drugs and alcohol as well as illicit drugs.

If the underlying purpose of drug testing is safety, there is no reason why drug testing should be limited to illicit drugs. In terms of the number of people who abuse them and the fatalities, injuries, and property damage caused by their effects in the workplace, alcohol and prescription drugs (often in combination) pose a much greater threat than illicit drugs. For example, a study published in 1989 looked at work-related fatalities in Harris County, Texas (Houston area) in 1984 and 1985. Drug and alcohol testing was performed at 173 of 196 autopsies. The results showed that 23 workers had a detectable blood alcohol content, 11 workers had detectable traces of prescription drugs with the potential to alter physical functions needed to avoid injury, and only one worker tested positive for marijuana.[139] In a 1988 survey of substance abuse in the construction industry, 85 percent of respondents (members of the American Subcontractors Association) said that alcohol was the most abused substance.[140]

There is valid employee consent before the testing and an opportunity to explain a positive test result.

An argument could be made that consent to drug testing is never voluntary (or valid) when employees are likely to be discharged or applicants not hired if they refuse. Nevertheless, if drug testing is essential to protect public safety in the face of a drug abuse problem by certain employees, and if the other criteria for testing are met, an employer ought to be able to make consent to drug testing a condition of employment. Employers, however, should not perform drug testing surreptitiously, such as by simply testing all urine samples obtained as part of a preemployment or periodic medical examination.

A related issue is whether applicants and employees should be given advance notice that a preemployment or periodic drug test will be performed. The obvious drawback to notice is that it permits individuals to abstain before being tested and then to resume drug use after the test. This drawback, however, may be outweighed by the following considerations. First, providing employees with notice improves employee acceptability of the program. It indicates that the purpose of the testing is to promote public safety and not to "catch" employees. Second, as to applicants, company resources will be saved because habitual drug users will not proceed further with their application. Third, individuals genuinely interested in obtaining or retaining employment may cease using drugs before the test and surveillance, supervision, and retesting may ensure that they do not resume drug use.

Test results are kept confidential.

Drug test results should be regarded in the same way as other medical records. Specifically, the data should be stored in the medical department (assuming there is one) and access should be limited to medical personnel. Supervisory and managerial employees should only be notified of the consequences of the results (e.g., employee A is medically unfit for work), but not the specific results. Other information essential to personnel actions should be provided only on a "need-to-know" basis. When an initial drug screen is positive and a confirmatory test is scheduled, no results should be released until after the confirmatory test. The failure to maintain confidentiality may lead to liability based on invasion of privacy, defamation, intentional infliction of emotional distress, or other torts.

Drug testing is only part of an overall drug abuse program, including education and rehabilitation.

Drug testing should be only one part, and indeed should be the least important part, of a comprehensive drug abuse program. The other two components of the program should be drug awareness and employee assistance.

Drug awareness programs are educational activities aimed at supervisors and employees. Supervisors need to be trained to recognize some of the "suspect changes in employee job performance and behavior that may portend a drug abuse problem."[141] They also need to be trained in how to respond to employees suspected of having a drug abuse problem.

Employees also should be involved in a separate drug education program. Although there are several different models of programs, all programs teach employees to recognize the signs of drug abuse in themselves, family, friends and coworkers. All programs also discuss the dangers of drug abuse and describe company and community services available for dealing with drug abuse.[142]

The other essential part of a drug abuse program is an employee assistance program (EAP). There are 8,000[143] to 10,000[144] EAPs today, giving about 20 percent of the work force access to such a program.[145] Most of the EAPs are in large companies. Some of the programs are run in-house, others are run on a contract basis. Both types of EAPs work the same way. An employee may voluntarily enter the program or may be referred by a supervisor. The employee contacts the EAP and works out an individual treatment program. Participation in an EAP is kept confidential. In some instances, employer discipline is waived on the condition that the employee completes the EAP.

7

Handicap Discrimination Law

Medical Information and "Handicaps"

The result of medical screening is to classify an individual or group of individuals as medically qualified or unqualified for employment. Besides the condition-specific legislation (e.g., genetic testing, AIDS testing, drug testing) already mentioned, the main laws prohibiting unreasonable medical disqualification are the federal and state handicap discrimination laws. This chapter, the first of three chapters largely devoted to legal issues, addresses a myriad of handicap discrimination issues raised by medical screening of workers.

The Rehabilitation Act of 1973 is the federal law prohibiting discrimination in employment on the basis of handicap. It was the first comprehensive effort to bring handicapped individuals within the mainstream of American life. Its expressed purpose, as restated in the 1978 Amendments, is "to develop and implement, through research, training, services, and the guarantee of equal opportunity, comprehensive and coordinated programs of vocational rehabilitation and independent living." Three sections of the Rehabilitation Act, sections 501, 503, and 504, pertain to employment and prohibit discrimination on the basis of handicap by the federal government, federal government contractors, and recipients of federal financial assistance.

In retrospect, it would seem logical that such antidiscrimination provisions would be passed in 1973, at the end of the Vietnam War. Congress traditionally has enacted vocational rehabilitation and handicap assistance legislation at the end of wars, when there is an increase in demand for services for the disabled. In addition, during the 1960s Congress had enacted sweeping laws proscribing discrimination in employment on the basis of race, color, religion, sex, national origin, and age. The movement for civil rights for people with disabilities was an outgrowth of these earlier civil rights efforts.

The legislative history surrounding the employment discrimination provisions of the Act, however, particularly section 504, reflect more happenstance than deliberation or historical imperative. As related by Edward Berkowitz in his book, *Disabled Policy*:

> "In late August 1972, during the long battle to enact a vocational rehabilitation law, a congressional staff member, no one knows which one, suggested putting a civil rights provision into the vocational rehabilitation law. According to Richard Scotch, who has made the closest study of the matter, the suggestion sent an aide to Senator Jacob Javits to look for the wording of Title VI [of the Civil Rights Act of 1964, prohibiting discrimination on the basis of race, color, or national origin by recipients of federal financial assistance]; when he brought the words back to the meeting, he created Section 504. Even though congressional debate on the rehabilitation law occasioned great publicity, Section 504 received the least possible mention in the committee reports and congressional hearings. It would not be an overstatement to say that Section 504 was enacted into law with no public comment or debate."[1]

Section 501, applicable to all federal departments, agencies, and other "executive instrumentalities" requires nondiscrimination, reasonable accommodation, and affirmative action for the "hiring, placement, and advancement" of individuals with handicaps.[2]

Section 503 provides that any contract in excess of $2,500 entered into with any federal department or agency shall contain a provision requiring that the contracting party take affirmative action to employ and promote qualified individuals with handicaps.[3] The term "individual with handicaps" is defined as "any person who (A) has a physical or mental impairment which substantially limits one or more of such person's major life activities, (B) has a record of such an impairment, or (C) is regarded as having such an impairment." "Major life activities" means functions such as caring for one's self, performing manual tasks, walking, seeing, hearing, speaking, breathing, learning, and working.[4]

Responsibility for enforcing section 503 is vested in the Office of Federal Contract Compliance Programs (OFCCP) in the Department of Labor. By regulation, the director of the OFCCP may seek to (1) withhold progress payments on the contract; (2) terminate the contract; or (3) bar the contractor from future contracts. The Labor Department also has awarded back pay to individuals who have been denied employment or advances in employment because of handicap. Individuals who believe they have been discriminated against may only pursue their administrative remedies through the OFCCP; most courts have held that there is no express or implied private right of action.[5]

Section 504 provides that no otherwise qualified individual with handicaps shall, solely by reason of handicap, be (1) excluded from the participation in, (2) denied the benefits of, or (3) subjected to discrimination under, any program or activity receiving federal financial assistance.[6] Unlike section 503, there is no monetary minimum amount of financial assistance required for coverage under section 504.

By regulation,[7] procedures for enforcement of section 504 by each federal agency must be the same as those used to implement Title VI of the Civil Rights Act of 1964. Also, unlike section 503, the courts have recognized a private right of action under section 504.[8]

The Rehabilitation Act has been amended several times since its passage in 1973. As discussed earlier, amendments in 1978 and 1988 clarified the Act's coverage of alcoholics and drug abusers and individuals with contagious diseases. The 1986 amendments changed the term "handicapped individual" to read "individual with handicaps" throughout the Act.[9] "This change was suggested by persons representing individuals with disabilities who testified . . . that by retaining the adjective 'handicapped' before the noun 'person' the legislation might be inadvertently adding to the stereotype that persons with handicaps are less worthy."[10]

Inspired by the federal law, every state has enacted a state handicap discrimination law, although the laws in Alabama and Mississippi only apply to public sector employees. The state laws differ from each other and the federal law in terminology and case law developments.[11] With regard to coverage, the states often exempt only small employers and therefore they often provide more comprehensive private sector coverage than sections 503 and 504 of the Rehabilitation Act.

Regulations promulgated to implement sections 503 and 504 prohibit employers from making preemployment inquiries about the existence, nature, and severity of handicaps unless the inquiry focuses on the ability to perform job-related functions.[12] In other words, in an application form or at a job interview an applicant may only be asked if he or she has any physical or mental impairment that would interfere with the ability to perform the job. Thus, an applicant may not be asked, for example, whether he or she has hypertension, epilepsy, diabetes, or other conditions. Similar regulations have been promulgated under state handicap laws.[13]

The role of medical examinations in the hiring process is often overlooked. Commonly, the applicant will be offered a job contingent on a satisfactory medical examination. At this point, there is no prohibition on a company physician or nurse inquiring about and testing for a series of medical conditions that only minutes before could not be asked about by the personnel officer. Although only job-related medical criteria will legally justify a refusal to hire, applicants often are not told of the reasons for their disqualification. In addition, the nonmedical personnel, who were barred from asking about specific medical conditions, may be given a detailed medical report.

It is hard to imagine that by having an applicant walk down the hall and give the medical information to someone in a white coat that the employer has satisfied the substantial policy interests of limiting the use of irrelevant medical criteria. Moreover, as increasingly sensitive medical information becomes available (e.g., HIV status, genetic markers), it will not be enough to limit the *use* of the information; the solicitation and disclosure of the information also must be controlled. If occupational health professionals will not restrict their medical inquiries to job-related information, then increased government regulation will be inevitable.

Handicap discrimination laws are important in diagnostic screening (Chapter 2) and in predictive screening (Chapter 3). Not surprisingly, the more difficult issues involve predictive screening. There are essentially two questions: (1) Are currently capable individuals considered "at risk" of future impairments covered under the definition of an "individual with handicaps"? and (2) If so, when may an employer consider future risks in deciding employability?

There have been very few cases under the Rehabilitation Act to raise the issue of future risks. In *OFCCP v. E.E. Black, Ltd.*,[14] George Crosby, a 31-year-old carpenter's apprentice, applied for a job with E.E. Black, Ltd., a general construction contractor in Honolulu. Crosby was required to submit to a preemployment medical examination, including a low-back x-ray, which revealed a lower back anomaly known as sacralization of the transitional vertebra. This is a congenital condition found in eight to nine percent of the population. Although its disabling long-term effects are in dispute in the medical profession, E.E. Black conceded that the condition did not affect Crosby's current capability to perform the duties of a carpenter's apprentice. In fact, Crosby was in excellent physical condition. He played football at the University of Hawaii and had tried out for several professional football teams. He had previously worked packing and moving furniture and had completed 8,000 hours in a carpenter's apprentice program—all without any problems. Nonetheless, relying on its medical officer's conclusions, E.E. Black determined that Crosby's spinal formation put him at risk of developing future back problems, and denied him employment. Crosby filed a complaint with the OFCCP, charging E.E. Black with violating section 503.

The Labor Department found in favor of Crosby and ruled that E.E. Black's use of preemployment medical examinations tended to disqualify handicapped applicants despite their current capability to perform the job. The Labor Department refused to define "impairment," as used in the definitional section of the Act, to be limited to permanent disabilities such as blindness or deafness. Instead, the term impairment was held to be "any condition which weakens, restricts or otherwise damages an individual's health or physical or mental activity"[15] resulting in a current bar to employment that the individual is currently capable of performing.

On judicial review, the United States District Court for the District of Hawaii agreed with the Labor Department that the Rehabilitation Act's coverage was intended to be broad, but it held that the Assistant Secretary of Labor's interpretation was overly broad.[16] According to the court, the Act's coverage is restricted to handicapped individuals who are "substantially limited" in pursuit of a major life activity. Thus, to be protected by the Act, an individual must have been rejected for a position for which he or she was qualified because of an impairment or perceived impairment that constitutes, for the individual, a substantial handicap to employment. Factors to be considered in determining whether an impairment substantially limits employability include the number and types of jobs from which the individual is disqualified, the location or accessibility of similar opportunities, and the individual's own job expectations and training.

Applying these factors, the court concluded that Crosby was subject to the protections of the Act. First, Crosby's back condition was found to be an impairment or, at least, was regarded as such by E.E. Black. Second, the impairment was found to constitute a substantial handicap to employment because Crosby would have been disqualified from all or substantially all apprenticeship programs in carpentry. Third, the court rejected E.E. Black's contention that Congress did not intend to protect job applicants denied employment based on the risk of future injury. The case was subsequently remanded to the Department of Labor[17] and later settled. E.E. Black gave Crosby $7,500 in back pay and promised not to exclude any apprentice carpenter solely on the basis of a radiological finding of a transitional lumbosacral vertebra.

State laws vary in their treatment of future risk. California's Fair Employment Practice Regulations specifically limit the degree to which future risk may be considered.

> "[I]t is no defense to assert that a qualified handicapped person has a condition or disease with a future risk, so long as the condition or disease does not presently interfere with his or her ability to perform the job in a manner that will not immediately endanger the handicapped individual or others, and the person is able to safely perform the job over a reasonable length of time. 'A reasonable length of time' is to be determined on an individual basis."[18]

This interpretation has been endorsed by case law in California.[19]

In *Brown v. City of Portland*,[20] a probationary police officer was discharged after a medical examiner's report of early degenerative disease in the knee led the police to conclude that he was likely to be incapacitated in the future. The Oregon Court of Appeals held that this was unlawful discrimination. "[O]nly the *present* risk of injury or incapacitation, not the risk of injury or incapacitation in the future, could be a proper basis for a discharge."[21]

The seemingly absolute approach of the Oregon court in *Brown* goes beyond the language of *E.E. Black*. The court in *E.E. Black* posed the situation where an individual had a 90 percent chance of suffering a heart attack within one month. The court suggested that screening out such an individual would be lawful under the Rehabilitation Act.[22]

Another important issue is whether minor physical and mental irregularities are "handicaps." In recent cases, a wide range of conditions have been alleged to be handicaps, including chronic lateness,[23] spider phobia,[24] small stature,[25] compulsive gambling,[26] and left-handedness.[27] Are these handicaps? Is it enough that the condition resulted in interference with a major life activity (a particular job)? Did the legislatures intend to protect these individuals or condone discrimination on such bases?

In *Forrisi v. Bowen*,[28] the United States Court of Appeals for the Fourth Circuit held that a telephone company employee, whose job required him to climb utility poles, was not a "handicapped individual" under the Rehabilitation Act because he suffered from acrophobia.

> "The Rehabilitation Act assures that truly disabled, but genuinely capable, individuals will not face discrimination in employment because of stereotypes about the insurmountability of their handicaps. It would debase this high purpose if the statutory protections available to those truly handicapped could be claimed by anyone whose disability was minor and whose relative severity of impairment was widely shared. Indeed, the very concept of an impairment implies a characteristic that is not commonplace and that poses for the particular individual a more general disadvantage in his or her search for satisfactory employment."[29]

To determine whether a particular impairment is a handicap to an individual, the courts have considered whether the impairment is a significant barrier to employment. This, in turn, depends on "the number and type of jobs from which the impaired individual is disqualified, the geographical area to which the individual has reasonable access, and the individual's job expectations and training."[30]

In *Chevron Corp. v. Redmon*,[31] Sheila Ann Carter Redmon applied for the job of maintenance helper with Gulf Oil Corporation (now Chevron Corporation). She was rejected because her corrected 20/60 vision in one eye fell below the company's minimum vision standard of 20/40. The Supreme Court of Texas held that Redmon's "minor visual problems" did not constitute a handicap under Texas law: "[T]he legislature was concerned with those physical and mental defects which are serious enough to affect a person's use of public facilities and common carriers, ability to obtain housing, and the ability to cross the street . . . . The legislature obviously was not concerned with minor physical or mental defects."[32]

The "future risk" and "minor condition" cases raise a particularly difficult problem in the context of predictive screening (for both occupational and nonoccupational illnesses). Medical risks that have a low likelihood of manifesting, are not severe, and will not occur for a long time represent the most unreasonable application of predictive screening. Yet, in these cases the courts are most likely to hold that the individual was not even covered under the statute.

Handicap discrimination cases have rejected "absolute" inter-pretations of federal and state statutes. Some future risks of illness will be considered so immediate as to justify exclusion. Not all minor conditions will be covered. Some jobs raise more substantial public safety interests. Consequently, in deciding whether to employ certain individuals and in adjudicating claims of discrimination, it is inevitable that lines will need to be drawn and distinctions must be made. In so doing, a framework for decisionmaking is essential.

A Framework for Medico-Legal Decisionmaking

Deciding whether individuals with current and potential impairments should be employed in specific jobs entails mixed questions of medicine, law, and personnel administration. These are more than intellectually provocative abstractions. Employment decisions must be made in thousands of real-life situations every day.

Two key questions that invariably arise are: (1) When medical opinions conflict, whose opinion should be given the most weight? and (2) What guidelines should employers (and courts) use to evaluate the legality of medical screening?

As to the first question, involving the appropriate deference in cases of conflict, there is no clear body of case law under handicap discrimination statutes. Nonetheless, courts will probably give greater deference to a treating physician than an examining physician and greater deference to an examining physician than a physician who has only reviewed records or seen test results. For example, in a recent New York case,[33] the court gave greater weight to the employee's treating physician, a specialist, than to the employer's examining physician, who had never before had contact with a patient who had multiple sclerosis. Similar decisions are common in Social Security and, to a lesser extent, workers' compensation cases.[34]

The theory behind giving greater weight to the testimony of treating physicians is that a treating physician is more experienced than a mere examining physician in determining the health status of a specific individual. Although it could be argued that the testimony of some treating physicians may be colored by undue sympathy for their regular patients, the countering argument is that some third-party examining physicians may be unduly sympathetic to the financial interests of the third parties who have retained their services.

Similarly, the opinions of physicians who have examined the individual are also likely to be given greater weight than the opinions of physicians who have merely reviewed medical records.

As to the criteria to be used in evaluating medical screening decisions, the following 10 factors should be considered. These factors are applicable to screening for occupational and nonoccupational illnesses and for diagnostic screening as well as predictive screening. Some factors, however, will not be relevant to every assessment.

Job-relatedness of the medical criteria underlying the screening process

The first step is to analyze the physical (and sometimes mental) demands of the job in order to develop relevant medical criteria. For example, if a job involves heavy lifting, then a healthy back would be a job-related medical criterion. If an applicant or employee had a back problem or was likely to develop one, then the individual could be denied employment at this position.

In *Carr v. General Motors Corp.*,[35] the plaintiff had undergone back surgery for a ruptured disk and was restricted by his own physician and the company physician from lifting more than 50 pounds. The Supreme Court of Michigan held that it was not unlawful to deny him a transfer to a job involving heavy lifting.

A similar result was reached in *Halsey v. Coca-Cola Bottling Co.*[36] The plaintiff serviced and repaired vending machines and was required to drive a truck to various locations in Iowa. As a result of macular degeneration of the retina he was unable to pass the state's required vision test and lost his operator's license. The Supreme Court of Iowa upheld the employee's discharge because the good vision (and driver's license) requirement was job related.

If the applicant or employee is "otherwise qualified" (meaning qualified despite the "handicap"), then the burden will be on the employer to prove that the disqualification was job related. For example, in *Micu v. City of Warren*,[37] the Michigan Court of Appeals held that the city had the burden of proving that its minimum height requirement of 5 feet 8 inches for firefighters was reasonably necessary to the operation of the "business."

Degree of correlation between the specific screening measures used and the job-related medical criteria

Medical criteria such as a healthy back, good vision, and mental stability are conclusions. The accuracy of the medical tests and procedures used in reaching these conclusions (especially as to future risks) needs to be considered carefully. Are the x-rays, laboratory tests, and other procedures medically accepted predictors of future illness? What is the predictive value of the test? (For a further discussion, see Chapter 3 under the heading "The Limits of Predictive Screening.")

In *Crane v. Dole*,[38] Robert Crane, an air traffic controller who wore a hearing aid, was denied a job as an aeronautical information specialist because of allegedly deficient hearing. The FAA employees responsible for testing his hearing had no experience whatsoever in either hearing or testing. They devised a test in which a series of 15 messages were read aloud at 100 words per minute without interruption and Crane was expected to copy the messages sequentially without error. In ruling that the FAA had violated the Rehabilitation Act, the district court found at least four serious deficiencies with the test: (1) In addition to testing hearing, the test measured skill in shorthand; (2) the test was not job related because an information specialist would never have to transcribe such long messages; (3) the conditions of the test were uncontrolled; and (4) the test was not validated to determine whether someone who was not hearing-impaired could pass. Only a game of "whispering down the lane" would appear to be less scientific.

In *Quinn v. Southern Pacific Transportation Co.*,[39] R. Brian Quinn, a railroad employee, was rejected for a position as a railroad hostler (train servicer) because he failed the Ishihara color vision test at a preemployment examination. Quinn, who had a mild red-green color deficiency, was able to pass the Farnsworth and Duochrome tests. The Oregon Court of Appeals held that the railroad failed to prove that passing the Ishihara test was essential to satisfactory performance.

Severity of the injury or illness

From a medical and human resources standpoint, it is illogical to screen out individuals based on the health risk of sneezing, tearing, a mild rash, or the like. From a legal standpoint, however,

such minor conditions may not be considered handicaps and therefore it would not be illegal to discriminate on the basis of either
having or being at risk of getting such a condition.

In *Chevron* (discussed in the previous section of this chapter)
and similar cases in which the defense is raised that the medical
condition is too trivial to constitute a handicap, the employer is in a
somewhat awkward position. In effect, the employer is arguing that,
for example, 20/60 eyesight in one eye is not a handicap because it
does not interfere with a major life activity (i.e., working) inasmuch
as no reasonable employer would deny employment on that basis.
Note: This is not the same thing as arguing that 20/40 vision is a valid
employment criterion, because issues such as safety need not be
considered if the individual is not "handicapped."

Severity of the consequences of the injury or illness

For both diagnostic screening and predictive screening cases, it
is important to determine the consequences of the individual's
handicap. This often relates closely to whether the individual is
"otherwise qualified" or is a threat to safety.

In *Jansen v. Food Circus Supermarkets, Inc.*,[40] Daniel Jansen,
a 39-year-old meatcutter who had worked without incident for eight
years, was discharged after suffering an epileptic seizure at work in
which he stood staring with a knife in his hand. In remanding the
case for further evidence, the Supreme Court of New Jersey stated
that the supermarket must prove and not assume that Jansen presented a danger. The court stated: "The failure to distinguish
between the risk of a future seizure and that of a future injury is
crucial. The assumption that every epileptic who suffers a seizure is
a danger to himself or to others reflects the prejudice that the Law
seeks to prevent."[41]

Absolute risk of future illness

Before screening out currently healthy individuals because of a
risk of future illness it is essential to determine the absolute risk. In
other words, what is the likelihood of the individual developing the
illness in question.

In *State ex rel. Gomez-Bethke v. Metropolitan Airport Commission*,[42] Roger Kumm applied for the job of airport maintenance
worker, which involved heavy lifting. He was rejected because a

preemployment back x-ray revealed hypertrophic degenerative changes at L5-S1 (fifth lumbar and first sacral vertebra) and an old compression fracture at L1. The Minnesota Court of Appeals upheld the refusal to hire because of medical testimony that Kumm had a 50 to 75 percent chance of becoming disabled due to a herniated disk. The court was unpersuaded by the fact that after being denied this job, Kumm secured a maintenance job with Republic Airlines involving heavy lifting and he performed the job without any problems for more than two years.

A contrary result was reached in *In re State Division of Human Rights (Granelle)*.[43] Peter Granelle, a police officer candidate, was denied appointment because a back x-ray revealed pre-spondylolisthesis and a widening of the lumbosacral angle. Although Granelle was asymptomatic, the police department relied on a nonexamining physician's estimate that Granelle had a 25 percent chance of developing a back disability within 10 to 20 years. The New York Court of Appeals held that the police department violated the state human rights law. "At best, there was speculation that a person with spondylolisthesis had a greater statistical probability of suffering low back disability than a person with normal back x-rays."[44]

Relative risk of future illness

In *Granelle* the candidate had a higher relative risk but there was inadequate evidence that the absolute risk was high. It is also possible to have a high absolute risk and a low relative risk. For example, a medical examination may indicate that an applicant for the job of coal miner, with a certain biochemical profile, has an 85 percent chance of suffering a lung impairment over the course of his working life. If all coal miners have an 80 percent chance of lung impairment, employment should not be denied on the basis of this slightly increased relative risk. Thus, to justify screening out an individual there should be both a high absolute risk and a high relative risk.

Latency period

Unless there is an overwhelming likelihood of the individual's contracting an extremely serious disease, such as cancer, from occupational exposures, illnesses with long latency periods should be disregarded in medical screening. For example, an individual aged 25 should not be denied employment as a bricklayer because of a heightened risk of developing arthritis at age 60. The courts have not yet addressed the issue of whether screening is lawful where it involves a nonoccupational illness with a long latency period. This issue would be of paramount importance if genetic testing were to become widespread.

Need for an individualized determination of fitness

In deciding whether an individual is fit for employment based on current health or future health risks the courts have disapproved of the use of broad, class-based screening. Instead, there must be an individualized determination of the medical condition of each individual applicant or employee. The courts have not yet addressed the issue of whether some individual test procedures are so expensive or have such low yields that requiring their use for individual decision-making is unduly burdensome.

In *Rozanski v. A-P-A Transport,*[45] two truck drivers were denied employment at the end of their 30-day probation periods because one had a small osteophyte or spur on his spine and the other had spondylolysis. The Maine Supreme Judicial Court held that it violated the state human rights act to deny employment to these asymptomatic individuals solely on the basis of an x-ray.

> "[D]efendant did not really assess either [man's] handicap and the relationship of that handicap to the truck driving job on an individualized basis . . . . No clinical examination was performed, no history taken by the [company] doctors. Such examination and history would have revealed the excellent physical condition of both plaintiffs . . . ."[46]

An example of a case where an individualized determination was made is *Pearson Candy Co. v. Huyen.*[47] The employer refused to hire Deborah Kanar to work on its assembly line because she had grand mal epilepsy. The company relied on reports of its own physician and Kanar's physician, both of whom recommended against hiring her because Kanar's history of seizures without warning and the dangerous machinery on the assembly line created a serious safety hazard.

Possibility of reasonable accommodation

Although reasonable accommodation is required under the Rehabilitation Act and many (but not all) state handicap laws, it is still not well settled what degree of accommodation is required. It is established, however, that accommodations are not reasonable if they are unduly burdensome or would cause undue hardship on the employer. In *Nelson v. Thornburgh*,[48] the court stated that, for purposes of section 504, whether accommodations would pose an undue hardship on an employer would be determined by: (1) the size of the program; (2) the type of operation and composition of the work force; and (3) the cost. In *Nelson*, the state of Pennsylvania was required to provide a half-time reader or its mechanical equivalent to enable a blind income assistance worker to perform the job.

In general, employers will probably be required to make facilities accessible, such as by adding ramps and widening doors,[49] and to allow the use of lead dogs, orthopedic aids, and mechanized equipment to help the employee perform the job.[50] Although employers may be required to make accommodations in assignments,[51] they probably will not be required to rewrite job descriptions to accommodate a single employee,[52] to modify equipment being used where doing so would be burdensome,[52] or to reassign personnel and alter workloads to accommodate one individual.[54]

Stutts v. Freeman[55] is an example of a case where the employer made little effort at accommodation. Joseph Stutts was refused entry into an apprentice program for heavy equipment operators at the Tennessee Valley Authority (TVA) because he had a low score on a written test. Stutts had dyslexia and consequently did badly on written tests, although non-written tests indicated he had above average intelligence, coordination, and aptitude to be a heavy equipment operator. When TVA was unable to obtain these other test results, it made no further efforts at accommodation (such as giving him an oral test) and simply rejected him. The United States Court of Appeals for the Eleventh Circuit held that TVA violated section 504 by failing to make reasonable accommodations.

A case in which the employer did a better job of accommodation is *Vickers v. Veterans Administration*.[56] Lanny Vickers was employed in the Supply Service Department at the Veterans Administration (VA) Medical Center in Seattle. Vickers, who was "unusually sensitive to tobacco smoke," brought an action under section 504 for damages and equitable relief requiring the VA "to make reasonable accommodations to his physical handicap by providing a work environment that is free of tobacco smoke."[57] The court held that Vickers was "handicapped" within the meaning of the Act because his hypersensitivity did in fact limit one of his major life activities, that is, his capacity to work in an environment which is not completely smoke free. Nevertheless, the court held that the VA was under no duty to provide an environment wholly free of tobacco smoke, and even if there were such a duty, the VA had satisfied it. Specifically, the VA had, among other things, separated smokers from nonsmokers in the office, installed two vents and an air purifier, and offered Vickers an alternative job.

A frequently litigated issue is whether employers have a duty to reassign employees who are no longer able to perform their jobs. In *School Board v. Arline*,[58] the Supreme Court addressed this issue: "Although they are not required to find another job for an employee who is not qualified for the job he or she was doing, they cannot deny an employee alternative employment opportunities reasonably available under the employer's existing policies."[59] Indeed, the employer may have a duty to assist a handicapped employee in obtaining an available position for which he or she is qualified.

Finally, the burden of proof with regard to reasonable accommodation rests with the employer. In *Prewitt v. United States Postal Service*,[60] the United States Court of Appeals for the Fifth Circuit explained the rationale:

> "The employer has greater knowledge of the essentials of the job than does the handicapped applicant. The employer can look to its own experience, or, if that is not helpful, to that of other employers who have provided jobs to individuals with handicaps similar to those of the applicant in question. Furthermore, the employer may be able to obtain advice concerning possible accommodations from private and government sources."[61]

Disclosure of all relevant information to the applicant or employee

The final consideration is not a legal mandate, but an ethical and policy concern. In Chapter 1 under the heading "Medical Screening and Employee Selection" it was suggested that applicants and employees should be informed of medical findings discovered in the course of an examination. The focus was on informing the individuals of the reasons for their exclusion and, where appropriate, the need for further medical care. Nevertheless, disclosures also should be made when the employer discovers a condition that it determines to be too minor to warrant exclusion. Especially as to conditions that may be aggravated by occupational exposures, considerations of individual autonomy demand that this information be conveyed to the applicant or employee. Thus, even if the employer deems the risks acceptable, the applicant or employee also should have the opportunity to make a similar, informed determination.

Employer Defenses: Safety and Cost

Several defenses may be raised to claims of discrimination in employment on the basis of handicap. For example, coworker preference and customer preference, although they are more explanations for discrimination than they are legal defenses, are sometimes raised. As noted in the AIDS discussion, Chapter 5, these defenses are unlikely to prevail.

The three key defenses to employment discrimination, job relatedness, business necessity, and bona fide occupational qualification, all have their origins in Title VII of the Civil Rights Act of 1964. Although the terms sometimes have been used interchangeably, there are differences. Job relatedness concerns whether an employer's criteria used in determining if an applicant or employee is qualified for employment bear a reasonable relationship to the demands of the job. For example, height and weight requirements[62] and standardized tests[63] have been evaluated under job relatedness.

Business necessity is somewhat broader and applies when a general employment practice is used whose purpose is not to determine ability to perform job requirements. For example, not hiring prior felons[64] or individuals whose wages were subject to garnishment[64] have been analyzed under business necessity. For both defenses, employers would have to prove that despite any possible discriminatory effects (along the lines of race, color, religion, sex, or national origin), the criteria were essential to the business and no other criteria with less of an effect would be possible to use.

Bona fide occupational qualification (BFOQ) is a statutory defense under Title VII, limited to religion, sex, and national origin. In effect, the employer is arguing that it is engaging in legitimate, noninvidious discrimination. For example, hiring only women to play the female parts in a movie would not be discriminatory. Being a woman would be a BFOQ for the part.

These three defenses all have been used in handicap discrimination cases. Often the defenses are closely related and are different ways of asking whether an individual is otherwise qualified. For example, is an applicant with a history of back spasms otherwise qualified for the job of furniture mover? Despite an adverse or disparate impact on individuals with handicaps, liability insurance considerations (not dropping expensive furniture) would be a business necessity in hiring decisions. Back strength testing procedures would be evaluated to see if they were job related. Being able to lift heavy furniture would be a BFOQ of the job.

The essence of these defenses, minus some of the legal intricacies, appears in the preceding section on medico-legal decision-making as well as the next section on specific conditions. Safety and cost, however, are defenses that deserve separate attention.

Safety

The most commonly raised defense in handicap discrimination cases is safety—of the employee with a handicap, of coworkers and customers, and of the public. The safety defense is likely to be taken quite seriously by the courts and even with less than compelling facts the courts have been willing to uphold the employer's action. Where safety is involved, the courts sometimes have shown little sympathy for plaintiffs' claims of discrimination. For example, in *Consolidation Coal Co. v. Ohio Civil Rights Commission*,[66] Ruth Rosset was denied employment as an underground coal miner because she failed a hearing test. In rejecting the claim that this was handicap discrimination, the court stated: "Is the Commission suggesting that . . . Consol should have put Rosset to work as an under-ground coal miner, one of the most if not the most hazardous of all occupations, and see how it works out! Underground Coal Mines are not social laboratories. Have we reached the point where every "social belch" has risen to the level of a justiciable controversy?"[67]

A reluctance to second-guess employers is especially evident where the individual with a handicap is responsible for public safety. For example, in *Ross v. Beaumont Hospital*,[68] a section 504 case, a surgeon with narcolepsy claimed that her discharge was handicap discrimination. The court, in rejecting this argument, indicated its view of the competing interests: "Where the lives of critically ill patients are at stake, public policy may dictate exclusion if there is any doubt concerning an individual's ability to serve such patients."[69]

In other cases where the person with a handicap had public safety responsibilities, the courts also have been highly deferential to the safety defense—perhaps too deferential. In *Dauten v. County of Muskegon*,[70] Alvina Dauten applied for the job of lifeguard and was rejected because she had a mild case of scoliosis, a common and rarely disabling lateral curvature of the spine. The county was concerned that she might suffer back spasms in trying to save a swimmer. The court agreed with the county. "Even if a lifeguard never has to attempt to save a life, her ability to do so is still perhaps the most important factor to be considered in making a decision to hire."[71]

The other main category of cases where there is a direct threat to public safety involves transportation workers. Again, the courts have given great weight to the public safety argument and, in some representative cases, have upheld employers who refused to employ a bus driver with hypertension (blood pressure of 160/80);[72] a bus driver with no measurable vision in his left eye;[73] and a taxi driver who was congenitally absent a right hand and forearm.[74]

If the safety risk is only to the individual or the danger to public safety is less immediate, the courts have reached less predictable results. In *Jansen v. Food Circus Supermarkets, Inc.*,[75] the New Jersey Supreme Court was unwilling to exclude categorically an epileptic meatcutter, but in *Father Flanagan's Boys' Home v. Goerke*,[76] the Nebraska Supreme Court upheld the discharge of an assistant family teacher with epilepsy who had not had a seizure in 10 years on the ground that he was a safety risk because part of his job involved driving the boys on activities. In deciding whether a possible safety risk is sufficient to exclude an individual, most courts have required the employer to show a "reasonable probability" of harm,[77] although some courts have adopted a less stringent "rational basis" test for common carriers.[78]

Cost

Cost already has been mentioned as one of the considerations in evaluating whether certain accommodations are reasonable. There are at least three other costs that may be raised as defenses in handicap discrimination cases: (1) liability for injuries and damages, to the employee and third parties, caused by an employee with a handicap; (2) lost productivity caused by absenteeism, turnover, and decreased efficiency; and (3) increased insurance and other health care costs.

The Rehabilitation Act and most state laws are silent on the issue of cost, although they implicitly recognize that equal employment opportunities for individuals with handicaps often means additional costs. It has been the job of the courts to decide whether the additional costs placed on employers are unreasonable. There have been only a few cases to raise this issue, but thus far, the cost defense has not been successful.

In *Higgins v. Maine Central Railroad*,[79] Maine Central attempted to justify its discharge of an epileptic employee on the ground that it was attempting to avoid potential liability for personal injury. The Supreme Judicial Court of Maine rejected this argument. "Merely because federal law and the hazards inherent in railroad operations subject the Defendants to a comparatively high risk of liability, the Defendants are not entitled to employ only the healthiest and least accident-prone segments of society."[80]

In *Laclede Cab Co. v. Missouri Commission on Human Rights*,[81] a taxi company refused to hire a man whose left hand had been amputated. The company claimed that its insurance would be jeopardized. Although the record did not contain any evidence on insurance cost, the Missouri Court of Appeals held that the man need not be hired, even if otherwise qualified, "if in fact the cost to insure him would be inordinately expensive."[82]

The issue of lost productivity caused by absenteeism was addressed in *Chrysler Outboard Corp. v. Department of Industry, Labor & Human Relations*.[83] Chrysler refused to hire an applicant who suffered from acute lymphocytic leukemia. The Wisconsin Court of Appeals rejected the argument that the fear of "future absenteeism" justified a refusal to hire.

The final cost concern, insurance and health care costs, is likely to be the most important as we move into an age of predictive screening for nonoccupational illness. Interestingly, the Pennsylvania Human Relations Act has a provision directly addressed to this issue: "Uninsurability or increased cost of insurance under a group or employe insurance plan does not render a handicap or disability job related."[84] There have been no cases, however, decided under this statutory provision.

In *State Division of Human Rights v. Xerox Corp.*,[85] Catherine McDermott, a computer programmer, applied for a job with Xerox. She was offered a position as a systems consultant, provided she passed a preemployment medical examination. The findings of the examination were unremarkable except that McDermott was obese;

she was 5 feet 6 inches and weighed 249 pounds. Xerox refused to hire her because "gross obesity posed a significant risk to short and long term disability and life insurance programs" administered by the company. The New York Court of Appeals, in holding that Xerox violated the New York Human Rights Act, rejected the cost defense. "[T]he company could not refuse to hire her because of the collateral effect her impairment, if it be that, might have on existing disability and life insurance programs."[86]

The cases decided by the courts so far involving the cost defense have been easy ones. The plaintiffs have been individual employees who were otherwise qualified, the defendants have been large corporations, and the costs have been speculative. Would a court find unlawful a refusal to hire by a small, marginal employer when the applicant already was receiving expensive dialysis treatments? Would it matter if the health care consumer were a dependent of the applicant or employee? How many people with AIDS does a small company have to employ? These and related questions are difficult indeed, and they are likely to arise with increasing frequency. For the moment, at least, the cost defense is more of a political argument for the legislatures than a legal argument for the courts.

Specific Medical Conditions

As the preceding sections of this chapter have shown, an employer's legal duty to employ a handicapped individual will depend on the jurisdiction (wording of state law and state judicial interpretations), the nature of the job in question, and the nature of the handicap. Consequently, it is often quite venturesome to predict the outcome of any given case. Over a decade of state and federal case law, however, has provided some guideposts on the way that certain handicapping conditions tend to be viewed by the courts. This information should be valuable not only to lawyers, but also to physicians and managers who are responsible for developing policies on hiring individuals with handicaps.

AIDS

For a discussion, see Chapter 5.

Alcoholism

Sections 503 and 504 of the Rehabilitation Act were amended in 1978 to exclude only those alcoholics "whose current use of alcohol . . . prevents such individual from performing the duties of the job in question or whose employment . . . would constitute a direct threat to property or the safety of others."[87] Although this provision does not apply to the federal government as an employer, the Comprehensive Alcohol Abuse and Alcoholism Prevention, Treatment and Rehabilitation Act[88] imposes certain obligations on the federal government. Federal employers must have alcoholism treatment programs and they may dismiss only alcoholic employees who have refused or repeatedly failed treatment.

The coverage of alcoholism under state handicap laws varies widely. In some states, alcoholics are expressly included; in other states they are expressly excluded; in still other states the statute is silent and the issue of coverage has been decided by the courts.[89]

Most cases of handicap discrimination based on alcoholism have involved current employees who have been dismissed from their jobs rather than applicants who have not been selected for a job. This may be a result of the complexity of detecting alcoholism and the denial of a drinking problem that is characteristic of the disease. Interestingly, the jurisdictions are divided on the issue of whether medical evidence must be introduced in a case alleging discrimination based on alcoholism.[90]

Two main legal issues predominate in handicap discrimination cases involving alcoholism: (1) whether the employer has satisfied its duty of reasonable accommodation; and (2) whether independent cause exists for the discharge.

In *Whitlock v. Donovan*,[91] a supervisory employee with 23 years of federal service was discharged for absences caused by alcoholism. The court held that even if an alcoholic has a relapse following treatment, the federal government must continue to make reasonable accommodations, such as allowing the individual to reapply after completion of treatment.

State court decisions involving private sector employees have held that it is unlawful to discharge an employee for absences caused by undergoing treatment for alcoholism.[92] Federal court cases involving federal employees, however, have upheld the discharge of alcoholic employees following repeated unsuccessful attempts at rehabilitation.[93]

In several cases involving alcoholism the courts have found a legitimate, nondiscriminatory basis for the discharge. For example, in *Blitz v. Northwest Airlines, Inc.*,[94] a pilot was lawfully discharged after he denied alcoholism, refused treatment, and lost his FAA medical certificate. Other cases upholding the discharge of alcoholics have involved intoxication on the job,[95] public intoxication,[96] criminal conduct caused by alcoholism,[97] falsifying an application form to deny a history of alcoholism,[98] and poor job performance unrelated to alcoholism.[99]

Amputations

Cases involving amputees have tended to confirm the principle that there must be an individualized determination of fitness. If an individual is able to safely and efficiently perform the job despite an amputation, then it will violate handicap discrimination laws to deny employment to such an individual. For example, in *Board of Trustees v. Human Rights Commission*,[100] Howard Laws, whose leg was amputated above the knee following a motorcycle accident, applied for a job with the University of Illinois as a sheet metal worker. Laws had successfully worked as a sheet metal worker for 20 years after his injury and he had climbed ladders and worked on scaffolds and roofs without any difficulty. The Illinois Court of Appeals held that the University acted illegally by rejecting Laws without giving him an opportunity to demonstrate his ability to perform the job.

In some jurisdictions, archaic laws remain on the books which prohibit the hiring of amputees for certain jobs. Such blanket exclusions are unlikely to be sustained if challenged in court.[101]

Safety concerns are often raised in defending an employer's refusal to hire an amputee. In *Boynton Cab Co. v. Department of Industry, Labor & Human Relations*,[102] the Supreme Court of Wisconsin upheld Boynton's refusal to hire Eli Godfried, who was congenitally absent a right hand and forearm from about three inches below the elbow. Despite the fact that Godfried had driven a taxi without incident for two other companies for approximately nine months, the court held that common carriers of passengers have a lesser burden in justifying safety-based employment standards.

In a more recent and better reasoned decision, *Laclede Cab Co. v. Missouri Commission on Human Rights*,[103] Matthew Williams, whose left hand had been amputated just above the wrist, applied for a job as a driver with Laclede. The Missouri Court of Appeals rejected Laclede's claim that hiring Williams could adversely affect its insurance (as discussed earlier) and held that, if qualified to safely drive a taxi, Williams could not be refused a job by Laclede.

Arthritis

Arthritis will be considered a handicap if it so severe that it substantially interferes with a major life activity.[104] Thus, rheumatoid arthritis has been held to be a handicap.[105] Minor osteoarthritis that does not interfere with normal activities will not be considered a handicap.[106] Refusals to employ individuals with arthritis for the jobs of bus driver[107] and postal worker[108] have been upheld where the arthritis prevented the person from performing the job in question.

Back Conditions

Cases involving back conditions have arisen from both pre-employment screening and disability evaluations after a current employee has suffered a back injury. The preemployment cases are often the most contentious. Because of the high cost of back injury cases (in terms of workers' compensation, disability, lost productivity, etc.), employers have used back x-rays and other techniques to screen out asymptomatic individuals who are considered at risk of future back problems. As discussed earlier,[109] these predictive screening measures have been repudiated in the medical literature. When challenged in a handicap discrimination case they also may be difficult to defend.

In *E.E. Black* it was held to violate section 503 of the Rehabilitation Act to refuse to hire an individual with asymptomatic sacralization of the transitional vertebra. Similar results have been reached in cases of asymptomatic spondylolisthesis,[110] asymptomatic spondylolysis,[111] asymptomatic scoliosis,[112] non-disabling spinal fusions,[113] and even where an applicant for a job with a railroad had a bullet lodged in his back.[114]

Preemployment back examinations have become increasingly sophisticated, although not necessarily more predictive or legally defensible. In *City of LaCrosse Police & Fire Commission v. Labor & Industry Review Commission*,[115] Daniel Rusch applied for a job as a police officer and was refused employment because he received a "B" rating on a Cybex machine back muscle strength test. The Wisconsin Supreme Court held that Rusch was covered under the state handicap law because he was perceived as having an impairment and the city failed to prove that he was unable to perform the job.

If the applicant is symptomatic, regardless of the condition, the courts are likely to uphold a refusal to hire. Employers have been successful in cases involving an applicant who had a laminectomy,[116] an unspecified "degenerative condition,"[117] spondylolysis,[118] and prior surgery to remove a spinal tumor.[119]

In light of the cases involving symptomatic applicants, it is not surprising that employers have prevailed in cases brought by current employees who have sustained back injuries. The courts have upheld the dismissal for excessive absences of a clerk who suffered a cervical and lumbar strain in a car accident,[120] the failure to rehire at her former position a flight attendant who had missed 18 months of work while recovering from two back injuries,[121] and the denial of a transfer to a job involving heavy lifting to a man who had back surgery for a ruptured disk.[122] In other back cases, employers have been sustained where they dismissed an employee who had falsified his employment record by failing to mention a prior back injury,[123] and where the courts ruled that "whiplash"[124] and a lumbar disk injury were not handicaps.[125]

The discharge of a truck driver with scoliosis, however, based on a "mere possibility" of future health problems was held unlawful by the California Court of Appeals in *Sterling Transit Co. v. Fair Employment Practice Commission*.[126] A temporary back sprain has been held to be a handicap, requiring the employer to make accommodations such as a straight back chair, use of an elevator, and coverage during regular breaks.[127]

Behavioral Conditions

The Supreme Court of Iowa has held that transsexualism is not a handicap under the state handicap discrimination law.[128] Transvestitism also has been held not to be a protected handicap under the Rehabilitation Act.[129]

Cancer

California[130] and Vermont[131] statutorily list cancer as a handicapping condition. In other states, cancer is evaluated in the same way as any other medical condition. Under the Rehabilitation Act, cancer is a handicap,[132] although legislation has been introduced in Congress to amend Title VII of the Civil Rights Act of 1964 to specifically include cancer as a proscribed basis for discrimination.[133]

There have been few cancer cases decided on the merits.[134] In perhaps the leading case, *Chrysler Outboard Corp. v. Department of Industry, Labor & Human Relations*,[135] the Wisconsin Circuit Court held that it was unlawful to refuse to hire an applicant with acute lymphocytic leukemia because the employer feared he would be unable to perform his duties in the future.[136] No case has yet raised the issue of whether an individual may be screened out based on an increased risk of developing cancer.

Dermatological Conditions

Contact dermatitis is the most common occupational disease.[137] It is seldom disabling, however, and therefore has not given rise to many handicap discrimination cases. In *Westinghouse Electric Corp. v. State Division of Human Rights*,[138] an 18-year-old high school student applied for a summer job as a general laborer. A preemployment examination revealed dermatitis in the femoral or intertriginous region and secondarily on parts of his body and limbs. Westinghouse refused to hire the applicant because chemical exposures in the plant would so exacerbate the dermatitis as to render him unable to perform his job. The New York Supreme Court, Appellate Division, upheld the company's action.

In *Shelby Township Fire Department v. Shields*,[139] the Michigan Court of Appeals held that pseudofolliculitis barbae is a handicap.

Diabetes

Diabetes is generally recognized as a handicap under federal and state law. Because the effects of the disease vary greatly among individuals, it is important to make an individualized determination of fitness based on sound medical evidence. Broad policies, such as a railroad's policy of refusing to hire any insulin-dependent diabetics as engineers,[140] may be held to violate handicap discrimination laws. In other cases, however, courts have upheld the FBI's policy of barring insulin-dependent diabetics as agents or investigators based on asserted health and safety concerns,[141] and a Maine law refusing to allow school bus drivers with diabetes.[142]

In *Bentivegna v. United States Department of Labor*,[143] the City of Los Angeles hired Philip Bentivegna as a "building repairer." Bentivegna had indicated on an application form that he had diabetes mellitus. Applicants with diabetes were required to demonstrate "control," meaning blood sugar levels below 150. Bentivegna was terminated when it was learned that his blood sugar was above 150. In holding that Bentivegna's termination violated section 504 of the Rehabilitation Act, the United States Court of Appeals for the Ninth Circuit found, among other things, that the city failed to prove a correlation between lower blood sugar levels and control of diabetes. The court, however, noted:

> "A requirement more directly tied to increased risk of injury, such as the exclusion of diabetics with demonstrated nervous or circulatory problems—some thing all physicians testifying in this case agreed would markedly increase the risks from injury—might present a different case if applied to applicants for a job that carries elevated risks of injury."[144]

Where employers have made individualized medical determinations about the employability of diabetics, they have been upheld in court.[145] This is especially true where employees are in hazardous jobs and had a prior hypoglycemic reaction at work.[146]

Drug Abuse

For a discussion, see Chapter 6 under the heading "Legal Challenges".

Epilepsy

It is well settled that epilepsy is a handicap under the Rehabilitation Act[147] and state handicap discrimination laws.[148] Indeed, discrimination based on irrational stereotypes and prejudices against people with handicaps such as epilepsy is precisely the reason for passage of handicap discrimination laws.[149]

As previously stated, employers are required to make an individualized determination of fitness and the failure to do so may lead to liability. For example, in *Kelley v. Bechtel Power Corp.*,[150] Paul Kelley was terminated from his position as a boilermaker mechanic at the Turkey Point, Florida, nuclear power facility when it was learned that he had epilepsy. In fact, Kelley had never had a seizure despite the diagnosis, and there was no evidence that he was unable to perform his duties safely. In finding a violation of the Florida Human Rights Act, the court stated: "It is unreasonable to deny a person employment because of a fear of recurrence of a condition [seizures] which that person has asserted he has never had . . . ."[151]

Epilepsy cases often involve the safety defense and several leading epilepsy cases were discussed earlier in this chapter under "Employer Defenses: Safety and Cost." In general, to justify a refusal to employ an epileptic because of safety concerns the employer must prove a reasonable probability of substantial harm.[152] For example, in one case a railroad excluded an epileptic welder by relying on general evidence that 10 to 30 percent of epileptics under medication will still have seizures.[153] The Wisconsin Supreme Court termed this degree of future risk "a mere possibility" and held that the railroad's action was illegal. In those cases where the individual was unable to perform the job, however, the courts have found for the employers.[154]

Employers also may be required to make reasonable accommodations for applicants and employees with epilepsy. In *Foods, Inc. v. Iowa Civil Rights Commission*,[155] Theresa Harkin was dismissed from her job as a cafeteria worker after having a seizure at work. The Supreme Court of Iowa held that the employer failed to meet its duty of reasonable accommodation. According to the court, Harkin could have been assigned to less hazardous tasks, such as washing dishes, bussing tables, and working on the serving line instead of working with hazardous equipment such as the deep fat fryer, meat slicer, and grill.

Hearing Impairments

Minimum hearing requirements have been upheld where they have been shown to be essential to job performance. This is especially true in hazardous jobs such as police officer[156] and coal miner.[156] Nevertheless, the method used to measure hearing must be scientifically valid[158] and the employer must satisfy its duty of reasonable accommodation.[159]

Heart Disease

Decisions regarding heart disease are among the most difficult judgments that occupational physicians have to make on employability.[160] Frequently, the decision involves a low risk of adverse outcome but a high severity of adverse outcome.[161] In heart disease cases employers usually have asserted either that the applicant or employee is unable to perform the job or the individual's employment would create a safety hazard to the employee or others.

For the most part, courts have deferred to the medical judgments of company physicians when the employers have concluded that an individual with heart disease would be unable to perform the job.[162] Thus, defendants have prevailed in handicap discrimination cases based on refusals to employ: as a Postal Service custodian a man with "heart disease;"[163] as a postal clerk a man with cardiovascular disease, an enlarged heart, and an abnormal electrocardiogram;[164] as a park technician with the Army Corps of Engineers a man who had undergone bypass surgery and had a pacemaker;[165] as a postal clerk a man with coronary artery disease;[166] and as a railroad clerk with the New York Transit Authority a man who had an unspecified heart condition.[167] Plaintiffs have been successful only where the employer discharged a school bus driver who had a history of heart disease without making an individualized determination of fitness;[168] and where the employer discharged an assembly line foreman, whose job was not strenuous, after he returned to work following a heart attack.[169]

Where the issue was safety, it was not a violation of the Rehabilitation Act for a longshoring company to refuse to hire a 63-year-old longshoreman who had undergone coronary bypass surgery.[170] On the other hand, in *Maine Human Rights Commission v. Canadian Pacific, Ltd.*,[171] an applicant was denied employment by Canadian Pacific because he had a heart murmur caused by a bicuspid aortic valve. The Supreme Judicial Court of Maine held that a "mere possibility" of sudden heart failure did not justify a refusal to hire.[172]

Hemophilia

In *Davis v. United States Postal Service*,[173] the court held that the Postal Service had no duty to accommodate a trainee with hemophilia and arthritis, who was unable to perform the job for which he was training, by reassigning him to a higher level position not otherwise available.

Hypertension

Some courts have held that hypertension is not a handicap, either because the affected individual did not seek medical treatment[174] or because the hypertension did not substantially interfere with a major life activity.[175] The majority rule, however, is that hypertension is a handicap.[176]

In *Mass Transit Administration v. Maryland Commission on Human Relations,*[177] Vance Simms was denied a job as a bus driver because his blood pressure of 160/80 exceeded the Transit Administration's maximum of 140/90. The Maryland Court of Special Appeals upheld the refusal to hire, noting the public safety risks posed by fainting, dizziness, and other side effects of hypertension.

A contrary result was reached in *American National Insurance Co. v. Fair Employment & Housing Commission.*[178] Dale Rivard was discharged as an insurance agent because of unspecified high blood pressure. The company claimed that the stressful nature of the job would expose Rivard to an excess risk of disability or death. The California Supreme Court held that the company failed to prove that Rivard was unable to perform the job or that his employment would endanger the health of himself or others.

Infectious Diseases

The leading infectious disease case, *School Board v. Arline,*[179] involving tuberculosis, is discussed in Chapter 5 under the heading "AIDS and the Workplace."

Learning Disabilities

For a discussion of an employer's duty of reasonable accommodation to an individual with dyslexia, see *Stutts v. Freeman,*[180] at page 138.

Miscellaneous Medical Conditions

In *State Division of Human Rights v. Leroy Central School District,*[181] Angela Giannavola applied to be a substitute school bus driver. The school district refused to hire her because she had both adrenal glands surgically removed and it was necessary for her to take daily hormone medication. The New York Supreme Court,

Appellate Division, held that because Giannavola was qualified to drive a school bus, the school district had violated the state human rights law in refusing to hire her.

In two cases involving employees with sarcoidosis,[182] the courts have held that the employers' duty of reasonable accommodation included assisting the employees in obtaining other positions after they no longer were able to continue in their present jobs.

Neurological Conditions

The most commonly litigated neurological condition (aside from epilepsy, which is discussed separately) is multiple sclerosis. In *Bayport-Blue Point School District v. State Division of Human Rights*,[183] the school district dismissed Laura Lynch from her job as a school bus driver after she was diagnosed as having multiple sclerosis. In holding that the school district had violated the New York Human Rights Act, the court relied on medical evidence that Lynch was qualified to continue driving and that "the symptoms of the disease come on gradually within a week or two and the weakness she experienced in her right side would never come on abruptly."[184]

A similar result was reached in *Carter v. Casa Central*,[185] a section 504 case, in which the United States Court of Appeals for the Seventh Circuit held that it was unlawful to discharge Joyce Carter, the director of nursing at a Chicago nursing home, because she had cerebellar ataxia caused by multiple sclerosis. Carter was otherwise qualified, and her job did not require her to walk or stand for prolonged periods of time.

In other multiple sclerosis cases the employers have prevailed where the affected individuals were unable to perform the job[186] or failed to establish that the challenged employment action was a result of handicap discrimination.[187]

In *Fitzgerald v. Green Valley Area Education Agency*,[188] Scott Fitzgerald applied for a job as a preschool teacher for handicapped children. He was denied the job because he had cerebral palsy and, despite having a driver's license, he would not be able to obtain a bus driver's license as a result of left side hemiplegia. The district court held that, as a recipient of federal funds under the Education of the Handicapped Act, the employer's duty "to take affirmative steps to accommodate for the handicap of a qualified applicant was greater than that imposed by section 504 on recipients of other types of federal aid."[189] The employer violated section 504 by failing to make any attempt to determine whether accommodations were possible that would permit the hiring of Fitzgerald, who in all other respects, was qualified for the position.[190]

Obesity

The weight of authority holds that obesity is not a handicap.[191] Among the reasons cited for such holdings are that the individual had not sought medical treatment for obesity,[192] concern for future absenteeism and disability caused by obesity was not handicap discrimination,[193] and obesity is not an "immutable condition" such as blindness.[194] Height and weight restrictions also may be considered job related.[195]

In some states obesity is a handicap.[196] In the leading case, *State Division of Human Rights v. Xerox Corp.*,[197] discussed previously, under the heading "Employer Defenses: Safety and Cost," the New York Court of Appeals broadly read the New York Human Rights Act to cover "a range of conditions varying in degree from those involving the loss of a bodily function to those which are merely diagnosable medical anomalies which impair bodily integrity and thus may lead to more serious conditions in the future."[198] The court rejected the argument that the statute should only apply to "immutable" and "involuntary" conditions.

Orthopedic Conditions

Besides back conditions, discussed previously, a number of other orthopedic impairments have been at issue in handicap discrimination cases. Employers have prevailed where they have been able to prove that an orthopedic impairment prevented the individual from performing the job. For example, it was not discriminatory to refuse to hire as a correctional officer a man who limped and wore a leg brace,[199] to refuse to hire as a firefighter a man who had knee surgery,[200] to demote a telephone lineman who injured his knee in a softball game and no longer could climb telephone poles,[201] to discharge a radial drill operator who developed lateral epicondylitis (tennis elbow) and could no longer perform the job,[202] and to discharge a letter carrier who injured his knee while being chased by a dog on his route.[203]

Plaintiffs have prevailed in the cases where they have been able to prove that despite an orthopedic impairment, such as wearing a leg brace[204] or having an injured knee,[205] they were otherwise qualified to perform the job. In addition, an employer was held liable for failing to make reasonable accommodation for an employee with chronic foot pain.[206]

Psychiatric Conditions

Individuals with well-documented, current psychiatric disorders are seldom able to prove that they are otherwise qualified. This is certainly the case with individuals who are paranoid schizophrenics,[207] manic depressives,[208] and those suffering from acute depression.[209] For individuals with less severe conditions, such as phobias and personality disorders, it may be difficult to establish that they are "handicapped" and subject to statutory protection.

Plaintiffs have been unsuccessful in proving allegations of discrimination based on acrophobia[210] and spider phobia.[211] In *Barnes v. Barbosa*,[212] Fletcher Barnes, a Chicago Transit Authority bus driver, was hospitalized with carbon monoxide poisoning. When he was released, he had a phobic reaction to carbon monoxide which prevented him from working on or around buses. The Illinois Court of Appeals held that Barnes was handicapped and that the transit authority's refusal to transfer him to another position constituted discrimination.

Compulsive behavior also has been asserted as a mental handicap. Although chronic lateness has been rejected as a handicap,[213] in *Rezza v. United States Department of Justice*,[214] the court held that it was possible that an FBI agent who was a compulsive gambler and went through a rehabilitation program could establish that he was covered under the Rehabilitation Act.

Renal Disease

In *Commonwealth v. Pennsylvania Human Relations Commission*,[215] the Supreme Court of Pennsylvania held that the state police academy could not refuse to admit an applicant who had only one kidney. The applicant was otherwise qualified and there was no evidence of a health or safety risk.

A similar result was reached in *Carrero v. New York City Housing Authority*.[216] The court held that the housing authority could not refuse to hire a housing police officer simply because he had kidney stones. The Illinois Court of Appeals, however, has held that having a transplanted kidney is *not* a handicap.[217]

Respiratory Conditions

Most respiratory conditions have been held to be handicaps, including asthma,[218] chronic bronchitis,[219] asbestosis,[220] sensitivity to tobacco smoke,[221] and carrying an erroneous diagnosis of an abnormal lung x-ray.[222] Chronic susceptibility to bronchitis has been held to be insufficiently disabling to be considered a protected handicap.[223]

Being covered by a federal or state statute, of course, is only one element of the case. For individuals who are unable to perform the job, the issue often becomes whether certain accommodations to respiratory conditions are reasonable. Although it is unsettled whether an employer must permit an employee to wear a respirator,[224] prohibiting all workplace smoking[225] and reassigning an asthmatic employee to a light duty position (in violation of collective bargaining agreement) have been held to be unreasonable.[226]

Stature

As with the obesity cases, individuals alleging handicap discrimination based on height and weight have not fared well. The first problem is to prove the existence of a handicap. For example, in *American Motors Corp. v. Labor & Industry Review Commission*,[227] AMC refused to hire Sharon Basile because, at 4 feet 10 inches, she was considered to be too small to perform the available jobs. The Wisconsin Supreme Court held that small stature is not a handicap. Similarly, in *Tudyman v. United Airlines*,[228] William Tudyman was denied employment as a flight attendant because, as a bodybuilder, his weight exceeded United's limits for a man of his height. The court held that Tudyman was not handicapped within the meaning of the Rehabilitation Act.

In *Dexler v. Tisch*,[229] Ilan Dexler, who suffered from achondroplastic dwarfism, applied for employment as a postal clerk through a program for the severely handicapped. The Postal Service refused to hire him because, at 53 inches tall, he would be unable to perform the job and accommodations such as a step stool would impair productivity and create safety hazards. The district court found that Dexler was handicapped and covered under the Rehabilitation Act, but it agreed with the Postal Service that accommodations needed to permit Dexler to perform the job would cause an undue hardship (and perhaps delay the mail?).

Vascular Conditions

In *Oesterling v. Walters*,[230] the United States Court of Appeals for the Eighth Circuit held that mild-to-moderate varicose veins did not affect major life activities and therefore was not a handicap under the Rehabilitation Act.

Vision Problems

Cases involving visual impairments may be divided into three categories based on the nature of the impairment: totally blind, reduced vision, and other medical conditions involving the eyes.

Clarke v. Shoreline School District,[231] illustrates how blindness may combine with other handicapping conditions to create truly formidable barriers to employment. Robert Clarke, a hearing-impaired teacher of handicapped special education students, developed retinitis pigmentosa, which left him legally blind. The combination of handicaps interfered with his ability to monitor student location and behavior in class, to see responses to verbal commands, to record information on student behavior, and to prepare for class. Despite the use of instructional assistants, Clarke was discharged because of his poor performance and the school district's concern for the welfare of his students.[232] The Supreme Court of Washington affirmed the discharge and held that Clarke was not otherwise qualified.

It should be remembered that in a leading handicap discrimination case initiated before passage of the Rehabilitation Act, *Gurmankin v. Costanzo*,[233] the United States Court of Appeals for the Third Circuit held that the policy of the School District of Philadelphia in refusing to assign blind school teachers to teach sighted students violated the equal protection clause of the fourteenth amendment.

Reasonable accommodation has been the key issue in other cases involving blind individuals. In *Nelson v. Thornburgh*,[234] the Pennsylvania Department of Public Welfare was held to have failed to accommodate a blind income maintenance worker by not providing him with at least a half-time reader. In *Carter v. Bennett*,[234] however, the United States Court of Appeals for the District of Columbia Circuit held that the Department of Education had satisfied its duty by furnishing readers, providing special equipment, and decreasing the employee's workload. According to the court, the government is not obligated to provide every accommodation requested.

The largest category of visual impairment cases involves individuals with partial sight. The cases are difficult to reconcile. A truck driver who was blind in one eye as a result of optic atrophy was held to be otherwise qualified[236] and individuals with severe vision problems secondary to sarcoidosis were owed a duty of reasonable accommodation.[237] On the other hand, a truck driver who lost his license because of macular degeneration was not otherwise qualified[238] and a bus driver who lacked stereopsis due to a displaced lens and cataractous cornea in his left eye was lawfully discharged because he was a threat to safety.[239]

Public safety officers often are required to meet rigorous visual acuity standards. In challenges brought by unsuccessful police applicants, the standards were struck down in Illinois[240] and Wisconsin;[241] they were upheld in Kansas[242] and Ohio.[243] In a Colorado case, wearing glasses was held not to be a handicap,[244] but glaucoma is a handicap in North Carolina.[245]

In other cases involving eye conditions, color blindness was held to be a handicap in Oregon,[246] but strabismus (crossed eyes) has been held not to be a handicap under the Rehabilitation Act.[247]

Other Conditions

In *de la Torres v. Bolger*,[248] Daniel de la Torres was discharged from his job as a Postal Service letter carrier because, among other things, he took too long to complete his rounds. De la Torres claimed that his slowness was caused by his left-handedness, which he asserted was a handicap. The United States Court of Appeals for the Fifth Circuit disagreed and held that being left-handed "is a physical characteristic, not a chronic illness, a disorder or deformity, a mental disability, or a condition affecting de la Torres' health."[249]

8

Labor and Employment Law

Constitutional Law

Even though handicap discrimination laws provide the most direct legal regulation of a wide range of medical screening practices, several other constitutional, statutory, and common law doctrines also are relevant to medical screening. This chapter deals with the legal issues related to job security, while Chapter 9 focuses on employee benefits and compensation for harm. These chapters demonstrate that our present system of medical screening laws is a patchwork of protections, regulations, and remedies, often working at cross-purposes and baffling to both employers and employees.

Applicants and employees who object to intrusive medical screening questions or procedures often will assert that certain employer practices are "unconstitutional." Knowing that, for example, criminal suspects are entitled to various constitutional protections, it comes as a surprise to many applicants and employees in the private sector to learn that federal constitutional guarantees are inapplicable to them.

"Nearly all of the Constitution's self-executing, and thus judicially enforceable, guarantees of individual rights shield individuals only from government action."[1] In the context of medical screening of workers, this means that federal constitutional protections are limited to public employees and private employees where medical screening is mandated by federal, state, or local governments. Specifically because of this limitation on constitutional protections, most legal challenges to workplace medical screening involve claims by public employees.

As discussed in Chapter 6, numerous lawsuits have been brought by public employees challenging government-mandated drug testing. A variety of constitutional arguments have been raised, but the most common claim is that the drug testing is an unreasonable search and seizure in violation of the fourth amendment.

Other medical screening practices also have been the subject of constitutional challenges. In *Gargiul v. Tompkins*,[2] Lorraine Gargiul, a tenured kindergarten teacher, took an extended sick leave because of a back ailment. When she sought to return to work, she was told that she had to be examined by the school district's physician, Dr. Paul Day. Gargiul submitted a certificate of good health from her own physician, but refused to be examined by Dr. Day because it was against her "creed" to be examined by a male physician. She offered to go, at her own expense, to any woman physician selected by the school board or recommended by a local medical society. The school board refused this offer and Gargiul was denied reinstatement.

The United States Court of Appeals for the Second Circuit held that, as a tenured teacher, Gargiul had a "property" interest in her job that, under the fourteenth amendment, could not be denied her without due process. (The fourteenth amendment prohibits the states from denying "life, liberty, or property" without due process of law.) According to the court, the school board's action was so arbitrary that it violated substantive due process.[3] In a concurring opinion, Judge Oakes wrote that he would have reached the same result by finding that the school board violated Gargiul's constitutional right to privacy.

Another illustrative constitutional case is *Grusendorf v. City of Oklahoma City*[4] (also discussed in Chapter 3 under the heading "Cigarette Smoking"). Greg Grusendorf was hired as a firefighter trainee by the city. He was required to sign an agreement not to smoke on or off duty during his first year of employment. Grusendorf had quit smoking, in order to improve his physical condition, about three months before being hired. After two months of work, during unpaid lunch time, another city employee observed him taking three puffs of a cigarette. When the incident was reported to the fire department, Grusendorf admitted the observed conduct and was discharged.

Grusendorf brought an action in United States district court, seeking declaratory, injunctive, and monetary relief. He alleged that the fire department rule, among other things, violated his rights to privacy and due process under the fourteenth amendment. The district court granted the city's motion to dismiss and the United States Court of Appeals for the Tenth Circuit affirmed.

According to the court, even assuming that Grusendorf had a liberty interest in smoking while off duty that was protected by the fourteenth amendment, the burden was on him to prove that the ban on smoking was irrational. The court specifically held, however, that the municipal regulation was a rational means of promoting good health. Although the court questioned the rationality of applying the rule only to trainees, it noted that Grusendorf failed to raise the issue of equal protection.

Courts considering the constitutionality of medical screening criteria that involve off-work activities (e.g., smoking, drinking, diet, hobbies), will find that analogous areas of public employment law have developed some generally instructive principles. First, restrictions on the work-time behavior of public employees (especially police and firefighters) are usually upheld even if there is some infringement upon the individual's freedom of expression, lifestyle, or similar interests.[5] Second, restrictions on off-work employee behavior usually will be upheld if the behavior interferes with or undermines the effectiveness of the individual or the governmental entity.[6] Third, restrictions on off-work behavior usually will not be upheld if there is an insubstantial employment-related governmental interest, especially where fundamental employee interests, such as freedom of expression, freedom of association, and the right of privacy, are implicated.[7] In the context of medical screening, it is not clear whether the courts will hold that economic interests (e.g., health insurance costs) are constitutionally adequate justifications.

Finally, even as to private sector applicants and employees, state constitutional law may afford a measure of protection. Unlike the federal Constitution, certain state constitutions apply to the acts of private individuals as well as governmental actions. The right of privacy, explicitly recognized in at least seven states,[8] including California,[9] may apply to private employment. Therefore, it could be argued that attempts by private employers to control the off-work activities of their employees violate the right of privacy protected by a state constitution. This theory has been used to challenge the drug testing of private sector employees.[10]

Common Law Actions for Wrongful Discharge

At common law, absent a statutory prohibition, an employer had virtually unfettered control in selecting its employees. The employer could hire or refuse to hire any person for any reason or no reason at all.[11] This right included the right to refuse to hire an individual because of the employer's opinion that the prospective employee was physically incapable of performing the job.[12] Once hired, the employee could be fired "at will" by the employer for any reason or no reason at all[13] and, again, this included the employer's belief that the employee could no longer perform the job because of his or her physical condition.[14]

During the last 15 years almost every jurisdiction has recognized one or more exceptions to the at-will rule. Some highly publicized cases, including some large recoveries, and a flood of law review articles, conferences, and debates have contributed to the impression that the at-will rule has undergone a major transformation. Although these developments are certainly significant, the changes have been more evolutionary than revolutionary. Only Montana has enacted a statute prohibiting wrongful discharge,[15] and wrongful refusal to hire cases are rare.

Wrongful discharge cases generally have been based on three theories. First, provisions in employee handbooks and manuals have been held to create implied contract rights in favor of the employees.[16] Many handbooks and manuals customarily contained statements that employees would not be fired without just cause. After several cases bound employers to these promises, numerous employers purged their handbooks and manuals of all language that could be construed as a promise of job security. Some now expressly provide that employment is at will.

Second, most jurisdictions have recognized the tort of wrongful discharge in violation of public policy.[17] The possibility of large awards for compensatory and punitive damages has focused attention on these tort actions, but public policy is not open-ended. It generally must be based on a clearly expressed policy, such as that embodied in a state statute, and is usually restricted to four main categories: (1) refusing to commit unlawful acts (e.g., perjury, falsification of public records); (2) exercising statutory rights (e.g., filing a workers' compensation claim); (3) performing public functions (e.g., serving on jury duty); and (4) reporting an employer's unlawful conduct (e.g., whistleblowing).

Third, a few jurisdictions have held that every employment contract contains an implied covenant of good faith and fair dealing, breach of which is actionable in contract or even tort.[18] Although this exception represents the application to employment law of a traditional contract doctrine,[19] it has been adopted by only a few courts. Moreover, its use in specific cases is often problematic. Good faith is subjective and therefore the absence of good faith may be difficult to prove except in the most compelling factual situations.[20]

Employee challenges to employer medical screening practices brought under common law theories have been infrequent and not often successful. The at-will exceptions only apply to discharges and even in discharge cases the use of medical criteria to decide on termination, even if ill-advised, is rarely considered wrongful.[21] Wrongful discharge cases related to medical screening have arisen in the following three ways: (1) the employee is discharged because of illness or a medical examination; (2) the employee is discharged for filing a claim under a group health insurance plan; and (3) the employee is not reinstated after a medical leave of absence. Although employees usually have not fared well in these cases,[22] there are some exceptions.

In *Hinthorn v. Roland's of Bloomington, Inc.*,[23] a clerk in the shipping department notified her supervisor that she had sustained a back injury and requested medical attention. Later that day, a company vice-president coerced her into resigning because she was "getting hurt too much—costing the company too much money." [24] The Supreme Court of Illinois held that Hinthorn had been constructively discharged in violation of the public policy exception to the at-will doctrine.

In *Price v. Carmack Datsun Inc.*,[25] however, the same court, the Supreme Court of Illinois, in a questionable and seemingly irreconcilable decision, held that the discharge of an employee for filing a claim under a group health insurance plan did not violate public policy because it was a purely private grievance and no "public" policies were implicated. (By contrast, it has been widely held that the discharge of an employee for filing a workers' compensation claim violates public policy.)[26]

The third type of wrongful discharge action is based on the employer's failure to reinstate an employee after a medical leave. Again, the majority of cases have upheld the discharge,[27] but there are some exceptions. For example, in *Coleman v. Safeway Stores,*

Inc.,[28] the Supreme Court of Kansas held that discharging an employee for absences caused by a work-related injury violates the public policy exception to the at-will rule.

Common law personal injury actions and actions involving dignitary torts (e.g., defamation, invasion of privacy) are discussed in Chapter 9. Another possible cause of action is negligence. In *Armstrong v. Morgan*,[29] an employee, upon being promoted, was requested to have a physical examination performed by a company-retained physician. The physician's report indicated that the employee was in very poor health, and as a result, the employee lost his job. According to the Texas Court of Civil Appeals, a negligence action against the physician stated a valid claim. "Dr. Morgan owed Appellant Armstrong a duty not to injure him physically or otherwise. If Dr. Morgan negligently performed the examination and as a result gave an inaccurate report of the state of appellant's health, and appellant was injured as a proximate result thereof, actionable negligence would be shown."[30]

A similar result was reached in *Olson v. Western Airlines, Inc.*[31] Robert Olson was denied employment by Western Airlines when Dr. Webster Marxer, a physician hired by Western to give Olson a preemployment examination, erroneously diagnosed Olson as being prediabetic. In reversing a granting of summary judgment for the defendants, the California Court of Appeals held that an action for negligence would lie against Western and Dr. Marxer.

Much of the recent wrongful discharge litigation based on medical screening has involved drug testing. In *Satterfield v. Lockheed Missiles & Space Co.*,[32] an employee was required to have a urine drug screen as a part of his annual physical exam. He was fired after an unconfirmed EMIT test showed positive for marijuana. In granting summary judgment for the company, the court rejected the various theories under which the plaintiff asserted that he was wrongfully discharged, as well as actions for intentional infliction of emotional distress and invasion of privacy. As demonstrated in Chapter 6, the results of an unconfirmed EMIT test are of dubious scientific value. Nevertheless, under common law principles employers are not liable either for using imprecise tests or for reaching erroneous conclusions.

Discharges for refusing to take a drug test also have been upheld in cases involving employees in such non-safety-sensitive jobs as a bulk plant operation warehouseman[33] and supervisory employee at a freight terminal.[34] Even the discharge of an individual seeking drug treatment has been held not to violate public policy. In *Moreland v. Department of Corrections*,[35] Bonnie Moreland, a nurse with the Illinois Department of Corrections, requested leave to enter a drug treatment program. After admitting "in confidence" to her supervisor that she had taken controlled substances from the hospital, Moreland was discharged. The Illinois Court of Appeals, holding that her discharge did not violate state policy, noted: "[W]e recognize the grave dangers that would arise if we hold that amnesty must be given to all drug abusers who confess to higher employees their misconduct which occurred when they were subject to drug abuse."[36]

A notable exception to these unsuccessful wrongful discharge cases is *Luck v. Southern Pacific Transportation Co.*[37] Barbara Luck, a computer operator in San Francisco, a position with no direct public safety implications, was fired after she refused to take a drug test in July 1985. The drug testing program was begun with no advance notice to employees only a few months before drug testing was severely limited by enactment of an ordinance in San Francisco. Luck was selected for testing at random and without any suspicion of drug use. She sued for wrongful discharge in violation of public policy, breach of the implied covenant of good faith and fair dealing, and intentional infliction of emotional distress. After a four-week trial, a San Francisco Superior Court jury awarded her $32,000 in compensatory damages, $180,000 in lost wages, and $273,000 in punitive damages, for a total of $485,000.[38]

Occupational Safety and Health Act

If, as is often asserted, the primary purpose of medical screening is to safeguard employee health, a key labor and employment law to consider is the Occupational Safety and Health Act.[39] The Act covers all private employment in the United States, an estimated five million workplaces and 75 million employees.[40] The purpose of the Act is "to assure so far as possible every working man and woman in the Nation safe and healthful working conditions . . . ."[41] The Occupational Safety and Health Administration (OSHA), the agency within the Department of Labor charged with enforcing the Act, is responsible for promulgating mandatory safety and health standards and ensuring employer compliance by conducting on-site inspections, issuing citations and abatement orders, and assessing civil penalties.

Medical examinations of workers are an important part of occupational health surveillance. OSHA's medical examination requirements (detailed in the discussion in Chapter 2 under "Medical Examinations"), however, are hazard-specific; examinations are only mandated when employees are exposed to substances such as lead, cotton dust, and coke oven emissions. OSHA has not promulgated a generic medical examination regulation with universal applicability. Moreover, even where medical tests are mandated, employers generally must merely perform certain tests. The use of additional medical tests and the ultimate decisionmaking about employability are not regulated by OSHA.

"Multiple physician review" and "medical removal protection and rate retention" are the two main exceptions to the rule of noninvolvement by OSHA in employers' medical fitness determinations. Both procedures have been challenged in court. In *Taylor Diving & Salvage Co. v. United States Department of Labor*,[42] the United States Court of Appeals for the Fifth Circuit struck down the medical examination provision of the commerical diving standard. The standard required medical examination of employees who were to be exposed to hyperbaric conditions. If the employee was found to be unfit by the examining physician selected by the employer, the employee could seek a second opinion. If the first two physicians disagreed, a third physician was to be selected by the first two physicians and that physician's determination would be dispositive. All costs were to be borne by the employer. (Similar procedures are often incorporated into collective bargaining agreement provisions dealing with, for example, return to work after a medical leave.) The Fifth Circuit held that the OSHA standard imposed a mandatory job security provision controlled by the third physician. "[T]he employer has no control over the third doctor's fitness standards, so that the employer is prevented from setting higher health standards for employees than the secondary examining doctors choose to set."[43]

In *United Steelworkers of America v. Marshall*,[44] the United States Court of Appeals for the District of Columbia Circuit reached the opposite result and upheld the multiple physician review procedure of the lead standard. The court relied on two findings in the record. First, lead diseases are often difficult to diagnose and multiple physician review increases the chances of a correct diagnosis.

Second, some company physicians have engaged in the unsound and harmful practice of prophylactic chelation to reduce the blood-lead levels of employees. The court distinguished *Taylor*, where employees would seek multiple physician review to obtain a finding of fitness, thus forcing the employer to retain employees considered unfit by its own physician and standards. In the lead standard, the multiple physician review procedure was to prevent excess exposure of "leaded" employees, and together with medical removal protection, the employer is not precluded from imposing more stringent health criteria.

OSHA's other method of regulating medical examinations and employment involves medical removal protection (MRP) and rate retention (RR) of previously exposed employees. When a periodic medical examination indicates that the employee is showing symptoms of the adverse effects of exposure to certain toxic substances, the employee is removed from further exposure—to a "safe" job if there is an opening—until it is medically advisable for the employee to return. If the new, safe position is at lower rate of pay, RR would require the maintenance of wage and benefit levels during the period of medical removal. Thus, MRP and RR attempt to protect employee health without a reduction in employee benefits, thereby shifting the economic burden to the employer and ultimately to the consumer.

MRP and RR provisions in OSHA health standards have become increasingly stringent. For example, the vinyl chloride standard provides for MRP, but not RR;[45] and the asbestos standard provides for MRP of employees for whom respirators are ineffective, but RR is required only if there is an available position.[46] The most sweeping MRP and RR provision is in the lead standard.[47] Employees whose blood-lead levels are above the specified limit or who show symptoms of lead disease must be removed until their blood-lead has returned to an acceptable level and their general health is good. The employer may transfer the employee to a nonlead plant or low-lead area of a plant, or may keep the employee in a high-lead area for a shorter work week. When an employee is removed in any way, the employee retains his or her earnings rate, seniority, and benefit levels for up to 18 months and upon return must be restored to his or her original job status.

In *United Steelworkers of America v. Marshall*,[48] the United States Court of Appeals for the District of Columbia Circuit upheld the validity of the MRP and RR provisions of the lead standard. In

American Textile Manufacturer's Institute, Inc. v. Donovan,[49] however, the Supreme Court struck down the MRP and RR provision of the cotton dust standard as promulgated and remanded the standard to the OSHA for further consideration. Although the Court did not decide the issue of whether OSHA has the statutory authority to promulgate *any* regulation containing MRP and RR, the Court held that OSHA failed to publish a statement of reasons (as required by section 6(e) of the Act) explaining why the MRP and RR provisions were needed to protect worker health and safety. According to the Court, "the Act in no way authorizes OSHA to repair general unfairness to employees that is unrelated to achievement of health and safety goals . . . ."[50] Therefore, any wide-ranging attempt by OSHA to improve employment terms and opportunities is likely to be held outside of OSHA's authority, but a standard with a documented need for MRP and RR to protect worker health is likely to be upheld.

A number of recent proposals have been made to give OSHA a larger role in developing workplace policies for cigarette smoking, drug testing, genetic testing, AIDS and infection control, and other difficult medical screening issues. It is questionable whether OSHA can be expected to assume such a role. First, the above-quoted language from the Supreme Court's decision in the *Cotton Dust* case makes it clear that OSHA's statutory mandate is limited to regulating working conditions by eliminating or reducing hazards. Job security and antidiscrimination protection are beyond the purview of the Act.

Second, historically OSHA has lacked the resources and political support necessary for effective regulation. From 1971 to 1988 OSHA promulgated only 24 new permanent health standards. Until new exposure limits for 376 substances were established in 1989,[51] OSHA's 450 health standards were based on 1968 scientific data. Even with these new standards, thousands of chemicals commonly used in industry are still not regulated at all.[52] It took 15 years of litigation and a court order before OSHA promulgated a standard requiring drinking water, hand washing facilities, and toilets for the nation's farmworkers.[53] In short, OSHA has been unable to deal effectively even with traditional workplace hazards.

An argument could be made, however, that OSHA is the most appropriate agency to regulate medical screening practices. OSHA has, or through NIOSH has, access to the scientific and medical expertise needed to regulate medical screening. In addition, unlike laws whose primary emphasis is antidiscrimination (e.g., the Rehabilitation Act, Title VII), the Occupational Safety and Health Act already contains provisions for rulemaking.

Even with an enlarged delegation of authority from Congress, however, OSHA would need more resources, personnel, and political support before attempting to take on an issue as complex as medical screening.

The National Labor Relations Act and Collective Bargaining

The National Labor Relations Act (NLRA) is the federal labor law guaranteeing employees "the right to self-organization, to form, join, or assist labor organizations, to bargain collectively through representatives of their own choosing, and to engage in other concerted activities for the purpose of collective bargaining or other mutual aid or protection . . . ."[54] Sections 8(a)(5), 8(b)(3), and 8(d) of the NLRA require the employer and union to bargain in good faith with respect to wages, hours, and other terms and conditions of employment.[55] These are referred to as "mandatory subjects of bargaining."[56] As to these subjects, neither the employer nor the union may make unilateral changes in conditions without first bargaining with the other side.

Medical examinations have been held to be a mandatory subject of bargaining. For example, in *Lockheed Shipbuilding & Construction Co.*,[57] the National Labor Relations Board (NLRB) held that Lockheed violated section 8(a)(5) of the NLRA by unilaterally implementing pulmonary function and audiometric tests for the purpose of denying employment to applicants and terminating employees who failed the tests. The issue of unilateral changes in conditions has been raised frequently when employers have instituted drug testing programs without prior bargaining.[58] The first Supreme Court case to address this issue involved the Railway Labor Act (applicable to railroad and airline employees), with the Court considering whether a railroad could unilaterally impose drug testing without prior bargaining.[59]

Most collective bargaining agreements contain broad arbitration clauses requiring arbitration of all disputes arising under the contract. Numerous arbitration cases have involved medical screen-

ing issues, including falsification of preemployment medical questionnaires,[60] drug and alcohol testing policies,[61] refusals to take
medical examinations,[62] compensation for time spent taking medical tests,[63] conflicts in medical opinions on employability,[64] return
to work and light duty work assignments,[65] and the denial of sick
leave or medical benefits.[66]

Chapter 7 under the heading "Specific Medical Conditions"
contains a discussion of the case law under federal and state handicap discrimination laws with regard to specific types of medical
conditions. It is interesting to compare those cases with some
recent, representative arbitration awards involving similar medical
conditions.

AIDS

Discharges of employees with AIDS have been set aside where
the employees were still capable of performing the job. Among the
jobs at issue have been plant machine operator[67] and nursing home
employee.[68]

Diabetes

An employer was upheld in sending an employee home for the
day without pay where diabetes-related medical conditions rendered the employee unable to perform the job safely.[69] A discharge
of an employee suffering from side effects of medication to control
diabetes was not upheld where the employee had a good work
record and a medical release to return to work.[70] In another case, a
diabetic employee was conditionally reinstated where his diabetic
seizures had been caused by emotional distress and a change in
medication.[71]

Epilepsy

Arbitrators have refused to reinstate employees with epilepsy
who worked in jobs having a safety component, such as truck
drivers[72] and a railroad trainman.[73] An employer was even upheld
in reclassifying a telephone equipment installer (whose job involved
driving, using power tools, and working at heights of 8 to 12 feet)
who suffered a seizure at work and was misdiagnosed as having
epilepsy when he actually had a toxic reaction to medication.[74] It is

not uncommon, however, for an arbitrator to order that an employee be given alternative work or reinstated when his or her health improved. [75]

Hearing impairment

An arbitrator upheld the transfer of a hearing-impaired steel mill employee out of a position in which hearing protection had to be worn. [76] The employee was considered to be a hazard to himself and other employees.

Heart conditions

A bus driver was discharged after suffering a heart attack. The arbitrator upheld the discharge, based on evidence of the driver's physical incapacity and the employer's legitimate concern for public safety. [77]

Obesity

Employers have been upheld where the employee was suffering from other medical conditions, such as hypertension, along with obesity. [78] On the other hand, arbitrators have held that it was improper to refuse to recall from layoff or discharge obese employees whose performance was not affected by their obesity. [79]

Psychiatric conditions

Arbitrators have shown a willingness to order the reinstatement of employees with psychiatric disorders contingent on the employee's continuing with treatment. [80] In one case an arbitrator reduced the discharge of an employee to a suspension where the employee, a compulsive gambler, was absent from work without leave for a four day trip to Las Vegas. [81] Even where an employer was justified in placing an employee on psychiatric leave, once the employee has recovered, it will be improper to deny reinstatement. [82] The discharge of a probationary employee was upheld, however, where the employee's acrophobia precluded his working on platforms, catwalks, and ladders which were 20 to 40 feet in the air. [83]

Vision impairment

Arbitrators have upheld strict vision standards for safety-sensitive jobs. For example, in a case involving an employee of a steel mill, the arbitrator held that the company's refusal to return an employee to work after an off-work eye injury was reasonable because good vision and depth perception were essential to safety.[84] In another case, the refusal to grant a medical waiver to an Air Force mechanic with poor vision was upheld.[85] On the other hand, an arbitrator ruled that a school of optometry had acted improperly in refusing to interview an otherwise qualified job applicant with a vision problem.[86]

Other conditions

Other arbitration cases have involved amputation,[87] asthma,[88] ataxia,[89] back problems,[90] body lice,[91] conjunctivitis,[92] Crohn's disease,[93] emphysema,[94] hernia,[95] lupus,[96] orthopedic impairments,[97] Parkinson's disease,[98] and stroke.[99]

In general, arbitrators have shown more latitude in dealing with employees with physical and mental impairments than have the courts in comparable handicap discrimination cases. They have ordered alternative work assignments, transfers, conditional reinstatement, and other remedies that go beyond what would be considered "reasonable accommodation" in handicap discrimination cases.[100] In *Kost Brothers, Inc.*,[101] a case involving an employee who had epileptic seizures at work, Arbitrator William J. Berquist listed nine factors to consider in determining whether an employee's medical condition creates an unreasonable risk of harm and therefore whether the employer had just cause for discharge:

"1. Length of service of the employee.
2. Whether the employer knew of the medical condition prior to the incidents.
3. The extent to which the condition previously interfered with the employee's job performance.
4. Whether the employee's condition previously had created a risk of harm to the employee or others.
5. The extent to which the condition is treatable and controllable by medication and by the employee.
6. The extent to which the employee has complied with his medical treatment regimen.

7. Whether the employee misrepresented the medical condition at the time of hiring and whether the employer reacted within a reasonable time after discovery of the misrepresentation.
8. Whether a medical incident on the job represents a threat to safety.
9. The social effect of the discharge or disqualification."[102]

Title VII and the ADEA

Title VII of the Civil Rights Act of 1964, as amended, prohibits discrimination in hiring, discharge, compensation, or other terms, conditions, or privileges of employment because of an individual's race, color, religion, sex, or national origin. It is the most comprehensive and important law prohibiting discrimination in employment. The Act applies to employers, labor unions, and employment agencies. To be an "employer" under the Act, an entity must have employed 15 or more persons for at least 20 weeks in either the current or preceding calendar year and be engaged in an industry affecting commerce. State and local government employees and certain federal government employees also are covered by Title VII.

The Age Discrimination in Employment Act (ADEA) prohibits age discrimination in the employment, discharge, promotion, or treatment of persons over the age of 40. The ADEA applies to every employer engaged in an enterprise affecting commerce that has 20 or more employees for each working day in each of 20 or more calendar weeks in the current or preceding calendar year. The ADEA also applies to employment agencies, unions, and state and local political subdivisions. Enforcement of both Title VII and the ADEA is vested in the Equal Employment Opportunity Commission (EEOC), but private actions also may be brought by aggrieved individuals.

Discrimination claims related to medical screening most commonly involve alleged sex discrimination. A wide range of employee health policies have been challenged, ranging from preemployment medical questionnaires to health benefits. The results have varied widely.

In *Wroblewski v. Lexington Gardens, Inc.*,[103] Judith Gail Wroblewski applied for a position with a new plant store in Glastonbury, Connecticut. She was required to complete a medical history form, including a section marked "women," which asked seven questions related to menstruation and reproductive health. She chose not to complete this section, although her private physician, who performed the preemployment physical exam, wrote "healthy female" in the section marked "physician's summary." When she was denied employment for refusing to complete the medical history, Wroblewski brought an action under the Connecticut employment discrimination statute, a state analog of Title VII. The Supreme Court of Connecticut held that the employer failed to justify the use of a facially discriminatory medical history form that did not ask male applicants questions about their urogenital health. Significantly, if detailed and arguably non-job-related health information had been required of both sexes, Wroblewski would have had no legal redress. [104]

Wroblewski involved intentional (disparate treatment) discrimination. In medical screening cases it is more common that the case will be brought on a different legal theory, disparate impact discrimination. In these cases, plaintiffs allege that they have been discriminated against because the employer has used a facially neutral selection criterion which has disparate impact along the lines of race, color, religion, sex, or national origin. [105]

Disparate impact theory has been used by women to challenge strength, agility, stamina, and other physical ability testing required of police officers, firefighters, and similar employees. Several principles have emerged from two decades of Title VII litigation. First, state "protective laws," seeking to limit the hours or nature of work performed by women are inconsistent with Title VII and therefore, under the supremacy clause of the Constitution, are invalid. [106] Second, minimum height and weight requirements have a disparate impact on women, and unless the employer can prove that these requirements are essential to the enterprise and cannot be replaced by less discriminatory criteria, they will be held unlawful. [107] Third, when a job includes heavy lifting and similar physical exertion, an employer cannot presume that only men are capable and must afford women an opportunity to demonstrate their ability. [108]

The most difficult cases concern whether physical ability standards having a disparate impact on women have been shown to be job related and essential. For example, in *Harless v. Duck*, [109] a class action lawsuit was brought to challenge the physical ability test used by the Toledo, Ohio, Police Department. Applicants were required to complete three of the following four tests: 15 push-ups, 25 sit-ups, six-foot standing broad jump, and 25-second obstacle course. The

United States Court of Appeals for the Sixth Circuit, while noting that physical abilities were undoubtedly essential to safe and effective police work, nevertheless concluded that "there is no justification in the record for the types of exercises chosen or the passing marks for each exercise."[110] Other cases considering different physical standards have reached varying results.[111]

The possible effects of workplace conditions on female reproductive health also have been a subject of Title VII litigation. The cases have involved fertility and pregnancy. Issues related to the exclusion of fertile women were discussed in Chapter 3 under the Heading "Reproductive Hazards." As to pregnancy, in 1978 Title VII was amended by the Pregnancy Disability Act (PDA) to prohibit discrimination in employment based on pregnancy, childbirth, or related medical conditions. The amendment provides in pertinent part:

"(k) The terms 'because of sex' or 'on the basis of sex' include, but are not limited to, because of or on the basis of pregnancy, childbirth, or related medical conditions; and women affected by pregnancy, childbirth, or related medical conditions shall be treated the same for all employment-related purposes, including receipt of benefits under fringe benefit programs, as other persons not so affected but similar in their ability or inability to work, and nothing in section 2000e(2)(h) of this title shall be interpreted to permit otherwise."

Based on this language, any treatment of women who are pregnant must be consistent with treatment accorded other persons. Because an employee's heightened risk of illness may justify excluding an employee from the workplace, a pregnant woman could be excluded, but only by applying the same standards used for nonpregnant persons with current or potential impairments.

There are three possible bases for excluding pregnant women: Continued employment could injure the woman, it could injure coworkers or the public, or it could injure the fetus. Different legal standards have been applied to each of these situations.

In *Khalifa v. G.X. Corp.*,[112] Tammy Englund, a pregnant hairstylist, began to suffer headaches when she gave permanents and her physician sent a note asking that she be relieved of these duties. She also had a family history of birth defects. The manager of the beauty shop placed Englund on involuntary medical leave of absence (rather than modifying her work assignments) until her physician wrote that it was safe for her to resume giving permanents. In an action brought under state law, the Minnesota Court of

Appeals held that the employer did not act unlawfully. In other cases, however, more harsh treatment of pregnant employees[113] or paternalistic exclusions[114] have been held to violate the fourteenth amendment or Title VII.

Where the concern is for coworker or public safety and health, the courts are more inclined to uphold the removal of pregnant employees. For example, in *Harriss v. Pan American World Airways, Inc.*,[115] the United States Court of Appeals for the Ninth Circuit upheld the airline's policy of requiring that female flight attendants take maternity leave immediately upon learning of their pregnancy. The court based its decision on evidence that a flight attendant's ability to perform her emergency functions might be impaired by fatigue, nausea and vomiting, or spontaneous abortion.

The involuntary removal of pregnant employees to protect fetal health will be upheld only where there is evidence of potential harm to the fetus and where pregnant employees are treated the same as other employees on medical leave of absence. In cases involving pregnant x-ray technicians, for example, hospitals have been found in violation of Title VII by terminating the employees rather than reassigning them or granting them a leave of absence in accordance with their own policies.[116]

Pregnancy-related health benefits also may be an issue. Under the 1978 amendment to Title VII, women actually disabled by pregnancy or childbirth must be afforded the same benefits and leave time as any other temporarily disabled employee. In *California Federal Savings & Loan Association v. Guerra*,[117] the Supreme Court considered the validity of a California law that extended preferential treatment to pregnant workers, by requiring employers to provide up to four months of unpaid pregnancy disability leave. The Court upheld the law, ruling that it was not preempted by the PDA. According to the Court, Congress intended the PDA to be "a floor beneath which pregnancy disability benefits may not drop—not a ceiling above which they may not rise."[118] The PDA provides that preferential treatment is not required, but it does not say that it is prohibited.

Claims of race or national origin discrimination could result from biochemical genetic testing for predisposition to occupationally related illness. Traits such as sickle cell trait, alpha$_1$ antitrypsin deficiency, and glucose-6-phosphate dehydrogenase deficiency are known to be more prevalent in certain racial and ethnic groups. These traits have been theorized to predispose individuals to specific occupational illnesses. Thus, biochemical genetic screening of workers to prevent these diseases would have a disparate impact on certain racial and ethnic groups.[119] The heavy legal burden to justify using the tests would rest with the employer and, consequently, for medical, legal, policy, and public relations reasons, the tests are not currently being used very widely.[120]

The racial and ethnic effects of screening for nonoccupational illnesses, however, also should be considered.[121] For example, screening out applicants and employees based on hypertension would have a disparate impact on blacks. Diabetes screening would have a disparate impact on Hispanics. If challenged under Title VII, would such screening be lawful? Despite an absence of case law, it is fair to say that such a lawsuit is possible.

In *Chaney v. Southern Railway*,[122] Willie F. Chaney, a black railroad employee, was discharged after his unconfirmed EMIT test was positive for marijuana. Chaney brought an action under Title VII, in which his expert witness testified that black people have a disproportionately high false positive rate on the EMIT test because the test misreads higher levels of the dark skin pigment, melanin, as ingested cannabinoid metabolites. Although there is little toxicological evidence to support this theory, if it could be proved, then the employer would have a difficult burden in proving the validity of the test. Such an argument could be used to challenge other forms of medical screening with a disparate impact along the lines of race, color, religion, sex, or national origin.

The final basis of discrimination to consider is age. An employer would violate the ADEA by refusing to hire older workers because of a belief that older workers have higher health care costs.[123] Medical risk determinations of individual older workers, however, may not be considered discriminatory.[124] It is not settled whether disparate impact discrimination theory is applicable to the ADEA.[125] If it is, predictive screening of individuals on the basis of prior occupational exposures or prior illnesses could have a disparate impact on older workers and thereby establish a prima facie case of age discrimination.

In defending a charge of age discrimination based on medical screening, the most important defense is safety. As in the handicap discrimination cases discussed in Chapter 7, the safety defense will be given careful consideration. In *Usery v. Tamiami Trail Tours, Inc.*,[126] the employer refused to consider applications from individuals over age 40 to be intercity bus drivers. In sustaining the employer's argument that age was a BFOQ, the United States Court of Appeals for the Fifth Circuit stated: "[S]afety to fellow employees is of such humane importance that the employer must be afforded substantial discretion in selecting specific standards which, if they err at all, should err on the side of preservation of life and limb."[127] Other age discrimination cases involving the safety defense have dealt with airline pilots, police officers, and fire fighters.[128]

9

Employee Benefits and Tort Law

Workers' Compensation and Unemployment Insurance

The financial consequences to employees of medical screening go beyond the mere loss of a paycheck. By assessing both employability and medical disability, medical screening affects an individual's eligibility for government and employer-provided income replacement and medical benefits. The first two sections of this chapter address these issues. The last two sections focus on tort actions by employees to recover for the reputational and emotional harms as well as the physical injuries that sometimes result from improper medical screening practices.

Workers' compensation is a term applied to an unconnected system of state and federal laws designed to compensate workers who suffer from a work-related injury or illness. Enacted in the early part of this century, each state has its own workers' compensation statute. In addition, separate federal laws have been enacted to cover federal government employees,[1] railroad employees,[2] longshore and harbor workers,[3] and sailors.[4]

Workers' compensation represents a compromise between employees and employers. Employees give up the right to bring common law personal injury actions in exchange for a system under which employees need not prove the fault of any party to be eligible for compensation. Employers give up common law defenses (e.g., assumption of risk, contributory negligence, fellow servant rule) in exchange for predetermined, limited liability. Eligible employees receive medical and disability benefits; there are no damages for "pain and suffering" or punitive damages. Theoretically, workers' compensation costs less to administer than the tort system and offers prompt and sure payments.

180

Benefits to claimants are employer funded and may be administered through a private insurance carrier, self-insurance, or a state fund. Under any system, an increase in claims means higher employer costs. This basic principle and a series of legal doctrines have the effect of encouraging employers to engage in increasingly detailed medical screening—both diagnostic and predictive—and to screen for occupational as well as nonoccupational illnesses.

A general rule of workers' compensation is that a claimant will not be denied compensation because of a preexisting allergy, weakness, disease, or susceptibility.[5] The courts have developed a series of doctrines to deal with the common situations where a compensable injury or illness is caused by the working conditions at two or more employers. These cases are sometimes referred to as cumulative exposure or successive disabilities cases. Under the "last injurious exposure rule," used in many states, the last employer is responsible for paying workers' compensation benefits and therefore has an incentive to screen out applicants with prior harmful exposures at a previous employer.

For example, in *Stovall v. Sally Salmon Seafood*,[6] Pamela R. Stovall worked for Sally Salmon for about one year. Her primary job was "shaking crab," which required her to strike her wrist against a pan or bench to loosen the crab meat from the shell. She also filleted fish and shucked oysters. Although the work caused pain and swelling in her wrist and hand, she never sought medical treatment. Shortly after leaving Sally Salmon, Stovall began working for Hallmark Fisheries as a black cod scraper. After only about six weeks of work, her wrist and hand were so painful that she sought medical treatment. The doctor diagnosed her condition as carpal tunnel syndrome, which required corrective surgery. The Supreme Court of Oregon held that, under the last injurious exposure rule, Hallmark (the second employer) was responsible for the entire workers' compensation payment—even though Stovall had only worked there six weeks and even though she had misrepresented on her application form that she had never had any hand, wrist, or arm trouble.[7] Only thorough medical screening could have prevented Hallmark's workers' compensation liability.

The combination of nonoccupational and occupational health factors may enhance the extent of a compensable illness. For example, when occupational lung disease is aggravated by synergistic or additive effects of tobacco smoke, all or part of the disease is usually compensable.[8] In addition, when occupational exposures aggravate a preexisting nonoccupational illness, the resulting condition is usually compensable.

For example, in *International Paper Co. v. Rogers*,[9] Dennis Wayne Rogers was hired as a chemical engineer by International Paper. Although a preemployment physical examination revealed asymptomatic spondylolisthesis, Rogers worked without incident for over three years. After suffering a back sprain at work, he was diagnosed as having probable nerve root pressure superimposed on the spondylolisthesis, which required surgery. The Alabama Court of Civil Appeals held that Rogers' injury was compensable.

> "[T]he employee never missed any work nor was he limited in any way in his activities prior to his accident. If a condition is aggravated by an accident occurring in the course of employment, the condition is still compensable even though the accident may not have caused the same injury in a normal person."[10]

As discussed in Chapter 7, the failure to hire Rogers, whose spondylolisthesis was asymptomatic, where his job did not require physical exertion, would probably be a violation of handicap discrimination laws. Yet, when he later suffered an injury on the job, the employer was responsible under workers' compensation. This fact could encourage some employers to undertake detailed medical screening, to base hiring and retention decisions on conservative medical assumptions, then not to disclose the reasons for a refusal to employ in the hopes that the individual will not file a discrimination claim.

Medical screening to reduce workers' compensation costs associated with nonoccupational causes also is encouraged by the difficulty in distinguishing between occupational and nonoccupational sources of illness. For example, Alzheimer's disease in a 61-year-old mechanic has been held to be a compensable, work-related illness where the man suffered a severe bump on his head at work 20 months prior to the onset of symptoms.[11] In another case,[12] a worker's widow was awarded death benefits following the worker's death from meningococcal septicemia. According to the medical testimony, he contracted the rare disease by merely kissing on the cheek a coworker who was a carrier of the organism *neisseria meningitis*.

Determining the source of an allergic or sensitizing reaction also may be difficult. In *Robinson v. SAIF Corp.*,[13] Maxine

Robinson suffered from a severe sensitivity to phenols, hydrocarbons, and formaldehyde. She was exposed to these chemicals both at her new mobile home, with its new carpet and furnishings, and at work. She worked at Struther's Furniture, in a hot, poorly ventilated showroom with low ceilings, which had new carpeting and wallpaper and which continually received new furniture. The Oregon Court of Appeals held that her illness was compensable.

> "Although the specific chemical cause of claimant's sensitivity is not conclusively established, she has shown by a preponderance of the evidence that the major contributing cause was her work environment at Struthers, which exposed her to concentrations of chemicals much greater than she was ordinarily exposed to outside the course of employment."[14]

Unemployment insurance laws provide income replacement to workers who have lost their job. Employers have similar incentives for aggressive medical screening to hold down unemployment insurance costs. Employees who are discharged for misconduct and employees who quit are ineligible for benefits. This is sometimes liberally construed in the case of medical conditions. For example, in *Casias v. Industrial Commission*,[15] the court held that unemployment insurance benefits could not be denied to an employee who had concealed a history of epilepsy on the employment application.

Employees who quit work because of job-related health problems also are entitled to unemployment insurance, even if the employees are particularly sensitive to the workplace environment.[16] Therefore, an employer that did not administer pre-employment allergy tests, for example, and hired an employee who was allergic to a substance in the workplace would be responsible for unemployment insurance benefits when the employee was forced to quit.

Drug testing also has created a contentious new area of unemployment insurance law. The issue is whether an employee who is discharged after a positive drug test or after refusing to take a drug test should be eligible for unemployment insurance. In *Glide Lumber Products Co. v. Employment Division*,[17] an employee was dismissed after he tested positive for marijuana in a random drug test. The Oregon Court of Appeals held that he could not be denied unemployment insurance benefits absent evidence of on-the-job intoxication or impairment. Merely testing positive on a drug test was not "misconduct connected with work" which would justify denial of benefits pursuant to the Oregon unemployment compensation law.

Glide Lumber may well represent the minority view, based on similar cases in other jurisdictions. For example, in *Texas Employment Commission v. Hughes Drilling Fluids*,[18] John Bodessa was discharged by Hughes for refusing to submit a urine sample for drug testing. The Texas Court of Civil Appeals upheld the denial of unemployment insurance benefits because Bodessa was fired for misconduct under a "reasonable" employer rule requiring random tests, which provided for employee privacy and confirmatory testing.

In 1987 Louisiana amended its unemployment insurance statute to provide for the disqualification of employees who test positive for drugs or who refuse to submit to drug testing.[19] The law also prescribes certain preconditions for drug testing, including: Sample collection must be with "due regard" for privacy; the chain of custody must be documented; confirmatory testing must be used; the marijuana cutoff may not be lower than 100 nanograms; and drug test results must be kept confidential.

The final unemployment insurance issue related to drug abuse concerns rehabilitation. In *Shaw v. Unemployment Compensation Board of Review*,[20] a bus driver who had tested positive for marijuana on two occasions was offered, as an alternative to discharge, a 30-day leave of absence for enrollment in a drug treatment program. When the employee refused he was discharged. The Pennsylvania Commonwealth Court upheld his disqualification from unemployment insurance benefits because his refusal to undergo drug treatment was "willful misconduct."

Regulation of Benefits

When Congress enacted the Employee Retirement Income Security Act (ERISA)[21] in 1974, it marked the beginning of a comprehensive federal effort to regulate employer-provided benefit plans, including pensions and health benefits. ERISA and similar laws have had and will continue to have important effects, direct and indirect, on the medical screening practices of many companies.

Some general provisions of ERISA are important to keep in mind. First, the law does not require employers to provide any benefits, but by conditioning an employer's tax deductions for benefit costs on compliance with ERISA, there is a strong incentive for every employers' program to comply. Second, ERISA protections apply to employees but not applicants. Third, ERISA preempts state regulation of qualified benefit plans.

Section 510 of ERISA[22] prohibits the discharge of an employee in order to deprive the employee of benefits under an employee benefit plan. In *Folz v. Marriott Corp.*,[23] John R. Folz had worked for Marriott for 18 years and was serving as general manager of the KCI Marriott in Kansas City, when he was terminated for supposedly poor performance. Only two months earlier, Folz, had notified Marriott that he had multiple sclerosis. The court found that Folz was discharged to deny him medical, sick leave, and long-term disability benefits. Folz was ordered reinstated, with full benefits, and awarded back pay of nearly $175,000.[24]

Another law regulating benefits, the Consolidated Omnibus Budget Reconciliation Act of 1985 (COBRA),[25] amended the Internal Revenue[26] and Labor[27] laws to encourage employers to offer a limited extension of health insurance benefits to employees and their dependents who have become ineligible for employer-provided health benefits. Employers of more than 20 employees who do not offer this extended coverage face losing their tax deduction for employee health benefits.

The COBRA amendments apply to employees and their dependents who are covered by employer-provided health plans. If an employee is terminated (for other than gross misconduct) or if an employee's hours are reduced to a level below coverage eligibility requirements, the employee may elect to extend coverage for up to 18 months. If health benefits for the employee or dependents are no longer available for certain other reasons, such as the death of the employee, coverage may be elected for up to 36 months. In either event, the employee or dependent electing continuation of coverage must pay for the coverage, even if it was previously paid for by the employer. The premiums, however, may be no more than 102 percent of the cost of covering employees who have remained eligible and continue in the plan.

The direct costs to employers of extending health coverage are minimal because the former employees or dependents pay the entire premium. Nevertheless, the indirect costs may be substantial because the former employees and dependents who elect to continue coverage are more likely to be unemployable, uninsurable, or to have medical conditions requiring use of the plan. Thus, both self-insured and experience-rated employers may be assuming additional costs.

According to a 1988 survey by Charles D. Spencer & Associates,[28] only 12.6 percent of qualifying employees elected to continue coverage and the average length of coverage was 6.51 months. (Spouses and dependents elected coverage at the rate of 36.6 percent for an average of 9.04 months.) Significantly, the average claims cost for individuals electing continued coverage pursuant to COBRA was much higher (135.97 percent) than for active employees. The average annual administrative cost per continuee was $139.

As a result of ERISA and COBRA, employers are, in effect, "stuck" with unhealthy employees and their dependents once the employee is hired. Because these laws do not apply to applicants, employers have an incentive to engage in detailed preemployment medical screening to identify individuals who are predisposed to illness and to refuse to hire them in the first place.

The final law affecting employer-provided health benefits, section 89 of the Internal Revenue Code,[29] was enacted as part of the Tax Reform Act of 1986.[30] Effective January 1, 1989, this provision, besides generating revenue, is designed to encourage employers to provide health care coverage to low- and middle-income workers. In essence, highly compensated employees must pay income tax on all health benefits not offered to all employees.

It is not clear whether section 89 will achieve its objective. Employers may extend some health benefits to all employees, but they also could elect to eliminate "premium" coverage, reduce all employees to minimum coverage, and give the highly paid employees the difference in cash, or they could simply let higher paid employees pay the additional tax. Faced with a new complex set of regulations, some employers might decide to eliminate health insurance altogether. Should this occur, section 89 will prove to have been counterproductive. Even if more generous health benefits, previously reserved only for executives, are extended to all employees, this could serve as another significant incentive for more detailed medical screening to prevent the hiring or retention of employees likely to use these costly health benefits.

Dignitary Torts

Medical screening often involves collecting sensitive information, and it may generate sensitive records. The negligent, wrongful, or intentional disclosure of this information or wrongful conduct in the screening itself may be damaging to an individual's reputation, employment opportunities, or emotional well-being. A variety of legal theories, including defamation, invasion of privacy, and intentional infliction of emotional distress (often referred to as dignitary torts) have been used in an attempt to redress alleged tortious conduct in medical screening.

An easy way to view the problem is to focus on the conduct giving rise to the lawsuits. There are three main types of cases: (1) disclosure of medical information by health professionals to management; (2) disclosure of medical information by management; and (3) wrongful conduct in the actual medical testing procedure.

An example of the first type of case, *Levias v. United Airlines*,[31] was discussed in Chapter 1 under the heading "Medical Records." A medical examiner's unauthorized disclosure of a flight attendant's gynecological condition to her flight supervisor and her husband was held to be an invasion of privacy. In a similar case, *Leggett v. First Interstate Bank*,[32] the Oregon Court of Appeals held that an employer's meeting with the employee's psychologist to discuss the employee's condition, without his consent, constituted an invasion of privacy.

In *Rogers v. Horvath*,[33] Helen Rogers, an employee of General Motors, injured her shoulder and filed a workers' compensation claim. She was examined by one of G.M.'s physicians, Dr. James Horvath. Dr. Horvath reported to G.M. and later testified at the workers' compensation hearing that there was nothing wrong with Rogers and that she was a malingerer. After her compensation claim was denied Rogers brought an action against Dr. Horvath. The Michigan Court of Appeals held that no cause of action would lie for malpractice in the absence of a physician-patient relationship and that Rogers failed to allege facts necessary to state a valid claim for fraud. Nevertheless, it held that she could proceed under the theory of libel.

To prevail in any one of these actions, the plaintiff must prove that the publication or dissemination of private information was extensive or that the action of the defendant was outrageous. Where this cannot be established, the defendant will win. For example, in *Valencia v. Duval Corp.*,[34] the court held that the conduct of a supervisor who telephoned an employee's physician to exchange medical information (including informing the physician of the employee's prior bout with the illness) was not sufficiently offensive to establish an invasion of privacy. The employee, who requested a medical leave, was required to submit a physician's report. Similarly, in *Bratt v. International Business Machines Corp.*,[35] IBM distributed memos stating that Robert Bratt was paranoid and had a mental problem. The United States Court of Appeals for the First Circuit held that this distribution was not an actionable invasion of privacy where only four managerial employees learned of the plaintiff's mental problem.[36]

The courts have held that when employees file workers' compensation claims or disability pension claims they waive their right of privacy pertaining to their medical condition, providing the investigation is reasonable and the information is not excessively disseminated.[37] In *Redmond v. City of Overland Park*,[38] the court upheld a release signed by a police officer which authorized disclosure of information by a psychiatrist to the police department. This holding is particularly significant in light of the increased use of releases or waivers in both the public and private sectors.

Another defense for employers is privilege. In *Davis v. Monsanto Co.*,[39] a psychologist treating an employee pursuant to a contract with Monsanto, concluded that the employee was "dangerous to the point of being suicidal to himself and homicidal toward his wife and others, and that he could easily be provoked into creating a life-threatening situation in the work place and other places."[40] The court held that the psychologist was privileged to disclose these findings to Monsanto, and therefore it was not an invasion of privacy under West Virginia law.

The most common type of disclosure of medical information by management involves communication of medical information to other employees. For example, in *Cronan v. New England Telephone Co.*,[41] Paul Cronan, a telephone repair technician alleged that he was required by his supervisor, Charles O'Brien, to disclose the reason for his medical absences. Cronan protested, but in fear of losing his job, he told O'Brien that he had been diagnosed as having ARC. Despite promising to keep the information confidential, O'Brien divulged this information to his supervisors who told other employees. "Company managers in large group meetings informed employees in locations where Cronan had previously worked and was presently working that he had AIDS. Shortly thereafter, Cronan received calls from co-workers who said that employees threatened to lynch Cronan if he returned to work."[42] Cronan did not return to work and sued the company. The Massachusetts Superior Court held that Cronan had alleged facts which, if proven, would establish a claim for invasion of privacy against New England Telephone.[43]

Disclosure of medical screening information to other employees may be privileged. In *Merritt v. Detroit Memorial Hospital*,[44] an employee brought a defamation action against his employer for publishing the results of a drug test to supervisory personnel. The employee had submitted to a drug test as part of an annual physical examination and had tested positive for morphine. The Michigan Court of Appeals held that the employer's communication of the drug test result to supervisory personnel was privileged. The court, in recognizing a qualified privilege in communications among employees with a need to know, observed that: "Employees responsible for hiring and firing are entitled to hear accusations of employee misconduct which warrant dismissal and preclude rehiring."[45] The privilege will be lost, however, if the disclosures are made with malice or are excessively disseminated.

A defamation action may be brought where a company official defames a former employee. Thus, a sports writer for the Chicago *Tribune* was entitled to sue the newspaper and the sports editor after the sports editor placed a memo in every employee mailbox in the sports department, which said that the plaintiff had been fired for, among other things, alcoholism.[46] Similarly, it has been held to be actionable for a former employer to write to a former employee's prospective employer that the employee "had some mental problems."[47]

Communications to other third parties also may give rise to an action for defamation. In *Houston Belt & Terminal Railway v.*

Wherry,[48] Joe Wherry, a railroad switchman, fainted after sustaining a knee injury on the job. In an attempt to establish the cause of the fainting, the company physician ordered a diabetes test and a drug test. The initial drug test result showed a "trace" of methadone, but a follow-up test showed the presence of a normal urinary compound whose chemical characteristics are similar to methadone. Wherry was later discharged for failure to report his accident in a timely manner. During the course of a Department of Labor investigation of the dismissal, the railroad wrote a letter to the Department of Labor stating that Wherry "passed out and fell" and that "traces of methadone" were present in his system. Wherry sued for libel. The Texas Court of Civil Appeals affirmed an award of $150,000 in compensatory damages and $50,000 in punitive damages based on this and other statements. The court stated, "We think the jury was entitled to conclude from the evidence that they made false statements in writing that he was a narcotics user when they knew better."[49]

Finally, liability may be based on the way in which the medical screening was conducted. In *Kelly v. Schlumberger Technology Corp.*,[50] the United States Court of Appeals for the First Circuit affirmed a jury award of $125,000 in damages for invasion of privacy and negligent infliction of emotional distress where a drilling rig employee was "disgusted" by a drug testing procedure in which he was forced to submit a urine sample under direct observation.

In a case filed in 1988, five flight crew employees of Comair, Inc., alleged that they were "shanghaied" to a hotel at the Greater Cincinnati International Airport, by an employee of the commuter airline, kept there for up to six hours, had their personal belongings searched, were denied use of telephones, were questioned repeatedly about their own and others' illegal drug use, and were coerced into giving urine samples in front of two witnesses.[51] Four of the five employees were suspended for a week despite negative drug tests and the fifth employee was discharged for refusing to cooperate. The employees sued, alleging false imprisonment, assault, defamation, invasion of privacy, intentional interference with employment, and intentional infliction of emotional distress. The Boone County, Kentucky prosecutor also filed criminal charges alleging 25 counts of false imprisonment against Comair executives.[52] Undoubtedly, the emotional distress felt by the five employees involved in the incident has since been shared by the Comair executives who, if convicted, could face prison terms.

Personal Injury Litigation

Improper medical screening practices have been alleged to be the cause of a variety of personal injuries. In tort actions to recover for these injuries the most formidable obstacle to overcome is the exclusivity bar of workers' compensation. In general, an injured employee's only recourse is to file a workers' compensation claim for any injury arising in the workplace. A growing list of exceptions to this rule has been recognized, however, and in actions against physicians, nurses, and other individuals and entities plaintiffs have asserted exceptions for independent contractors, coemployees, "dual capacity," and intentional torts. Although the intricacies of these exceptions are beyond the scope of this book, it is important to explore the factual circumstances giving rise to the lawsuits.

As in more traditional medical malpractice cases, an injury caused during the course of an employer-mandated medical examination would establish liability on the part of the examining physician as well as the employer. Not surprisingly, these situations are rare.[53] A more common allegation is that in conducting a medical examination the physician failed to diagnose a serious illness and the delay in treatment aggravated the individual's condition or reduced the likelihood of successful treatment.

In *Coffee v. McDonnell-Douglas Corp.*,[54] Robert Coffee applied for the position of pilot and was given a series of pre-employment medical tests, including a blood test. The blood test showed an extremely high sedimentation rate suggestive of an inflammatory condition or serious disease. The blood test report, however, was never read and Coffee was hired. Seven months later Coffee became ill and was hospitalized, at which time he was diagnosed as suffering from multiple myeloma. The Supreme Court of California affirmed a judgment for Coffee against McDonnell-Douglas, holding that the company physician's failure to discover the inflammatory condition constituted actionable negligence.

Other cases have alleged a negligent failure to diagnose lung cancer,[55] a brain tumor,[56] and a heart attack.[57] The cases have arisen from preemployment, annual, post-injury, and disability evaluation examinations.

Another theory on which plaintiffs have sued is that a negligent medical assessment resulted in an improper job placement, including improperly returning an employee to work after an injury. Employees have alleged, for example, that they: aggravated a back injury by being returned to work too soon by a physician employed by a workers' compensation insurance carrier,[58] suffered a miscarriage by being compelled to work under stressful conditions,[59] and were forced to continue work after sustaining a burn injury.[60] Actions against employer-salaried physicians and employers for improper job placement will normally be found to be barred by workers' compensation,[61] but actions against independent contractor physicians are more likely to be successful.[62]

The relationship of medical screening, job placement, and occupational hazards is illustrated by the case of *Becker v. R.E. Cooper Corp.*[63] Janeen Becker, a 26 year-old factory worker was exposed to toxic levels of carbon monoxide produced by a truck inside the plant where she worked. The ventilation system inside the plant was inadequate and violated the city building code. Becker had an undiagnosed, dormant case of multiple sclerosis, which was activated by her exposure, resulting in her becoming a paraplegic.[64] In a suit against her employer and the truck company, a jury awarded her $4.8 million in damages. While, in theory, one purpose of tort law is to encourage safety measures, a case such as this one might encourage companies to engage in detailed medical screening to exclude "vulnerable" workers.

Another line of cases is based on the alleged fraudulent concealment from employees of work-related illnesses detected by company physicians in the course of a medical examination. Although an action for contracting the disease in the first place would be barred by workers' compensation, fraudulent concealment cases seek to recover for aggravation of the condition caused by a delay in obtaining treatment.

In *Delamotte v. Unitcast Division of Midland Ross Corp.*,[65] David Delamotte was given periodic chest x-rays by his employer beginning in 1952. Although the x-rays revealed a progressively worsening case of silicosis, it was not until 1972 that he was informed of his condition and advised to consult his own physician. The Ohio Court of Appeals held that an action based on fraudulent, malicious, and willful concealment was not barred by workers' compensation.[66] Similar results have been reached in cases involving asbestos-related diseases,[67] lead poisoning,[68] and other medical conditions.[69]

Besides providing medical examinations, some company physicians and nurses become involved, to varying degrees, in the actual treatment of employees, from first aid to ongoing care. A number of lawsuits have alleged malpractice in treatment. For example, employees have alleged that: A physician aggravated the employee's knee injury by reusing on at least five occasions the same hypodermic syringe;[70] improper treatment of an employee's leg injury necessitated subsequent surgery;[71] and a company nurse sent an employee back to work after he had suffered a stroke.[72] In all of these cases, personal injury actions were barred by workers' compensation because the exclusive remedy for harms caused by coemployee negligence is to file a workers' compensation claim. Similar results have been reached where plaintiffs alleged that a company was negligent in failing to maintain a post-employment medical surveillance program[73] and in failing to provide transportation to a hospital for emergency treatment.[74]

In some cases of alleged negligent treatment the courts have held that the plaintiffs have stated a legally cognizable claim. For example, plaintiffs have been permitted to proceed with claims that a company physician failed to diagnose torn ligaments in the plaintiff's wrist and returned him to work, which caused a permanent disability;[75] that a hospital employee who had sustained a broken hip a month earlier was forcefully pushed into a wheelchair, which further aggravated the injury;[76] and that a company physician over-prescribed painkilling drugs for an injury, causing the employee to become addicted.[77] The disparate results reached in these cases is caused by wide differences among the states in whether they recognize exceptions to the workers' compensation exclusive remedy principle.

In all of the cases discussed in this section thus far, the plaintiffs have been employees who were subject to medical screening or treatment. There are two other potential classes of non-employee plaintiffs. First, the children of exposed employees may sue for birth defects caused by parental exposures. Although fear of this kind of lawsuit is a major reason why companies have adopted the fertile female exclusionary policies discussed in Chapter 3 under the heading "Reproductive Hazards," there have been very few such cases. Unsuccessful lawsuits have been brought based on chromosomal damage allegedly caused by maternal exposure to ethylene oxide,[78] birth defects allegedly caused by maternal exposure to lead,[79] and birth defects allegedly caused by paternal exposure to lead.[80]

The litigation surrounding the birth defects of children of male workers exposed to the pesticide DBCP in Lathrop, California, described in *Medical Screening of Workers*, remains ongoing in the courts.[81] Other cases of fetal harm have involved more traditional hazards, including a pregnant waitress who fell at work and suffered a miscarriage,[82] and a pregnant employee of a sawmill whose request for light duty work was denied and she gave birth to twin girls who died within 12 hours of their birth.[83]

Finally, personal injury lawsuits may be brought by third parties, including members of the public, who allege that negligence in medical screening (through omission or commission) caused their injuries. Cases involving DOT examinations[84] and drug usage[85] already have been discussed. In *Homer v. Pabst Brewing Co.*,[86] Randall Hendricks, a night shift brewing supervisor for Pabst, reported to the plant medical department with severe cramps, nausea, and diarrhea. The nurse on duty gave Hendricks some Kaopectate and, after a nap in the medical department, he was sent back to work. Still sick at the end of his shift, Hendricks lost consciousness while driving home and crashed into Virgil Homer, the plaintiff, causing permanent injuries. A jury award of over $525,000 against Pabst for negligence was reversed by the United States Court of Appeals for the Seventh Circuit, which held that: "Pabst has not assumed a duty to unidentifiable members of the general public by undertaking to provide occupational temporary health care to its employees."[87]

10

Health Insurance

Employers and Health Insurance

Employer-provided group health insurance became common during World War II because such fringe benefits were not subject to wartime wage and price controls. Thus, employees (often union members bargaining collectively) were given health insurance coverage when increasing wages was not possible. Perhaps the most attractive feature to employees of health insurance as an employer-provided fringe benefit was the tax-favored treatment of benefits. Employer contributions to a group plan were and still are deductible to the employer as a business expense and, more important, are excluded from the taxable income of the employee. Consequently, health insurance provides a greater after-tax gain to employees than comparable (taxable) wage payments.

From the 1950s through the 1970s, the scope of coverage of health benefits expanded from hospital care to a wide range of medical, dental, and other benefits. Coverage also was extended to retirees and workers' family members. In his book, *America's Health Care Revolution*, Joseph A. Califano, Jr., former Secretary of Health, Education and Welfare, chronicled the growth of employee health benefits funded by Chrysler Corporation. This growth, representative of many large corporations, is illustrated in Table 10–1.

Although Chrysler has been in the forefront of efforts to reduce health care costs, the general trend of increasing the scope of employee health benefits has continued in the 1980s. For example, between 1980 and 1986 the percentage of medium and large companies providing vision care benefits nearly doubled— from 21 percent to 40 percent.[1]

Today, 85 to 90 percent of Americans covered by health insurance are covered by group health insurance[2] and 68 percent

Table 10–1

The Growth of Chrysler Corporation's Health Benefits Plan, 1941–1979

1941 Hospitalization plan with employees paying all costs through payroll deductions

1950 Chrysler pays half the costs and extends coverage to cover physicians' fees

1953 Retirees added to plan, but they pay all costs

1961 Chrysler pays all costs for employees and their dependents; half the costs for retirees and their dependents

1964 Full health coverage for retirees and their dependents; first-dollar coverage for employee outpatient psychiatric care

1967 Prescription drug plan added for employees and dependents

1973 Dental coverage for employees and dependents

1976 Dental coverage for retirees and dependents; eyeglasses for employees; hearing aids for employees and retirees

1979 Eyeglasses for retirees

Source: Adapted from J. Califano, America's Health Care Revolution 13–15 (1986). Copyright 1986, Random House, Inc. Reprinted by permission.

are covered under employer-provided plans.[3] The availability of health insurance through an employer not only represents a tax saving to employees, but, for many workers, it is their only opportunity to obtain health insurance. Without employer-funded or employer-subsidized group health insurance, many lower paid workers would be unable to afford the premiums on an individual health insurance policy or would be uninsurable because of their medical condition.

In short, health insurance is now a highly prized and expected fringe benefit. In a 1988 Gallup poll, 73 percent of Americans said employers should be required to provide all their employees with health insurance. For less educated (84 percent among those without a high school degree), younger (82 percent of those under age 30), and lower paid respondents (79 percent with a household income under $20,000), the percentages were even higher.[4]

The most obvious problem facing employer-provided health benefits is cost. In 1987, health care expenditures in the United States amounted to $498.9 billion, or about 11.2 percent of the nation's gross national product.[5] In 1988, the total cost was $544 billion. Employer health costs in 1988 were $2,354 per employee and they increased over 1987 levels by 18.6 percent.[6] Some industries had even larger increases. For example, health care costs in the Energy/Petroleum industry increased 40.3 percent, to $3,110.[7]

There are several factors causing the sharp increase in the costs of employer-provided health care. First is the increase in health care costs generally. Technology is a major factor. For example, 20 years ago a patient's diagnosis might be based on a $15 x-ray; today that x-ray is $50 and may be followed up with a $400 CAT scan and a $1,000 MRI. In medicine, miracles often have large price tags. Second is the increased coverage of company health plans, which now often include substance abuse treatment, mental health treatment, and long-term care. Third is demographic changes, meaning more retirees in the health plan. Fourth is increased utilization per subscriber.

It is also important to consider the changing method of funding employer health benefits. During the 1970s many larger corporations with rising health costs realized that, with a stable work force, increases in experience-rated premiums were predictable by simply applying an inflation factor. Insurers actually were eliminating very little risk. "In effect, the employee groups covered by large corporations had grown to such a size as to render of little value the essential function of insurance—i.e., reducing the risk by pooling independent exposures."[8]

The result was a growing use of self-insurance, whereby employers directly assume responsibility for health care expenses rather than by purchasing health insurance. Some self-insured companies still contract with commercial insurers or other service companies for claims processing or to purchase "stop loss" insurance to limit their liability for large claims. By 1987, 49 percent of all companies and 75 percent of *Fortune* 100 companies were self insured.[9]

Employers obtain several advantages from self-insurance. They save the profits of the commercial insurers; they are able to use and retain earnings on amounts paid to insurers and held as claims reserves; and they pay no taxes on premiums. Most important, in an era of increasing state regulation of health insurance, self-insured plans are exempt from state insurance laws and regulations, including state high-risk insurance pools. These latter laws, enacted in at least 15 states in the 1980s, provide a fund to enable medically uninsurable individuals to obtain health insurance at subsidized rates.

In *Metropolitan Life Insurance Co. v. Massachusetts,*[10] the Supreme Court addressed the issue of whether a Massachusetts state law, which mandated that all group health insurance policies issued in the state include coverage for mental illness, is preempted by ERISA. The Court held that under ERISA the states were free to regulate insurance policies, even those purchased by employers under an ERISA-qualified plan. Nevertheless, the states may not regulate a self-insured ERISA plan. The Court stated: "We are aware that our decision results in a distinction between insured and uninsured plans, leaving the former open to indirect regulation while the latter are not. By so doing we merely give life to a distinction created by Congress . . ., a distinction Congress is aware of and one it has chosen not to alter."[11]

The Massachusetts statute at issue in the *Metropolitan Life* case is quite typical. Since the early 1970s, laws enacted in every state have mandated the inclusion of various substantive terms in group health insurance contracts. There are now over 700 such mandates.[12] Alcoholism, drug abuse, home health care, maternity, mental health, newborn care, outpatient surgery, and nursing home benefits are some of the more common provisions. While the Supreme Court's decision may have been a reasonable statutory interpretation of ERISA, the result is to create a tripartite health benefits system. Large companies are the most likely to be self-insured and not subject to state regulation; medium-sized companies are the most likely to purchase a group health insurance contract regulated by state law; and small companies are the most likely not to offer any health insurance.

Health Care Cost Containment

As health benefits expenditures have risen, companies have actively searched for ways to reduce costs or at least control increases. Although past efforts have varied in their effectiveness, it is clear that the cost containment battle has just begun. There are four basic ways in which an employer can limit exposure for employee health benefits: (1) limit who is covered; (2) limit the conditions that are covered; (3) limit the level of coverage; and (4) limit the method of coverage.

Who Is Covered

The three main groups of people covered by employer benefit plans are employees, retirees, and dependents of employees and retirees. With regard to employees, as discussed in Chapter 9 under the heading "Regulation of Benefits," effective January 1, 1989, employers are not permitted to discriminate among employees in the health benefits that are offered. Thus, in theory, all employees will have access to the same health benefits. The important issue of the effect of health insurance underwriting considerations on employee selection is discussed in the following section, "Health Insurance Underwriting."

Whether retirees are covered by employer health benefit plans seems to be based largely on the size of the employer. This is indicated in Table 10–2.

The health benefits coverage of retirees also tends to vary by industry. Utilities provide benefits to 95 percent of retirees under age 65 and 84 percent of retirees age 65 and over; by contrast, health services employers provide benefits only to 31 percent of retirees under age 65 and 29 percent of retirees age 65 and over.[13] Sixty-three percent of all employers require contributions from retirees under age 65, and 53 percent require contributions from retirees age 65 and over.[14] Although amounts of contributions vary (from 25 percent to 100 percent),[15] most employers offer the same level of benefits to retirees as current employees.[16]

Retiree health care costs (especially when expressed as the cost per employed worker) are increasing at a tremendous rate because of several factors. First, workers are retiring at a younger age. In 1978, 19 percent of retirees chose to retire at age 65.[17] By 1986, fewer than five percent of employees waited until they were 65 to retire.[18] Because of Medicare payments, the average employee retiring at age 65 uses $32,000 of health care benefits.[19] For employees retiring at age 55, the average cost is $55,000 per retiree.[20]

Table 10–2

Percentage of Employers Providing
Retiree Health Benefits, by Employer Size

| Employer Size by | % of Retirees by Age | |
Number of Employees	under age 65	age 65 and over
<500	39	37
500–999	66	58
1000–2499	75	63
2500–9999	86	79
10000–39999	89	82
>40000	96	90
All	64	57

Source: Adapted from A. Foster Higgins & Co., Inc., Foster Higgins Health Care Benefits Survey 1987, at 52 (1987). Reprinted by permission.

Second, retirees are living longer. In 1987, the life expectancy of a male at age 65 was 14.7 years; for a female, 18.9 years.[21] By 2030, life expectancy for a male at age 65 will be 16.8 years and for a female, 22.1 years.[22]

Third, the ratio of workers to retirees continues to decline. In 1960 there were 5.1 workers for each retiree; in 1987 the ratio was 3.3 workers for each retiree; by 2005 the ratio will drop to 3:1; and by 2020 the ratio will be 2:1.[23] At some companies the ratio is worse than that already. For example, Bethlehem Steel now has 33,000 active employees and 70,000 retirees and surviving spouses.[24]

Finally, increases in Medicare costs, including the deductible amounts, mean that the company's share of health care is continuing to expand. The Medicare deductible in 1985 was $400; by 1988 it had increased 40 percent, to $560. Many companies pay part or all of this amount.

The prospect of increasing retiree costs has led to action by the government and by employers. In 1988 Congress enacted the Retiree Benefits Bankruptcy Protection Act.[25] The legislation had its origins in 1986, when LTV Corporation filed for Chapter 11 bankruptcy reorganization. Congress was concerned that 78,000

LTV retirees might lose their health benefits. The new law prevents an employer from unilaterally terminating a health plan when it files for reorganization and places the retirees in a stronger position to maintain their plan or recover from a company through bankruptcy proceedings. The funding for such a plan, however, is not guaranteed.

Another important development relates to the accounting method used by companies in stating their retiree health obligations. Currently, most companies show in their earnings reports only what they actually pay out for health care in any given year. The Financial Accounting Standards Board, the main accounting standards body, is considering requiring this future obligation to be expressed on financial statements, beginning in 1991 or 1992. With an estimated $402 billion in unfunded health benefits liabilities,[26] the pressure to reduce costs and improve the balance sheet will intensify.

Already, companies have begun to restrict retiree health benefits. Besides the usual cost containment measures (discussed later in this section), some companies have taken even more dramatic steps. For example, at TRW, Inc., the company no longer guarantees the level of the benefits, but only guarantees a certain dollar contribution by the company each year. If costs increase and the company does not increase its contribution, then retirees would be forced to pay more of the share.[27] Other companies announcing cuts in retiree benefits include Metropolitan Life Insurance, General Motors, and Singer.[28]

What Is Covered

Another way of reducing expenditures is to reduce or eliminate coverage for certain medical conditions or certain types of medical care. Long-term care, prescription drugs, psychiatric care, drug and alcohol treatment, dental plans, and other elements of employee health benefits are possible targets for reduced coverage or elimination. Although some employer-purchased health insurance contracts may be regulated by the states, self-funded plans can eliminate any or all of the health benefits employees are currently offered.

In August 1988, Circle K Corporation, the nation's second-largest convenience store chain, with about 26,000 employees, announced that it was discontinuing medical benefits for illnesses resulting from "personal life-style decisions," including AIDS, alcohol and drug abuse, and self-inflicted wounds.[29] As a self-funded employer, there was no legal prohibition on Circle K implementing such a policy. Nevertheless, the public outcry following the announcement[30] led the company to suspend the policy only a week later[31] and to cancel the plan a month later.[32]

Circle K adopted the measure because its 1987 cost for medical care for nine employees with AIDS was $500,000.[33] Undoubtedly, the public furor was related to the emotional and political reaction that accompanies the AIDS issue. It is not clear that there would be a public outcry if an employer were to discontinue coverage for recreational injuries, cosmetic surgery, drug and alcohol abuse, or some other category of medical care.

It is also ironic that the controversy over limiting some benefits would involve an employer such as Circle K. Convenience store employees, like fast food and other low-paid employees in the service sector, often receive no health benefits at all. Undoubtedly, Circle K would not have made front page news if it had announced that the company's financial position did not permit it to continue to offer *any* employee health benefits.

How Much Is Covered

Employers have implemented a variety of cost containment measures. Table 10–3 lists some of the case-management techniques used to control costs.

Besides case-management techniques, employers have initiated cost-sharing programs whereby employees are responsible for an increasing percentage of health costs.[34] These programs have been adopted for two reasons. First, if more costs are borne by employees, then obviously fewer costs are borne by the employer. Second, utilization rates decrease sharply when employees are responsible for more than a de minimis contribution. Therefore, fewer costs are incurred. Table 10–4 indicates the substantial growth in cost sharing from 1982 to 1987.

Method of Coverage

Third-party payers, including the government, commercial insurers, and employers have recognized that free-choice indemnity plans are much more expensive than other delivery systems.

Table 10–3

Techniques for Controlling Employee Health Benefit Costs, by Percentage of Companies Using Them

Outpatient surgery	89%
Preadmission testing	76
Home health care	71
Alcohol abuse program	67
Drug abuse program	63
Extended care facilities	58
Non-surgical outpatient care	56
Hospice care	54
Mandatory surgical second opinion	45
Voluntary surgical second opinion	45
Monitoring medical services and care	36
Generic drug program	27
Employee assistance program	26
Birthing alternatives (non-hospital maternity care)	25
Disability rehabilitation	23

Source: Slater, Bottom Line Medicine, Wall St. J., Apr. 24, 1987, at 8D (based on data from Wyatt Co., 1986). Reprinted by permission.

According to the Health Insurance Association of America, from 1984 to 1987 the percentage of commercial health insurance business with "free choice" (employee has total control over the selection of a physician) decreased from 96 percent to 40 percent.[35] Health maintenance organizations (HMOs) and preferred provider organizations (PPOs) have been increasing.[36]

HMOs tend to be offered by larger employers. In 1987, 62 percent of all employers and 94 percent of employers with 40,000 or more employees offered HMOs.[37] In 1987, 29 percent of all eligible employees elected to enroll in an HMO.[38] The cost for an HMO is likely to be lower than for other health care delivery systems, although the "gatekeeping" function of HMOs may limit patient access to health care. Consequently, there is concern about "adverse selection" in HMO utilization, in which younger,

Table 10-4

Health Benefit Cost-Sharing Measures
Used by Major Companies, 1982 and 1987

Cost-Sharing Measures	% Use by Year	
	1982	1987
Plans requiring employee contributions	38	47
Plans requiring employee contributions for dependents	53	58
Deductibles of $100 or less	86	30
100% reimbursement for hospital room and board	80	32
100% reimbursement for surgery	39	15

Source: Adapted from Hewitt Associates, Salaried Employee Benefits Provided by Major U.S. Employers in 1987 (1988). Reprinted by permission.

healthier employees opt for low premium HMOs and older, less healthy employees opt for more expensive health care systems.

PPOs also are growing in popularity (at least with employers). From 1986 to 1988 the percentage of employers with PPO contracts increased from 15 percent to 29 percent.[39] In 1987 PPOs had average discounts of 14.7 percent on hospital charges and 13.9 percent on physician's fees.[40] PPOs, however, were the least popular of the three main methods of health care delivery. According to the Foster Higgins Health Care Benefits Survey, 86 percent of employers reported that their employees were satisfied with an indemnity plan, 80 percent were satisfied with HMOs, and 75 percent were satisfied with PPOs.[41] Increasingly, flexible benefits plans are giving employees the choice of health care delivery system (at varying employee costs) as well as other fringe benefits. In fact, 82 percent of employers now offer flexible medical benefits.[42]

Finally, it must be understood that many of the corporate strategies for "cost containment" are, in reality, merely strategies for cost shifting. For example, some companies are paying employees (e.g., $25/month) who opt out of employer-sponsored coverage to be covered under their spouse's policy. Nevertheless, reducing one employer's obligations by increasing the obligations of other employers, individuals, government, or charities is a zero-sum game. Access and cost issues related to health insurance are not individual problems of employers and employees, but societal problems.

Health Insurance Underwriting

The problem with employer-provided health insurance is not that it is employer funded. The problem is that because employer costs are indirectly or directly related to utilization rates, employers increasingly are acting as health insurance underwriters. The growth of self insurance has operated to magnify this problem.

If employers are acting as health insurance underwriters and not merely as health insurance providers, it is valuable to look at how commercial health insurance companies actually go about the process of medical underwriting. Some employers already have begun using underwriting techniques in deciding employability and thus eligibility for employer benefits. If we look at health insurance medical underwriting we may be getting a glimpse of the workplace medical screening of the future.

Health insurance is either individual or group. An individual health insurance contract runs between the insurance company and the insured individual. On the other hand, a group health insurance contract runs between the insurance company and a sponsor (usually an employer) that is the insured party. These contracts are continuous and survive the membership of any particular members of the group.

Group health insurance is generally issued without a medical examination or other evidence of insurability. (This is a particularly attractive feature for many individuals.) Insurers have found that medical examinations are not cost effective; they are only interested in whether the group as a whole is insurable. In a large group of employed persons (and their dependents), it is presumed that the overall risk for the group is close to average.

By contrast, applicants for individual insurance are not part of a well-defined, homogenous, and generally healthy group. Because of the potentially great differences in health status and potential risks presented to insurers by individual applicants, insurers evaluate individuals by applying medical underwriting criteria.

In 1988 the Office of Technology Assessment of the U.S. Congress (OTA) issued a detailed study of health insurance underwriting, *Medical Testing and Health Insurance*. The study surveyed the practices of commercial insurers, Blue Cross/Blue Shield plans, HMOs, and employers. While the underwriting process varies among insurers and among the classes of insurance products, there is a trend toward increased testing in all categories.

For individual health insurance, a health history questionnaire is generally required and is the most important step. Depending on what is indicated, an attending physician statement, physical exam, and blood and urine screening may be required. The underwriting process also may consider non-medical factors, such as those listed in Table 10–5.

Interestingly, most insurers considered all of the factors except place of residence and sexual orientation to be very important or important. Most employers have not yet begun to consider these factors in deciding employability.

The applicant's health history questionnaire or attending physician's statement (for which the applicant will be required to sign a release) may indicate that the individual has a particular medical condition. Table 10–6 indicates the effect that this information may have on insurability.

It may be valuable to contrast Table 10–6 with the handicap discrimination case law discussed in Chapter 7 under the heading "Specific Medical Conditions." Even as to the most serious conditions, such as AIDS or leukemia, for which commercial health insurers will deny coverage, an employer may violate handicap discrimination laws by refusing to employ an individual with such a condition. If cost containment pressures encourage employers to engage in "preemployment medical underwriting," it is not clear what the effect will be on handicap discrimination laws.

Finally, the questionnaire, attending physician's statement, or medical examination may indicate the need for blood and urine testing. Millions of these tests are performed annually. Table 10–7 shows some of these tests and their purpose.

Some mention should be made of the testing for prescription drug use. This is done for two reasons: (1) to indicate the level of patient compliance with medically prescribed treatment, or (2) as evidence that an applicant is undergoing treatment for a medical

Table 10-5

The Importance of Nonmedical Factors in Individual Underwriting by Commercial Health Insurers

Underwriting factor (n = 61)	Very important	Relative Importance Important	Unimportant	Never used
1. Age	38%	48%	10%	5%
2. Type of occupation	30	48	18	5
3. Avocation (e.g., race car driving)	15	64	15	7
4. Financial status	16	43	33	8
5. Health endangering personal habits (e.g., drug abuse)	93	5	—	2
6. Health enhancing personal behavior (e.g., non-smoking)	10	56	15	20
7. Illegal or unethical behavior	72	21	3	3
8. Place of residence	5	21	34	39
9. Sexual orientation	2	7	21	70

Source: Office of Technology, U.S. Congress, Medical Testing and Health Insurance 64 (1988).

Definitions: Very Important—Critical to underwriting process; can affect acceptance/rejection.
  Important—Always considered but will never by itself affect acceptance/rejection. It may, however, influence coverage limits (e.g., exclusions or waiting period) and/or premium.
  Unimportant—Rarely affects acceptance/rejection, coverage limits, or premium—unless in conjunction with other more important factors.
  Never used—Never considered.

Table 10–6

Risk Classification by Commercial Health Insurers

Higher premium	Exclusion waiver	Denial
Allergies	Cataract	AIDS
Asthma	Gallstones	Ulcerative colitis
Back strain	Fibroid tumor (uterus)	Cirrhosis of liver
Hypertension (controlled)	Hernia (hiatal/inguinal)	Diabetes mellitus
Arthritis	Migraine headaches	Leukemia
Gout	Pelvic inflammatory disease	Schizophrenia
Glaucoma	Chronic otitis media (recent)	Hypertension (uncontrolled)
Obesity	Spine/back disorders	Emphysema
Psychoneurosis (mild)	Hemorrhoids	Stroke
Kidney stones	Knee impairment	Obesity (severe)
Emphysema (mild to moderate)	Asthma	Angina (severe)
Alcoholism/drug use	Allergies	Coronary artery disease
Heart murmur	Varicose veins	Epilepsy
Peptic ulcer	Sinusitis, chronic or severe	Lupus
Colitis	Fractures	Alcoholism/drug abuse

Source: Office of Technology Assessment, U.S. Congress, Medical Screening and Health Insurance 60 (1988).

condition he or she has not divulged on the medical question-naire. The most common medications tested for are drugs to treat cardiovascular diseases such as hypertension and heart disease (e.g., diuretics and beta-blocker drugs) and diabetes (e.g., hypo-glycemic or blood-sugar-lowering drugs). Prescription drug screening could be very easily incorporated into a preemploy-ment medical examination.

According to the OTA study, each year there are about 2.24 million applications filed for individual health insurance.[43]

Table 10–7

Tests Commonly Ordered by
Commercial Health Insurers

Type of Test	Common diagnostic use
Blood screens	
I. *Diagnostic screens*	
Glucose	Diabetes
Bun/creatinine	Kidney function
Uric acid	Kidney stones
Alkaline phosphatase	Liver function
Bilirubin total	Gall bladder and liver function
SGOT/SGPT	Hepatitis (alcoholic), liver function
GGTP	Liver function
Total protein	General health
Albumin	Liver function
Immunoglobulin	Immunodeficiency, infection
Cholesterol	Circulatory disorders
Triglycerides	Circulatory disorders
HDL	Circulatory disorders
Chol/HDL chol ratio	Circulatory disorders
ELISA/ELISA/Western blot	HIV infection
T-Cell subset	HIV infection, immune system
Urine screens	
I. *Diagnostic screens*	
Microscopic analysis:	
White blood cell count	Infection, cancer
Red blood cell count	Anemia
Casts (granular, hyaline)	Kidney disorders
Protein	Kidney disorders, hypertension
Glucose	Diabetes
Specific gravity	Kidney function
II. *Prescription drug screens*	
Oral hypoglycemics	Diabetes
Beta-blocker	Hypertension, coronary disease
Thiazide diuretics	Hypertension
III. *Drug abuse screens*	
Barbiturates	
Cocaine	
Nicotine	

Source: Office of Technology Assessment, U.S. Congress, Medical Testing and Health Insurance 75 (1988).

There are 446,000 attending physicians' statements[44] and 94,000 physical examinations.[45] In 1986 the Home Office Reference Laboratories (which performs testing for about 80 percent of insurers in the United States and Canada) performed 128,129 HIV tests.[46] The Medical Information Bureau, a databank for more than 700 insurance companies, which facilitates the sharing of underwriting information,[47] adds this new information to previous applications and claims filed. The result is a massive computerized medical data system. Employer access to this data would raise serious questions of confidentiality and public policy.

According to OTA, each year about 164,000 applicants are denied individual health insurance coverage by commercial insurers.[48] A variety of state laws have been enacted to prohibit discrimination in health insurance based on blindness, deafness, prior exposure to DES, sickle cell trait, sexual orientation, and other factors.[49] As mentioned earlier, however, these laws do not apply to self-insured employer plans. It is difficult to estimate how many of the 164,000 applicants denied individual health insurance would be denied employment.

Finally, in discussions of medical underwriting, there is rarely any mention made of dependents. Unquestionably, a covered dependent can accumulate just as many medical bills as an insured employee. According to one study, among patients whose annual medical expenses were $25,000 or higher, the male spouses of female employees were the most overrepresented group.[50]

Health Promotion and Wellness Programs

In the last decade numerous companies have begun or expanded worksite health promotion and wellness programs. These voluntary programs encourage employees to stop smoking, lose weight, exercise, reduce stress, and generally adopt more healthful lifestyles. Although large employers are more likely to offer such programs, the Department of Health and Human Services estimates that two-thirds of the nation's worksites with 50 or more workers have at least one health promotion activity. (See Table 10-8.)

Health promotion and wellness programs further two important goals: improve the health of employees and save money for

Table 10–8

Wellness Programs at Worksites
With 50 or More Workers

Activity	Companies Offering
Smoking control	36%
Health risk appraisals	30
Back care	29
Stress management	27
Exercise/physical fitness	22
Off-the-job accident prevention	20
Nutrition education	17
High blood pressure control	17
Weight control	17

Source: U.S. Department of Health and Human Services, Public Health Service, Office of Disease Prevention and Health Promotion, National Survey of Worksite Health Promotion Activities (1987).

the companies in health care costs, absenteeism, disability costs, and similar ways. There is a large and growing body of literature devoted to assessing the effectiveness of health promotion programs—who uses them,[51] the health benefits,[52] and the economic benefits.[53] By most accounts, these programs have been successful. For example, in a survey of corporate wellness programs, the Health Research Institute reported per-employee medical care cost savings of $49.74 per month for companies with wellness programs.[54] For every dollar spent on wellness programs the companies saved $3.44 on medical costs.[55] Table 10–9 indicates the specific benefits of wellness programs.

It is hard to be critical of programs that encourage smoking cessation, weight loss, and the like. Yet, there are two potential problems with health promotion and wellness programs. The first relates to the type of data used in health promotion programs and health risk assessments. For example, Focus Technologies of Washington, D.C., received $1 million from the Equitable Life Assurance Society to develop a program of risk assessment involving "high tech" biochemical tests, including genetic testing.[56] It is not clear that the science supports these risk analyses. Moreover,

Table 10–9

The Benefits of Wellness Programs, by
Percentage of Programs Reporting Specific Benefits

Type of program	Benefit				
	Improved Health	Reduced Costs	Increased Productivity	Improved Morale	None
Nutrition	59.6%	5.8%	25.5%	20.7%	7.2%
High blood pressure control	57.5	13.6	31.8	15.0	0.9
Physical fitness	53.5	4.7	26.0	37.4	8.6
Weight control	53.2	6.4	29.6	34.4	12.0
Health risk appraisal	47.1	14.3	24.2	14.2	8.3
Smoking control	40.9	7.9	16.4	9.0	10.2
Stress management	20.2	4.2	46.5	30.0	7.8
Back care	26.3	40.7	24.3	—	3.2
Off-the-job accident prevention	19.8	24.9	23.3	—	4.6

Source: U.S. Department of Health and Human Services, Public Health Service, Office of Disease Prevention and Health Promotion, National Survey of Worksite Health Promotion Activities (1987).

detailed "lifestyle" questions, a part of some risk assessments, raise concerns about confidentiality.

The second problem with health promotion and wellness programs is the potential for discrimination. Although participation in such programs is now voluntary, it is possible that employees who refuse to stop smoking or to exercise regularly may face adverse employment consequences. "A fine line exists between using incentives to facilitate health behavior changes at the worksite and bringing about changes through manipulation or coercion."[57]

Efforts already are underway to tie employer health insurance costs to employee lifestyle. Prudential Insurance Company has developed a program, "Health Sketch," in which employer costs are based in part on how employees answer more than 50 questions on family health history, stress management, and seatbelt use.[58] According to Delaware Insurance Commissioner David Levinson, "It just isn't fair for the person who leads a clean life style to subsidize the debauchery of those who don't."[59]

Some companies pay cash subsidies to employees who adopt healthy lifestyles or who file few health insurance claims.[60] Rewarding well employees, however, may be viewed as penalizing employees who are ill. Moreover, rating employees and applicants based on their likely consumption of health care resources encourages employers not to hire or retain an employee with a large family, with a sick child or spouse, or with a history of illness in the family. As a policy matter, wellness should be encouraged—but not at all costs.

Mandated Benefits

About 37 million Americans under age 65 have no health insurance coverage, public or private.[61] Nearly two-thirds of these people (24 million) are workers or dependents of workers.[62] The number is growing. From 1980 to 1987 the number of uninsured Americans rose by 7.3 million,[63] as more people began working in the retail and service sectors. These jobs are often part-time, at smaller companies, at low wages, and without health insurance. Insurers usually individually underwrite small firms with fewer than 10 employees and, consequently the rates are often 10 to 40 percent higher than for large companies. Even small companies that want to offer health insurance often are unable to obtain coverage at all or cannot afford to pay the increasingly expensive premiums.[64]

Employees working for these small companies are hardly able to obtain the health insurance for themselves. These workers are usually too poor to afford to buy individual health insurance (even more expensive than group health insurance) but not poor enough to qualify for Medicaid.

The first legislative efforts to address the problem were at the state level. In 1974 the Hawaii Prepaid Health Care Act was passed.[65] Under the law, employers in Hawaii are required to provide employees who work 20 hours or more per week with health insurance covering hospital, surgical, diagnostic, maternity, substance abuse, and mental health services. When the law took effect in 1975, the uninsured rate in Hawaii was 11.7 percent. By 1987 it had declined to about five percent, comprised of the unemployed and part-time and seasonal workers.[66]

In 1988 Massachusetts enacted universal health insurance legislation to provide coverage for the state's 600,000 uninsured.[67] Massachusetts goes beyond Hawaii in providing health insurance to all residents, not just those who have jobs, although this latter feature is to be phased in by 1992. Employers must pay $1,680 per worker each year to a state fund unless the employer provides health benefits. Employee contributions of 25 to 30 percent are "recommended" by the law, but employee contributions may not exceed 50 percent and, for employees earning less than $4.19 per hour, no employee contributions are permitted. The law also limits copayments to 20 percent, deductibles to $500 per family, and total out-of-pocket payments to $3,000.

In 1989 the state of Washington also began an experimental program to provide health insurance to working people who cannot afford it.[68] Unlike Massachusetts, Washington does not require employer contributions. The state will pay up to 90 percent of the cost of insurance for families whose incomes are less than double the poverty level. Individual contributions range from $7.50 to $38 per month, depending on family size and income. The pilot project involves just 30,000 people in two counties, but if successful, it may be implemented on a statewide basis.

At the federal level, the proposed Minimum Health Benefits for All Workers Act,[69] sponsored by Senator Edward Kennedy and Representative Henry Waxman, would require employers of employees who work 17.5 hours per week or more to provide minimum health insurance coverage. Employee contributions would be limited to 20 percent, and for workers earning $4.19 per hour or less, zero. The deductibles, copayments, and out-of-pocket limits would be the same as in Massachusetts. The annual cost for each employee is estimated to be $1,168. There are no provisions for the unemployed.

Not surprisingly, this proposed legislation has been quite controversial. Among the reasons for the legislation, supporters of the bill have argued the following: First, it is unconscionable that the richest nation on earth should not assure basic health care to its people. As Governor Dukakis said when he signed the Massachusetts law: "As an American, I don't want my country to stand alone with South Africa as the only two industrialized nations in the world that do not provide basic health security for their citizens."[70]

Second, universal health insurance may be more efficient. Preventive medicine in areas such as prenatal care costs much less money than neonatal care of high risk babies. A study by the National Academy of Sciences estimated that every additional dollar spent for prenatal care saves at least $3 by reducing the need for intensive care and long-term institutional care of babies born with physical or mental defects. Moreover, office visits of insured people are far less costly than emergency room treatment (for the same medical conditions) of the uninsured.

Third, employers and taxpayers are currently subsidizing the coverage of the uninsured (and their employers) indirectly and inefficiently. Hospitals with high levels of uncompensated care pass along those costs to paying customers in the form of increased charges. With DRGs and PPOs, hospitals are now more limited in their ability to pass on these costs.

Fourth, some companies now maintain a competitive advantage by reducing health benefits. At hearings on the Kennedy bill, Robert L. Crandall, Chairman and President of American Airlines, testified that employee benefits is one of the few airline costs that is not fixed. At Continental Airlines, the employees pay $360 to $600 per year for family health insurance; at American, after their first year of work they pay nothing. At Continental, deductibles are between $300 and $900 per person; at American they are $100. Continental eliminated all medical benefits for retirees, thereby creating a "nearly irresistible pressure" on competitors to reduce retiree costs. Mandated benefits, according to Mr. Crandall, would eliminate this unfair competition.[71] Some large corporations also favor mandated benefits because they are now providing health insurance to spouses of their employees who work for smaller companies that do not provide health insurance.

Opponents of the legislation also have raised a number of arguments, including the following: First, it would drive small employers out of business. If small employers paying minimum wages to workers were forced to pay for health insurance, it would amount to increased costs of 19 percent for full-time employees and 39 percent for half-time employees.[72]

Second, by increasing per-employee compensation, employers will hire fewer workers and thus unemployment will rise. Dr. Karen Davis, a health economist at Johns Hopkins University, however, testified that even if 100,000 to 120,000 jobs are lost as a direct result of higher labor costs, at least 100,000 new jobs will be created in the health sector due to increased demand.[73] Few people have addressed the issue of whether labor-intensive operations would be likely to move offshore.

Third, mandated benefits will result in lower wages. Faced with these additional costs, companies will reduce wages or, at least, eliminate any wage increases. Indirectly, some of the lowest paid workers may be paying for health insurance from their own paychecks.

Fourth, increased labor costs will be passed on to consumers. This will result in higher prices or reduced market share for domestic companies.

Fifth, there is a general philosophical opposition to government-mandated benefits. According to Senator Orrin Hatch, the Kennedy bill is "socialism, pure and simple."[74]

The foregoing sample of arguments, pro and con, hardly begins to scratch the surface of this complicated social, political, and economic issue. In all of the debates, however, one important issue has been overlooked. That issue is the effect that mandated employer-provided health insurance is likely to have on medical screening practices by employers. If large numbers of employers that previously had not provided health insurance are suddenly required to do so, they would be under tremendous pressure to hire and retain only individuals who were likely to keep insurance rates low by being low users of health benefits.

In this scenario, discrimination against people considered to be health insurance risks could become rampant—based on their current or future health or the health of their dependents. As Diana Chapman Walsh observed in her book, *Corporate Physicians*:

> "The ability to identify 'high-cost users' of health care gives employers a scientific tool they can use to conduct witch hunts. It also raises equity questions since behavioral risk factors, like most illnesses, are concentrated in lower socioeconomic and educational strata. Moreover, if high-cost employees (for example, those who drink, smoke, or overeat) are to be a target of cost-reducing interventions, what about high-cost spouses or children? What about

large families, or families that ski or engage in other high-risk sports? Where is a company to draw the lines?"[75]

The most plausible avenue of legal redress for unfair employment practices would be under state and federal handicap discrimination laws, but for a variety of substantive and procedural reasons discussed already, it is highly unlikley that these laws would be effective. In addition, the issue of discrimination based on the health of dependents would undoubtedly be beyond the purview of these laws, which prohibit discrimination against employees. As explored in the following chapter, medical screening based on presumed health benefits utilization could lead to a series of regrettable social and economic consequences.

11

In Search of Medical Screening Policy

Medical Screening and Employment Policy

Referring to the drug testing of applicants and employees, one management lawyer recently stated: "In the nonpublic sector, employers have the right to do whatever they damn please—and they are going to do it."[1] The accuracy of this statement cannot be questioned; the implications, however, must be.

The employment relationship is based on contract. In theory, employers and employees are both free to bargain over conditions of employment and, if no agreement is reached, either side is free to decline to enter into or to withdraw from a contract. In reality, at least for large companies, the employers establish all conditions of employment. Except for top executives, there are no negotiations. The applicant or employee accepts the conditions or looks for another job.

The economic leverage (some would say coercive power) of employers is formidable. It is neither new nor difficult to understand. To illustrate, during the Great Depression, New York enacted legislation designed to eliminate the fraudulent and oppressive practices of many employment agencies, which preyed on desperate unemployed workers. In upholding the constitutionality of the legislation, the court stated:

> "Unemployed working persons who are under the necessity of jobs to sustain themselves and their dependents are unable as a class to protect themselves . . . . There is no equality between the parties under the circumstances. One is in a position to exact, and necessity has deprived the other of any ability to resist."[2]

Although times have changed, workers remain vulnerable. Despite the assertions of some libertarians,[3] the notion of equality in bar-

218

gaining between employers and the vast majority of employees is widely viewed as "romantic fantasy."[4]

Today, a superior bargaining position allows some companies to use intrusive medical inquiries or to make specific health criteria conditions of employment. Employees usually acquiesce. For example, in 1978 five women at the Willow Island, West Virginia, plant of American Cyanamid Company underwent surgical sterilization in order to keep their jobs in the inorganic lead pigments department. Because of fears that lead exposure during the early stages of an unsuspected pregnancy could cause birth defects, the company adopted a policy that all women were presumed fertile and, regardless of marital status, contraception, or other similar factors, all fertile women were considered potential mothers. Consequently, no fertile women were employed.[5] OSHA issued citations to the company under the Act's "general duty clause," but the citations were vacated on the ground that American Cyanamid's "fetal protection" policy was beyond OSHA's jurisdiction. Indeed, Judge Robert Bork's opinion for the United States Court of Appeals for the District of Columbia Circuit, affirming the vacating of the citations, became a *cause celebre* during his Supreme Court confirmation hearings. A Title VII sex discrimination claim filed by the five women against American Cyanamid (after they later lost their jobs) was settled out of court.

Another example, this time of an onerous medical screening program, involves Georgia Power Company, which set up a special drug hotline in 1984 so that employees could anonymously report coworkers suspected of using drugs. The accused workers would then be required to undergo drug testing. In early 1985, an employee named Susan Register, who had previously reported safety violations to the Nuclear Regulatory Commission, was one of two employees who was told she had been "hotlined" and ordered to submit to drug testing.

> "[Register was] forced by a nurse to drop her pants to her ankles, bend over at the waist with her knees slightly bent, hold her right arm in the air, and with her left hand angle a specimen bottle between her legs. She sobbed and shook, wet herself, and vomited. She was fired for insubordination: refusal to take another test."[6]

Although these are extreme examples, the fact that such events could occur in America raises deeply troubling questions. How can a society that gives a panoply of rights (e.g., presumption of innocence, right to be free of unreasonable searches and seizures, due process of law) to suspects charged with the most heinous crimes give so few rights to workers? How can a society with such avowed concerns for autonomy and privacy be so unconcerned about autonomy and privacy in the workplace? How can employment policies such as these be justified? Is there a logical basis for granting fewer rights to private sector employees than to public sector employees?

The preceding questions are indeed difficult, even in the context of the two examples presented. But the problem is more complicated. Autonomy and privacy are only two of the concerns raised by medical screening. Some of the tests used by employers may be harmful—psychologically or physically. Genetic testing, psychological testing, and HIV testing, especially if performed without counseling of the individual, have a tremendous potential for psychological harm. Chest x-rays, back x-rays, and other diagnostic and predictive screening procedures of dubious efficacy may actually create health risks to the individual. Nevertheless, there is no clearly established legal right for an applicant or employee to refuse (without jeopardy) even a medical procedure, such as bronchoscopy, that may be painful or dangerous.[7]

Finally, there is the potential for discrimination. In the early part of this century medical screening was used as a way of ousting union sympathizers and other "undesirables." Today, the possible abuse of medical screening practices remains a source of concern.

> "[T]he actual history of risk-based occupational screening is among the most inglorious chapters of American medicine. Workers, particularly workers who belong, by reason of race or gender, to groups previously victimized by occupational discrimination, have reason to worry that fitness and risk evaluations may be instruments of covert discrimination."[8]

In general, the law has not acted to regulate medical screening to protect privacy interests, to give workers greater autonomy in decisionmaking regarding workplace health risks, or to prevent the use of harmful tests and procedures. Legal intervention has been limited to efforts to redress discrimination. In fact, the anti-discrimination laws affecting medical screening are limited, condition-specific, and vary widely. Moreover, to a great extent, they are local and state laws because the cities and states have replaced the federal government in the forefront of legislative action to protect employees. Four states restrict genetic testing,[9] 10 states prohibit HIV testing,[10] and nine states regulate drug testing.[11] Federal action in the area of "right to know" laws, polygraph protection, and related areas came about long after the states began to act.

In several areas, such as drug testing, both the federal and state governments have enacted legislation. Concurrent state and federal regulation of employment, however, creates problems. Besides the obvious variations among jurisdictions, there is the recurring legal question of whether state laws are preempted by federal legislation. Furthermore, the state and federal laws related to medical screening have fostered inconsistent policies. Some laws, including workers' compensation and ERISA, encourage preemployment medical screening. Other specific statutes (e.g., HIV testing) and handicap discrimination laws prohibit some forms of medical screening. This inconsistent, piecemeal legislative approach, dealing with working conditions, benefits, and discrimination separately, is unlikely to be effective in formulating a comprehensive medical screening policy in an age of rapid technological change.

A number of important aspects of medical screening need to be addressed through legislation, regulation, or professional standards. First, medical inquiries of employees should be limited to job-related information. Second, medical examination and testing procedures need to be limited to those that are safe and of proven efficacy. Third, applicants and employees should be told of all medical procedures and laboratory tests in advance, they should be given all test results, and they should be told when any employment decision is based on medical information. Fourth, the intra-company and extra-company disclosure of medical records must be controlled and confidentiality assured. Fifth, comprehensive, consistent, and predictable handicap discrimination legislation should be enacted. The proposed Americans with Disabilities Act,[12] for example, would prohibit discrimination on the basis of handicap by any employer covered by Title VII.

In contemplating any possible new regulation of the workplace, however, it is essential to consider the legitimate interests of employers in safety, efficiency, productivity, and cost containment. Restricting employer prerogatives to screen out workers could cause higher production costs, decreased productivity, reduced wage levels, higher prices, unemployment, and other adverse consequences. Certainly, each new employment regulation brings added administrative costs. As explored in the following section, however, the failure to control excessive workplace medical screening may impose substantial economic and noneconomic costs on society as a whole.

Medical Screening and Social Policy

In an article on genetic testing, "Listen to Your Genes," TRB of the *New Republic* conceptualized the issue as follows:

"It is sound human instinct that finds it just too galling for your fate in life to be determined by some test over which you have no control. But what exactly is the concern here? Is it that the tests might be wrong? Or that they might be right? Is it (1) that you might not actually get cancer despite a genetic predisposition; or (2) that a genetic predisposition shouldn't be held against you, whether it leads to cancer or not?"[13]

Most challenges to medical screening have focused on TRB's first concern, the accuracy of the screening tests. Polygraphs, back x-rays, unconfirmed drug tests, and biochemical genetic tests have been challenged as being inaccurate. Even handicap discrimination laws are premised on the idea that an otherwise qualified individual should not be discriminated against on the basis of a handicap that is irrelevant to job performance—not that a handicap affecting job performance should be overlooked on policy grounds. Increasingly, however, accurate predictive tests, from HIV tests to recombinant DNA techniques, will raise the more difficult question of whether predictive screening should be prohibited for reasons of public policy.

Should an individual's employment opportunities be determined by an increased risk of future illness that may never eventuate and, even if it does, is years away? What companies would be most likely to adopt personnel policies of attempting to hire only "perfect" workers? If it is jobs at larger companies and the higher paid jobs at smaller companies that require the new screening procedures, employees who are medical risks could be concentrated in low paying, dead-end jobs. At the present time, these are also the jobs that tend not to offer health insurance as an employee benefit. What would be the economic and social implications of such a trend?

Although it may be economically efficient for an individual company to refuse to employ an individual who is likely to develop a serious illness in the future, it may not be efficient for society. An individual at age 20 who is unemployable because he will develop

Huntington's disease at age 40 should not be a ward of the state for the 20 years he remains healthy and potentially productive, yet unemployed. Taxpayers will end up paying more to support this individual than any company will save. And this does not even consider the human costs.

Social scientists and public health analysts have long known of the negative health consequences of unemployment in terms of alcoholism, suicide, child abuse, and other manifestations. The effects of biological unemployability could be even worse. Could such medical screening satisfy the ethical concerns for autonomy, privacy, justice, and benevolence? Would we want to live in a society that, in effect, tells the parent of a child with Tay Sachs, spina bifida, cystic fibrosis, muscular dystrophy, or some other serious illness that your child's illness makes you unemployable? Can we deny jobs and health insurance to those who need them most?

To be fair, besides the "horror stories" of workplace medical screening, one also should consider its potential to do good. Supporters of medical screening, particularly in the medical community, assert that workplace medical screening promotes public health. It leads to the early detection and treatment of disease and, through wellness and health promotion programs, supports behavioral changes that help to prevent illnesses. The argument is appealing. It is difficult to oppose medical check-ups and health promotion; it is less difficult to oppose them when they are employer-initiated, employer-controlled, and related primarily to cost containment. As discussed in Chapter 10, there is too great a potential to use health risk appraisals more coercively.

In many respects, the question of whether employers should be engaged directly in health promotion and nonoccupational wellness programs is a part of the larger question of the role of employers in promoting social policies or solving social problems. Since at least the New Deal, the workplace has been used as a vehicle for social policy. For example, in enacting the Fair Labor Standard Act's minimum wage provision,[14] Congress sought to increase consumer spending and stimulate the economy out of the Great Depression. But employment policies, ranging from the Davis-Bacon Act (prescribing wage levels on government construction)[15] to wage/price controls generally were limited to economic policy. Even Title VII attempted to promote equal employment opportunity and thereby realign income levels and living standards skewed by race.[16]

In recent years, the workplace has been used increasingly as a way of solving larger, often noneconomic, social problems. There are a number of examples of this phenomenon. The Immigration Reform and Control Act of 1986[17] is premised, at least in part, on the theory that employer sanctions for hiring undocumented workers will decrease the demand for undocumented workers and ultimately stem the flow of illegal immigration. Public sector and private sector drug testing is an attempt to decrease the demand for illegal drugs by making drug users unemployable. The United States is now attempting to end delinquent child support at the plant gate, provide child care at the plant gate, supply health insurance at the plant gate, and encourage wellness at the plant gate. The question is: At what cost?

It may be that, like public schools and the military, the large numbers of people passing through the employment system make it an ideal point to effect social policy. Nevertheless, there are economic and social costs in using the workplace as the first line of attack in dealing with societal ills. Employers are not well suited to substitute for the Drug Enforcement Administration, the Immigration and Naturalization Service, or the Public Health Service. They are also not well suited to be health insurance underwriters.

Medical Screening and Health Policy

With 68 percent of Americans obtaining their health insurance through their employer, it is clear that employers have been assigned a pivotal role in our nation's health policy. This role should not be overlooked, and neither should the role of medical screening in employment policies. If the current trend continues, medical screening could determine who is employed, which could determine who is insured, which could determine who has access to quality health care.

Increasingly detailed medical screening and consumption-based cost containment strategies place great strains on employers, employees, and society. For employers: Health care costs continue to rise but the law prohibits discrimination against otherwise qualified individuals with handicaps. In addition, employers offering health insurance are subsidizing employers that do not offer health insurance by covering spouses working for other companies, by paying higher provider charges (to offset more uncompensated care), and by paying higher taxes (to support the medically indigent). For employees: There is more medical screening and potential for employer intrusion into personal health and lifestyle. At the same time, health benefits provide less coverage, less freedom of choice, higher copayments, and higher deductibles. For society: People who are the worst health risks and the lowest paid tend to be uninsured and require government assistance. The total number of uninsured continues to rise.

The most important recent attempt to deal with this problem has been the proposal to require all employers to provide health insurance. Indeed, this proposal was one of the keystones of the domestic platform of Michael Dukakis in the 1988 presidential campaign. George Bush's victory over Dukakis, however, does not mean that the issue of mandated, employer-provided health insurance is dead. Congressional supporters of universal health insurance are apparently convinced that the only politically feasible way of extending health insurance coverage to the 24 million workers now without it (and eventually to the additional 13 million uninsured who are unemployed) is to mandate employer health benefits. This legislative legerdemain, health insurance without government involvement or expenditure, reflects a probably accurate but nonetheless cynical view of the American public: Only a social program offering something for nothing (i.e., no new taxes or increases in the budget deficit) has a chance of gaining sufficient public support.

Despite their public rhetoric, both proponents and opponents of mandated benefits know that "there is no free lunch." The costs of mandated benefits ultimately will be borne by consumers, shareholders, and employees—if not taxpayers as well. The fact that mandated benefits constitute an indirect health insurance tax has caused strong opposition to the concept. Yet, besides the "pernicious economic consequences" of mandated benefits,[18] there could be pernicious civil rights consequences. Requiring employers to provide health insurance could trigger an unprecedented wave of medical screening and risk-based exclusions from employment. This discrimination may be invidious, stigmatizing, ubiquitous, and long term. One possible consequence could be the creation of an underclass of medically unemployable individuals requiring increased government transfer payments for income support. Moreover, the negative effects could include invasions of privacy, breaches of confidentiality, and the psychological despair of those permanently excluded from the American work force and the American dream.

Mandated benefits, if enacted, will only hasten a trend that already has begun. It is hardly surprising that if employers are increasingly functioning as health insurance underwriters that they should behave increasingly the way health insurance companies behave by excluding medical risks. The simplest way of reversing this trend of medical screening and discrimination is to remove the economic incentive for employers to screen out high risk employees. In short, employers need to get out of the business of health insurance underwriting.

Changing the role of employers in the health insurance system will involve major structural changes. It would be presumptuous to propound and impossible to predict the details of a system that would emerge from public debate and congressional deliberations. There certainly is no shortage of proposals.[19] The foreign model most widely mentioned as a possibility in the U.S. is the Canadian system.[20] Before 1966 the U.S. and Canadian systems were virtually the same. In 1966 Canada enacted the Medical Care Insurance Act. Under this law, each Canadian province runs its own health insurance plan. Some provinces charge a modest premium to people who can afford it, but most are financed only by tax revenues of the provinces and the federal government. Except for a few procedures, such as cosmetic surgery, provincial health insurance pays all the costs of treatment by any physician or hospital in Canada, with patients having freedom of choice. An important feature is that unlike Great Britain, where the government provides direct care, the Canadian government only provides insurance.

The attraction of the Canadian plan is that it is less costly than the U.S. health system—about 8.5 percent of GNP in 1988, compared with 11.5 percent in the United States.[21] As a direct purchaser of health care services, the Canadian government has more leverage to control health care costs. According to Alan Morson, Vice Chairman of Toronto's Crown Life Insurance Company: "In Canada, the costs are a lot less because the government is controlling them. In the U.S., nobody is controlling them."[22] By most statistical measures, such as life expectancy and infant mortality rates, Canadians receive good health care.[23] Critics, however, point to a shortage of hospital beds and diagnostic equipment (e.g., CAT scans) as well as delays in services. According to Michael A. Walker, Executive Director of the Fraser Institute in Vancouver:

"Cardiac-bypass queues grow and patients die before their turn; hip replacements and cataract operations join a growing list of corrections that are triaged, ostensibly because more serious operations must be performed, but in reality because the resources are being used to continue first-dollar insurance coverage for sniffles and splinters . . . ."[24]

To some Americans, the Canadian model may be viewed as increasing the access to health care of the lower class while reducing the access to health care of the middle class. (Presumably, the upper class, which is capable of paying fees for services, is largely unaffected by most changes in the health insurance system.) It could be argued, however, that middle class access to health care continues to erode under the present system.

Regardless of the merits of the Canadian system, it deserves to be studied. As to the best system for the United States, it is easier to discuss general characteristics than specifics. Any effective health insurance system needs to address the following three issues: (1) The method of funding; (2) the method of administration; and (3) the method of underwriting risks.

With regard to funding, there are two main possibilities. The simplest and most direct method would be to impose a health insurance surcharge on individual income taxes. The amount of tax due would be based on income and number of dependents, up to a maximum tax, such as in Social Security withholding. Individuals with low or no incomes would have a negative income tax and would be entitled to the same health insurance coverage as taxpayers. The windfall to corporations (from being relieved of health insurance costs) and the burden on individuals (from paying for health insurance in taxes) could be equalized by raising corporate tax rates and lowering individual tax rates. This adjustment would also factor in the individual's loss of health insurance as a pretax benefit.

The obvious problem with this method of funding is that it utilizes the income tax system as a way of generating the money. It also appears to be giving a break to corporations. Thus, any new health insurance system is not likely to adopt such an approach, but is more likely to resemble the current system (as well as mandated benefits proposals) by being jointly funded by employers and employees, with a maximum employee contribution. In the Kennedy-Waxman bill, employee contributions would be limited to 20 percent of the premium charges. For the lowest paid employees, the insurance would be solely funded by employers. One of the problems that would still need to be addressed, however, is how to fund health insurance for the unemployed. One proposal, suggested by Dr. Uwe Reinhardt, a health economist at Princeton University, is to use federally subsidized HMOs for the unemployed poor to be funded by a surcharge on federal income taxes.

The most politically feasible method of administration also would be similar to the present system. It would retain much of the current structure and would rely on commercial health insurers, Blue Cross/Blue Shield plans, and the other customary entities of our health system. Under any funding mechanism, employees and the unemployed could receive vouchers or credits for health insurance. They could use these vouchers to purchase health insurance from a commercial insurer, Blue Cross/Blue Shield plan, or an HMO. Employees could elect the plan that best suits their needs and wants, such as opting for higher copayments to have a freedom-of-choice plan.

To eliminate the incentives for discrimination, the method of underwriting would have to be dramatically different. Individual losses could not be assigned directly or indirectly to a particular employer. Accordingly, self insurance would have to be prohibited, as would the experience rating of employers. There would be no individual underwriting. One way of removing unfairness from insurers would be to pool all losses of all insurers within the state. Thus, each state would have a statewide risk pool.[25] In this way, an individual who used health care would not be a direct cost to the employer or the insurer. It is an open question whether, under such a system, states could continue to mandate that certain provisions be contained in health insurance policies, such as alcohol and drug abuse treatment, psychiatric services, and prenatal care.

The new health insurance system also will need to confront the difficult problem of cost containment. An increased demand for health services may have an inflationary effect.[26] Providing access while discouraging over-utilization will be difficult. Waste, fraud, and abuse must be carefully controlled. Moreover, with an aging population requiring more medical care per capita and the development of increasingly expensive medical technology, limitations on access to certain medical procedures (e.g., organ transplants, hip replacements) may be necessary.[27] Revising the basic system will not eliminate these difficult health allocation choices and indeed may call greater attention to them.

In 1965 when Medicare and Medicaid were enacted "[w]e arrived at a social contract that if the government would take care of the old and the poor, the private sector would take care of the working."[28] Obviously, the contract has been breached by government as well as some segments of business and is being renegotiated. Under the new contract, the lines between public and private sector responsibilities may be less clearly drawn. It is time to consider the characteristics and consequences of new proposals for cooperative public-private national health insurance systems.

Some Final Thoughts

A silver lining to the dark cloud of drug testing and HIV testing in employment may be that they have alerted the public to the importance and omnipresence of workplace medical screening. Some forms of medical screening, such as back x-rays and psychological screening, have been used for years. Other forms of medical screening, such as genetic testing or using lifestyle in health risk appraisals, are newly emerging. For employees, all types of medical screening raise concerns about privacy, confidentiality, autonomy, and nondiscrimination.

The laws regulating medical screening, to the extent they exist at all, reflect a collection of well-meaning but inconsistent policies. Separate laws, agencies, procedures, and remedies apply to working conditions, benefits, discrimination, and health insurance. In practice, the laws have tended to encourage medical screening, despite economic, ethical, and social considerations that send clear warning signals. If restraint in implementing medical screening is needed, the restraint surely will not come from science, which will not stop to wait while policy makers ponder legal and policy issues. The challenge is to use science wisely—carefully anticipating new technology and planning our responses to emerging discoveries. If we fail to appreciate the consequences of new scientific developments, they will inevitably overwhelm us.

Finally, universal health insurance may soon be a reality in the United States. If, as has been shown, changes in workplace medical screening affect health insurance and health policy, then changes in health policy and health insurance will affect workplace medical screening. Health policies should not be adopted if they will provide irresistible economic pressures for employers to engage in needless and deleterious medical screening to control employee health costs.

Notes

Chapter 1

1. D. Walsh, Corporate Physicians 39 (1987).
2. Bureau of National Affairs, Recruiting and Selection Procedures 17 (1988).
3. Ricklefs, *Pre-Hiring Physicals Are Gaining at Small, Cost-Conscious Firms*, Wall St. J., Jan. 3, 1989, at B2, col. 3.
4. Chapman, *The Ruckus Over Medical Testing*, Fortune, Aug. 19, 1985, at 57, 58.
5. Fowler, *Drug Testing Common for Job Seekers*, N.Y. Times, Jan. 19, 1988, at 47, col. 1.
6. Allstate Insurance Co./Fortune Magazine Survey (Jan. 1988).
7. Bureau of National Affairs, Inc., Basic Patterns in Union Contracts 127 (11th ed. 1986).
8. U.S. Chamber of Commerce, Employee Benefits 1986 (1988).
9. A. Foster Higgins & Co., Foster Higgins Health Care Benefits Survey 1987, at 7 (1987).
10. *See, e.g.*, J. Califano, America's Health Care Revolution: Who Lives? Who Dies? Who Pays? 11–35 (1986) (describing efforts to contain costs by Chrysler, Johnson & Johnson, and other companies).
11. A. Foster Higgins & Co., Foster Higgins Health Care Benefits Survey 1988, at 12–13 (1988).
12. Ricklefs, *supra* note 3.
13. Himmelstein & Pransky, *Preface* (to *Symposium on Worker Fitness and Risk Evaluations*), 3 Occup. Med.: State of the Art Revs. ix (1988).
14. D. Walsh, *supra* note 1, at 140.
15. Block, *How Will We Be Remembered?*, 29 J. Occup. Med. 605, 606 (1987) (citing American Board of Medical Specialties Record, 1985).
16. Kirchner, *1995: Which Specialties Will Prosper?*, 1 Med. Econ. 5, 8 (Review Series 1985).
17. Crowley & Etzel, *Graduate Medical Education in the United States*, 260 J.A.M.A. 1093, 1094 (1988).
18. American Occupational Medical Association, personal communication, May 16, 1988.
19. OSHA Access to Exposure and Medical Records Standard, Preamble, 45 Fed. Reg. 35,223 (1980) (citing testimony of Dr. Alan A. McLean of AOMA).
20. American Board of Preventive Medicine, personal communication, May 16, 1988.
21. Zoloth, Michaels, Lacher, et al., *Asbestos Disease Screening by Non-Specialists: Results of an Evaluation*, 76 Am. J. Pub. Health 1392, 1394 (1986).
22. *See* Ilka, *Necessity and Adequacy of the American Occupational Medical Association Code of Ethics*, 1 Seminars in Occup. Med. 59, 60 (1986).
23. National Academy of Sciences, Role of the Primary Care Physician in Occupational and Environmental Medicine 3 (1988).

24. Levy, *The Teaching of Occupational Health in United States Medical Schools: Five Year Follow-up of an Initial Survey*, 75 Am. J. Pub. Health 75, 79–80 (1985).

25. 45 Fed. Reg. 35,212 (1980), *codified at* 29 C.F.R. §1910.20 (1988).

26. For a further discussion, see M. Rothstein, Occupational Safety and Health Law §193 (2d ed. 1983 and 1988 Supp.).

27. H.R. 162, S. 79, 100th Cong., 1st Sess. (1988).

28. For a further discussion, see M. Rothstein, Medical Screening of Workers 4–8 (1984).

29. Himmelstein, *Worker Fitness and Risk Evaluation in Context*, 3 Occup. Med.: State of the Art Revs. 169, 170 (1988).

30. Weinstein, *The Dilemma of Medical Privacy in the Work Place*, 8 Am. Coll. of Physicians Observer No. 7 (July/Aug. 1988), at 1, 16.

31. *See* Rothstein, *Legal Issues in the Medical Assessment of Physical Impairment by Third-Party Physicians*, 5 J. Legal Med. 503 (1984).

32. *See, e.g., Keene v. Wiggins*, 69 Cal. App. 3d 308, 138 Cal. Rptr. 3 (1977); *Rogers v. Horvath*, 65 Mich. App. 644, 237 N.W.2d 595 (1975); *Johnston v. Sibley*, 558 S.W.2d 135 (Tex. Civ. App. 1977).

33. *See, e.g., Lotspeich v. Chance Vought Aircraft*, 369 S.W.2d 705 (Tex. Civ. App. 1963). *See also Peace v. Weisman*, 186 Ga. App. 697, 368 S.E.2d 319 (1988) (using both "treatment" and "benefit" theories).

34. *Brown v. United States*, 419 F.2d 337, 341 (8th Cir. 1969).

35. *Baker v. Story*, 621 S.W.2d 639 (Tex. Civ. App. 1981).

36. *LoDico v. Caputi*, 129 A.D.2d 361, 517 N.Y.S.2d 640 (App. Div. 1987); *Lotspeich v. Chance Vought Aircraft*, 369 S.W.2d 705 (Tex. Civ. App. 1963).

37. *Beadling v. Sirotta*, 41 N.J. 555, 197 A.2d 857, 860 (1964).

38. *Hoover v. Williamson*, 236 Md. 250, 203 A.2d 861 (1964).

39. Brown, Krieder & Lange, *Guidelines for Employee Health Services in Hospitals, Clinics and Medical Research Institutions*, 25 J. Occup. Med. 771 (1983).

40. *See Peace v. Weisman*, 186 Ga. App. 697, 700–03, 368 S.E.2d 319, 322–25 (1988) (dissenting opinions).

41. Derr, *Ethical Considerations in Fitness and Risk Evaluations*, 3 Occup. Med.: State of the Art Revs. 193, 207 (1988).

42. American Occupational Medical Association, Code of Ethical Conduct for Physicians Providing Occupational Medical Services, Principle 6 (1976).

43. Ilka, *Necessity and Adequacy of the American Occupational Medical Association Code of Ethics*, 1 Seminars in Occup. Med. 59, 62 (1986). *Accord*, Deubner, *Ethics*, 2 Seminars in Occup. Med. 177, 180 (1987). *See also* Watterson, *Occupational Medicine and Medical Ethics*, 34 J. Soc'y Occup. Med. 41 (1984).

44. Ratcliffe, Halperin, Frazier, et al., *The Prevalence of Screening in Industry: Report of the National Institute for Occupational Safety and Health National Occupational Hazard Survey*, 28 J. Occup. Med. 906, 907 (1986).

45. *Id.* at 909.

46. *Id.* at 910.

47. Goldman, *General Occupational Health History and Examination*, 28 J. Occup. Med. 967, 970 (1986).

48. Weinstein, *supra* note 30.

49. Lappe', *Ethical Concerns in Occupational Screening Programs*, 28 J. Occup. Med. 930, 933 (1986).

50. *See* Joseph & Rachlin, *Use and Effectiveness of Chest Radiography and Low-Back Radiography in Screening*, 28 J. Occup. Med. 998 (1986); *Chest X-Ray Examinations in Occupational Medicine*, 25 J. Occup. Med. 773 (1983).

51. *See* Himmelstein & Anderson, *Low Back Pain: Risk Evaluation and Preplacement Screening*, 3 Occup. Med.: State of the Art Revs. 255 (1988).

52. *See* Robbins, *Psychiatric Conditions in Worker Fitness and Risk Evaluation*, 3 Occup. Med.: State of the Art Revs. 309 (1988).

53. Hanks, *The Physical Examination in Industry: A Critique*, 5 Archives Envtl. Health 365, 370 (1962).

54. *See, e.g.*, Rothstein, *Medical Screening and Employment Law: A Note of Caution and Some Observations*, 1988 U. Chi. Legal F. 1.

55. Office of Technology Assessment, United States Congress, Medical Testing and Health Insurance 60 (1988).

56. American Occupational Medical Association, Code of Ethical Conduct for Physicians Providing Occupational Medical Services, Principle 7 (1976).

57. D. Walsh, *supra* note 1, at 147.

58. *See* Ilka, *supra* note 43, at 62.

59. *See* D. Walsh, *supra* note 1, at 147.

60. Mass. Gen. Laws Ann. ch. 149, §19A (West 1982).

61. 29 C.F.R. §1910.20 (1988).

62. *See* Rothstein, *supra* note 31.

63. 27 Ohio App. 3d 222, 500 N.E.2d 370 (1985).

64. *See also* Bratt v. *IBM*, 392 Mass. 508, 467 N.E.2d 126 (1984) (mental disorder); *Cronan v. New England Tel. Co.*, 41 FEP Cases 1273 (Mass. Super. Ct. 1986) (AIDS); *Houston Belt & Terminal Ry. v. Wherry*, 548 S.W.2d 743 (Tex Civ. App. 1976), *appeal dismissed*, 434 U.S. 962 (1978) (drug usage).

65. 715 P.2d 74 (Okla. 1986).

66. Cal. Civ. Code §§56 to 56.37 (West Supp. 1988).

67. *See, e.g.*, Vt. Stat. Ann. tit. 21, §516 (Supp. 1987).

68. Neb. Legis. Bill No. 582 (Jan. 29, 1988).

Chapter 2

1. American Medical Association, Guides to the Evaluation of Permanent Impairment vii (2d ed. 1984).

2. Goldman, *General Occupational Health History and Examination*, 28 J. Occup. Med. 967, 969 (1986).

3. *Id.*

4. *Id.* at 968.

5. *Id.*

6. Schilling, *The Role of Medical Examination in Protecting Worker Health*, 28 J. Occup. Med. 553, 554-55 (1986).

7. *See* Frank, *The Occupational History and Examination*, in Environmental and Occupational Medicine 21, 22–25 (W. Rom ed. 1983).

8. Freudenheim, *Debate Widens Over Expanding Use and Growing Cost of Medical Tests*, N.Y. Times, May 30, 1987, at 9 col. 1 (estimate of National Blue Cross and Blue Shield Association).

9. *Id.*
10. *Doctors' Fee Schedules Tied to Ordering of Medical Tests*, N.Y. Times, Apr. 24, 1986, at A14 (citing 1986 study by Harvard School of Public Health).
11. *See* Pinckney & Pinckney, *Unnecessary Measures*, The Sciences, Jan./Feb. 1989, at 21.
12. Griner & Glaser, *Misuse of Laboratory Tests and Diagnostic Procedures*, 307 New Eng. J. Med. 1336 (1982).
13. R. Galen & S. Gambino, Beyond Normality: The Predictive Value and Efficiency of Medical Diagnoses 3 (1975).
14. Bogdanich, *The Pap Test Misses Much Cervical Cancer Through Labs' Errors*, Wall St. J., Nov. 2, 1987, at 1, col. 6, 16, col. 1.
15. Spletter, *13 Common Medical Tests Yield Mixed Results*, Hippocrates, May/June 1987, at 86.
16. Clinical Laboratory Improvement Amendments of 1988, H. Rep. 100-899, 100th Cong., 2d Sess., at 10 (1988).
17. Pinckney & Pinckney, *supra* note 11, at 22.
18. *Medical Tests Put to Music*, Wall St. J., June 17, 1987, at 25, col. 3.
19. Bogdanich, *Medical Labs, Trusted as Largely Error-Free, Are Far From Infallible*, Wall St. J., Feb. 2, 1987, at 7, col. 1.
20. H. Rep. 100-899, *supra* note 16, at 11.
21. Pub. L. 100-578, 102 Stat. 2903 (1988), *amending* 42 U.S.C. §263a (1988).
22. Finn, Valenstein & Burke, *Alteration of Physicians' Orders by Nonphysicians*, 259 J.A.M.A. 2549, 2550 (1988).
23. 856 F.2d 467 (2d Cir. 1988).
24. *Mental Stress: "Occupational Injury" of 80s That Even Pilots Can't Rise Above*, 259 J.A.M.A. 3097 (1988).
25. *See* A. Foster Higgins & Co., Inc., Foster Higgins Health Care Benefits Survey, 1987, at 19 (1987).
26. Tsai, Bernacki & Reedy, *Mental Health Care Utilization and Costs in a Corporate Setting*, 29 J. Occup. Med. 812 (1987).
27. *Id.*
28. Weybrew, *Psychologic Screening of Job Applicants*, 1 Seminars in Occup. Med. 141, 144 (1986).
29. *See* Robbins, *Psychiatric Conditions in Worker Fitness and Risk Evaluation*, 3 Occup. Med.: State of the Art Revs. 309, 312–13 (1988).
30. 49 Fed. Reg. 30,726 (1984) (proposing to add 10 C.F.R. §73.56).
31. Personal communication, June 22, 1988.
32. *Handwriting Analysis*, 37 BNA Bull. to Management No. 19 (May 8, 1986).
33. *Id.*
34. Robbins, *supra* note 29, at 314 (citing Sandra Hurd).
35. Office of Technology Assessment, United States Congress, Scientific Validity of Polygraph Testing 8 (1983).
36. *Id.* at 41.
37. Robbins, *supra* note 29, at 314.
38. 29 U.S.C. §§2001–2009 (1988).
39. *See* Polygraph Protection Act of 1985: Hearing on S. 1815 Before the Senate Comm. on Labor and Human Resources, 99th Cong., 2d Sess. 1 (1986) (opening statement of Sen. Hatch).

40. *See* D. Lykken, A Tremor in the Blood 1–4 (1981).
41. *See* Note, *Lie Detectors in the Workplace: The Need for Civil Actions Against Employers*, 101 Harv. L. Rev. 806, 811-12 (1988).
42. D. Lykken, *supra* note 40, at 199.
43. Gorman, *Honestly, Can We Trust You?*, Time, Jan. 23, 1989, at 44.
44. *See, e.g..*, *State v. Century Camera, Inc.*, 309 N.W. 2d 735 (Minn. 1981). *See generally* Decker, *Honesty Tests—A New Form of Polygraph?*, 4 Hofstra Lab. L.J. 141 (1986).
45. Or. Rev. Stat. §659.330(2) (Supp. 1987); W. Va. Code Ann. §21-3-17 (Michie 1985).
46. For a further discussion of these and related questions, see Rothstein, *Substantive and Procedural Obstacles to OSHA Rulemaking: Reproductive Hazards as an Example*, 12 B.C. Envtl. Affairs L. Rev. 627 (1985).
47. *Phelps Dodge Corp.*, 11 OSHC 1441, 1983 OSHD para. 26,552 (1983), *aff'd*, 725 F.2d 1237 (9th Cir. 1984).
48. 30 U.S.C. §§801–962 (1982).
49. *Id.* §843(a).
50. 49 C.F.R. §§391.41 to −.49 (1987). The Act provides that the initial x-ray should be taken as soon as possible after commencement of employment. The implementing regulations add that in no event may this be later than six months after commencement. 42 C.F.R. §37.3(b)(1) (1987).
51. *Id.* §391.43.
52. 14 C.F.R. §§67.1 to −.31 (1988).
53. Ill. Ann. Stat. ch. 122, §24-5 (West Supp. 1988); Ind. Admin. Code 410, §2-12; S.D. Codified Laws Ann. §§13-43-3, 13-43-3.1 (Supp. 1988); Wis. Stat. Ann. §143.16 (West 1974 & Supp. 1987).
54. Ind. Code Ann. §20-9.1-3-2 (Burns 1985); Iowa Code Ann. §321.375 (West 1985); Mich. Comp. Laws Ann. §257.316a (West 1977 & Supp. 1988); Tenn. Code Ann. §49-6-2108 (Michie 1983).
55. Ind. Code Ann. §16-1-22-16 (Burns 1983).
56. Iowa Code Ann. §189A.6 (West 1987).
57. 838 F.2d 850 (6th Cir. 1988).
58. 10 C.F.R. §§1046.11 to −.13 (1988).
59. 606 S.W.2d 521 (Tenn. 1980).
60. State of California and San Bernardino County, Medical Standards Project (4th ed. 1987).

Chapter 3

1. *Mesothelioma: Has Patient Had Contact With Even Small Amount of Asbestos?*, 257 J.A.M.A. 1569 (1987).
2. Woodard, Friedlander, Lesher, et al., *Outbreak of Hypersensitivity Pneumonitis in an Industrial Setting*, 259 J.A.M.A. 1965 (1988).
3. Ratcliffe, Halperin, Frazier, et al., *The Prevalence of Screening in Industry: Report From the National Institute for Occupational Safety and Health National Occupational Hazard Survey*, 28 J. Occup. Med. 906, 910 (1986).
4. Brownson, Chang, & Davis, *Occupation, Smoking, and Alcohol in the Epidemiology of Bladder Cancer*, 77 Am. J. Pub. Health 1298 (1987).

5. Albrecht & Bryant, *Polymer-Fume Fever Associated With Smoking and Use of a Mold-Release Spray Containing Polytetrafluoroethylene*, 29 J. Occup. Med. 817 (1987).

6. Barone, Peters, Garabrant, et al., *Smoking as a Risk Factor in Noise-Induced Hearing Loss*, 29 J. Occup. Med. 741 (1987).

7. Hertz & Emmett, *Risk Factors for Occupational Hand Injury*, 28 J. Occup. Med. 36 (1986).

8. *See* Guidotti, *Exposure to Hazard and Individual Risk: When Occupational Medicine Gets Personal*, 30 J. Occup. Med. 570 (1988).

9. *See* L. Speroff, R. Glass, & N. Kase, Clinical Gynecologic Endocrinology & Infertility 467 (3d ed. 1983).

10. Guidelines for Studies of Human Populations Exposed to Mutagenic and Reproductive Hazards 71 (A. Bloom ed. 1981) (450,000 spontaneous abortions per 3,000,000 births); Fabro, *Reproductive Toxicology: State of the Art, 1982*, 4 Am. J. Indus. Med. 391 (1983) (600,000 spontaneous abortions per 3,000,000 births). *Cf.* Carr & Gedeon, *Population Cytogenetics of Human Abortuses*, in Population Cytogenetics 1–9 (E. Hook & I. Porter eds. 1977) (as many as 60% of all conceptions end in spontaneous abortion). According to the National Center for Health Statistics, in 1979, 32,969 fetuses died in utero. National Center for Disease Statistics, 2A Vital Statistics of the U.S. (1985), section 3 at 2 (1984) (table 3–1) [hereinafter cited as Vital Statistics].

11. Fabro, *supra* note 10, at 391.

12. U.S. Department of Health and Human Services, Health, United States 248 (1983). "Of all infant deaths, two-thirds occur in those weighing less than 5.5 pounds (2,500 grams) at birth. Infants below this weight are more than 20 times as likely to die within the first year. Low birth weight is sometimes associated with increased occurrence of mental retardation, birth defects, growth and development problems, blindness, autism, cerebral palsy and epilepsy." U.S. Department of Health, Education, and Welfare, Healthy People: The Surgeon General's Report on Health Promotion and Disease Prevention 24 (1979).

13. Fabro, *supra* note 10, at 391.

14. Wilson, *Environmental Effects on Development—Teratology*, in 2 Pathophysiology of Gestation 269–320 (Assali ed. 1972). It has been estimated that 20% of birth defects are caused by known genetic transmission, 5% by chromosomal aberration, and 6–10% by environmental factors (e.g., radiation, infections, maternal metabolic imbalance, and drugs and environmental chemicals.) *Id.*

15. Vital Statistics, *supra* note 10, section 2, at 4 (table 2–4).

16. *See* Wilson, *supra* note 14.

17. Sever, *Reproductive Hazards of the Workplace*, 23 J. Occup. Med. 685, 686 (1981).

18. Messite & Bond, *Reproductive Toxicology and Occupational Exposure*, in Developments in Occupational Medicine 64–69 (C. Zenz ed. 1980). In addition, each year about 1,000 new chemicals are introduced into American industry. For most of the 63,000 chemicals in common use in this country there is little or no information concerning their effects on reproduction. *See* Williams, *Firing the Woman to Protect the Fetus: The Reconciliation of Fetal Protection With Employment Opportunity Goals*

Under Title VII, 69 Geo. L.J. 641, 661 (1981), and authorities cited therein.

19. Office of Technology Assessment, U.S. Congress, Reproductive Health Hazards in the Workplace 37 (1985).

20. *See* Rosenberg, Feldblum & Marshall, *Occupational Influences on Reproduction: A Review of Recent Literature*, 29 J. Occup. Med. 584 (1987).

21. Personal communication, July 3, 1984, quoted in Rothstein, *Substantive and Procedural Obstacles to OSHA Rulemaking: Reproductive Hazards as an Example*, 12 B.C. Envtl. Affairs L. Rev. 627, 650 (1985).

22. For a further discussion, see M. Rothstein, Medical Screening of Workers 62–66 (BNA Books 1984).

23. Warshaw, *Employee Health Services for Women Workers*, 7 Preventive Med. 385, 387 (1978); Welch, *Decisionmaking About Reproductive Hazards*, 1 Seminars in Occup. Med. 97, 99 (1986).

24. Welch, *supra* note 23.

25. Introduction to Proposed Interpretive Guidelines on Employment Discrimination and Reproductive Hazards, 45 Fed. Reg. 7514 (1980), *withdrawn*, 46 Fed. Reg. 3916 (1981).

26. Reid, *Reproductive Health: What Will the Future Hold?*, Occup. Hazards, Apr. 1988, at 45, 46.

27. *See* Lewin, *Companies Found to Ignore Reproductive Risks to Men*, N.Y. Times, Dec. 15, 1988, at 45, col. 1.

28. Stellman, *The Effects of Toxic Agents on Reproduction*, Occup. Health & Safety, Apr. 1979, at 36, 40.

29. W. Ganong, Review of Medical Physiology 359 (13th ed. 1987).

30. Hunt, *Occupational Radiation Exposure of Women Workers*, 7 Preventive Med. 294, 304 (1978).

31. Paul, *Reproductive Fitness and Risk*, 3 Occup. Med.: State of the Art Revs. 323, 336 (1988).

32. 697 F.2d 1172 (4th Cir. 1982).

33. *Id.* at 1190.

34. Cal. Gov't Code §2945.5 (West Supp. 1988).

35. Conn. Pub. Act 81-382 (1982).

36. Equal Employment Opportunity Commission, Policy Guidance on Reproductive and Fetal Hazards (1988).

37. *Hayes v. Shelby Mem. Hosp.*, 726 F.2d 1543, *rehearing denied*, 732 F.2d 944 (11th Cir. 1984); *Zuniga v. Kleberg County Hosp.*, 692 F.2d 986 (5th Cir. 1982).

38. 9 Ill. Hum. Rts. Comm'n Rep. 5 (1983).

39. *Id.* at 21.

40. *See, e.g.*, Meier, *Companies Wrestle With Threats to Workers' Reproductive Health*, Wall St. J., Feb. 5, 1987, at 23, col. 4; Reid, *supra* note 26.

41. *See e.g.*, Special Report, *Reproductive Hazards and the Pregnant Worker: Technology and Work Force Changes Create New Concerns*, 17 Occup. Safety & Health Rep. (BNA) 97 (1987).

42. Trost, *Corporate Prenatal-Care Plans Multiply, Benefiting Both Mothers and Employers*, Wall St. J., June 24, 1988, at 21, col. 3. *See also* Freudenheim, *In Pursuit of the Punctual Baby*, N.Y. Times, Dec. 28, 1988, at 25, col. 3.

43. *See, e.g.*, Hadler, *Occupational Illness: The Issue of Causality*, 26 J. Occup. Med. 587 (1984).
44. Ames, Magaw & Gold, *Ranking Possible Carcinogenic Hazards*, 236 Science 271, 277 (1987).
45. Tierney, *Not to Worry*, Hippocrates, Jan./Feb. 1988, at 29, 34 (remarks of Marvin Legator of the University of Texas Medical Branch in Galveston).
46. *Id.* (remarks of Samuel Epstein of the University of Illinois).
47. *Id.* (remarks of Devra Lee Davis of the National Academy of Sciences).
48. Kerr, *Indoor Radon: The Deadliest Pollutant*, 240 Science 606 (1988).
49. Richards, *New Study Strengthens Suspected Links Between Electromagnetism and Cancer*, Wall St. J., July 16, 1987, at 31, col. 4 (quoting David Carpenter). *See* Modan, *Exposure to Electromagnetic Fields and Brain Malignancy: A Newly Discovered Menace?*, 13 Am. J. Indus. Med. 625 (1988); Speers, Dobbins & Miller, *Occupational Exposures and Brain Cancer Mortality: A Preliminary Study of East Texas Residents*, 13 Am. J. Indus. Med. 629 (1988).
50. Schatzkin, Jones, Hoover, et al., *Alcohol Consumption and Breast Cancer in the Epidemiologic Follow-Up Study of the First National Health and Nutrition Examination Survey*, 316 New Eng. J. Med. 1169 (1987).
51. Gwinn, Webster, Lee, et al., *Alcohol Consumption and Ovarian Cancer Risk*, 123 Am. J. Epidemiology 759 (1986) (heavy drinking).
52. Kolonel, Yoshizawa & Hankin, *Diet and Prostatic Cancer: A Case-Control Study in Hawaii*, 127 Am. J. Epidemiology 999 (1988).
53. Tornberg, Holm, Carstensen, et al., *Risks of Cancer of the Colon and Rectum in Relation to Serum Cholesterol and Beta-Lipoprotein*, 315 New Eng. J. Med. 1629 (1986).
54. Claude, Kunze, Frentzel-Beyme, et al., *Life-Style and Occupational Risk Factors in Cancer of the Lower Urinary Tract*, 124 Am. J. Epidemiology 578 (1986).
55. Cantor, Blair, Everett, et al., *Hair Dye Use and Risk of Leukemia and Lymphoma*, 78 Am. J. Pub. Health 570 (1988).
56. Miller, Silverman, Hoover, et al., *Cancer Risk Among Artistic Painters*, 9 Am. J. Indus. Med. 281 (1986).
57. Dubrow, *Malignant Melanoma in the Printing Industry*, 10 Am. J. Indus. Med. 119 (1986).
58. Milham, *Increased Mortality in Amateur Radio Operators Due to Lymphatic and Hematopoietic Malignancies*, 127 Am. J. Epidemiology 50 (1988).
59. Hodgson & Parkinson, *Respiratory Disease in a Photographer*, 9 Am. J. Indus. Med. 349 (1986).
60. Goldsmith, *Paler is Better, Say Skin Cancer Fighters*, 257 J.A.M.A. 893 (1987).
61. E. Calabrese, Ecogenetics: Genetic Variation in Susceptibility to Environmental Agents 288–90 (1984).
62. U.S. Department of Health, Education, & Welfare, Healthy People—The Surgeon General's Report on Health Promotion and Disease Prevention 121 (1979). *See also Smoking-Attributable Mortality and Years of Potential Life Lost—United States, 1984*, 36 Morbidity & Mortality Weekly Rep. 693 (1987).

63. Committee on Passive Smoking, National Research Council, National Academy of Sciences, Environmental Tobacco Smoke: Measuring Exposures & Assessing Health Effects 250, 257 (1986) [hereinafter Environmental Tobacco Smoke].

64. Staff Memo of Office of Technology Assessment, U.S. Congress, Smoking-Related Deaths and Financial Costs 32 (1985) [hereinafter Financial Costs].

65. Staff Paper of Office of Technology Assessment, U.S. Congress, Passive Smoking in the Workplace: Selected Issues 15 (1986) [hereinafter Passive Smoking].

66. Berke, *Surgeon General Raises Estimate of Smoking Toll*, N.Y. Times, Jan. 11, 1989, at 11, col. 1.

67. Warner, *Health and Economic Implications of a Tobacco-Free Society*, 258 J.A.M.A. 2080 (1987).

68. Bureau of National Affairs, Where There's Smoke: Problems and Policies Concerning Smoking in the Workplace 7 (2d ed. 1987) (citing 1985 Report of the Surgeon General) [hereinafter Where There's Smoke].

69. Texas Heart Institute, *Cardiovascular Disease Cause and Prevention*, THI Today 12 (Winter 1987) [hereinafter *Cardiovascular Disease*].

70. *Id. See also* Environmental Tobacco Smoke, *supra* note 63, at 262.

71. Financial Costs, *supra* note 64, at 1–3, 43.

72. *Id.* at 43.

73. Environmental Tobacco Smoke, *supra* note 63, at 269; Financial Costs, *supra* note 64, at 43.

74. Council on Scientific Affairs, American Medical Association, *A Physician's Guide to Asbestos-Related Diseases*, 252 J.A.M.A. 2593, 2596 (1984).

75. Passive Smoking, *supra* note 65, at 15–16.

76. Advisory Committee to the Surgeon General, U.S. Department of Health and Human Services, The Health Consequences of Using Smokeless Tobacco (1986); Council on Scientific Affairs, American Medical Association, *Health Effects of Smokeless Tobacco*, 255 J.A.M.A. 1038 (1986).

77. Where There's Smoke, *supra* note 68, at 8.

78. Environmental Tobacco Smoke, *supra* note 63, at 2, 45.

79. *Id.* at 2; Passive Smoking, *supra* note 65, at 9, 16.

80. Passive Smoking, *supra* note 65, at 16. *See* Fielding & Phenow, *Health Effects of Involuntary Smoking*, 319 New Eng. J. Med. 1452 (1988).

81. Passive Smoking, *supra* note 65, at 28; Environmental Tobacco Smoke, *supra* note 63, at 8, 172–77.

82. Environmental Tobacco Smoke, *supra* note 63, at 8.

83. Where There's Smoke, *supra* note 68, at 8. *See also* Environmental Tobacco Smoke, *supra* note 63, at 176–77.

84. Environmental Tobacco Smoke, *supra* note 63, at 8.

85. Among the states are the following: Arizona, Connecticut, Florida, Maine, Minnesota, Montana, Nebraska, New Hampshire, New Jersey, Rhode Island, Utah, Vermont, and Wisconsin. Among the cities are the following: Chicago, Cincinnati, Houston, Los Angeles, New York, Philadelphia, and San Francisco.

86. Where There's Smoke, *supra* note 68, at 17.

87. *See, e.g.*, Reibstein, *Forced to Consider Smoking Issue, Firms Produce Disparate Policies*, Wall St. J., Feb. 10, 1987, at 41, col. 4.

88. Where There's Smoke, *supra* note 68, at 17.

89. Where There's Smoke, *supra* note 68, at 7.
90. Environmental Tobacco Smoke, *supra* note 63, at 10, 107, 186–87, 188–89, 202–03, 216, 272–76; Passive Smoking, *supra* note 65, at 23, 30; Humble, Samet & Pathak, *Marriage to a Smoker and Lung Cancer Risk*, 77 Am. J. Pub. Health 598 (1987).
91. Where There's Smoke, *supra* note 68, at App. G-5 (based on survey in R. Carlson, Toward A Smokefree Workplace (2d ed.), published by Group Against Smoking Pollution, Summit, N.J.). It is not clear how many of these companies that refuse to hire smokers will discharge current employees who refuse to stop smoking.
92. *Id.*
93. Blackwell, French & Stein, *Adverse Health Effects of Smoking and the Occupational Environment*, NIOSH Current Intelligence Bull. No. 31, 40 Am. Indus. Hygiene A.J. A38 (1979), cited in Omenn, *Predictive Identification of Hypersusceptible Individuals*, 24 J. Occup. Med. 369, 373 (1982); Blackwood, *Health Risks of Smoking Increased by Exposure to Workplace Chemicals*, Occup. Health & Safety, Feb. 1985, at 23.
94. Where There's Smoke, *supra* note 68, at App. G-5.
95. *See Concern Warns It Will Dismiss All Who Smoke*, N.Y. Times, Jan. 21, 1987, at A16, col. 1 (city ed.); *Employees of USG Unit Are Told to Stop Smoking*, Wall St. J., Jan. 21, 1987, at 4, col. 3. *Cf. Manufacturer Now Says Smoking Won't Mean Automatic Dismissal*, N.Y. Times, Jan. 29, 1987, at B7, col. 1 (city ed.).
96. Brown, McCarthy, Marcus, et al., *Workplace Smoking Policies: Attitudes of Union Members in a High-risk Industry*, 30 J. Occup. Med. 312 (1988).
97. Some of the laws also include police officers and other public employees. Ala. Code §§11-43-144(b) and (c); §36-30-20, §36-30-23 (1977 & Supp. 1988) (firefighters, police); Cal. Lab. Code §§3212, 3212.2, 3212.5 (West Supp. 1987) (police, sheriff's office, district attorney's staff of inspectors or investigators, firefighters, game wardens, corrections employees, state hospital security, youth authority); Conn. Gen. Stat. Ann. §§5-145a, 7-433a (West 1972 & Supp. 1988) (police, firefighters, security personnel at universities, aeronautics employees, corrections officers); Fla. Stat. Ann. §§112.18, 185.34 (West 1987) (police, firefighters); Ga. Code Ann. §47-7-102 (1986) (firefighters); Hawaii Rev. Stat. §88-77(b) (1985 & Supp. 1987) (police, firefighters, sewer workers); Ill. Rev. Stat. ch. 108 1/2, paras. 5-154.1, 6-151.1 (West 1987) (police, firefighters); La. Rev. Stat. Ann. §33.2581 (West 1988) (firefighters); Md. Gen. Prov. Code Ann. art. 101, §§64A(a)(1) and (2) (1985 & Supp. 1988) (police, firefighters); Mass. Gen. Laws Ann. ch. 32, §94 (West 1983 & Supp. 1988) (police, firefighters, corrections officers, crash crews at Logan Airport); Mich. Comp. Laws Ann. §418.405 (West 1985 & Supp. 1988) (police, firefighters); Minn. Stat. Ann. §176.011.15 (West 1987) (police, firefighters, conservation officers, department of natural resources forest officers); Mo. Ann. Stat. §87.005 (Vernon 1971 & Supp. 1988) (firefighters); Neb. Rev. Stat. §18.1723 (1987) (police, firefighters); N.H. Rev. Stat. Ann. §281:2 (V-a) (1987) (firefighters); N.J. Rev. Stat. Ann. §34:15-43.2 (West Supp. 1988) (firefighters); N.Y. Gen. Mun. Law §207-k (McKinney 1986 & Supp. 1988) (police, firefighters); N.D. Cent. Code §65-01-02(12)(d) (1985) (police, firefighters); Ohio Rev. Code Ann. §742.37(c)(4) (Page Supp. 1985) (police, firefighters); Okla. Stat.

Ann. tit. 11, §49-110 (West 1978 & Supp. 1988) (firefighters); Ore. Rev. Stat. §§656.802(1) and (2) (1985) (firefighters); S.C. Code Ann. §42-11-30 (Law. Co-op. 1985) (firefighters); Tenn. Code Ann. §§7-51-201(a)(1) and (b)(1) (Supp. 1988) (law enforcement officials, firefighters); Tex. Civ. Stat. Ann. §6243e-3 (Vernon Supp. 1988) (firefighters); Vt. Stat. Ann. tit. 21, §601 (11)(c) and (e) (1987 & Supp. 1988) (police, firefighters); Va. Code Ann. §65.1-47.1 (Supp. 1987 & Supp. 1988) (police, firefighters); Wis. Stat. Ann. §891.45 (West Supp. 1987) (firefighters).

98. Gold, *One State Says No Smoking for Police and Fire Depts.*, N.Y. Times, Oct. 2, 1988, at 14, col. 1.

99. Where There's Smoke, *supra* note 68, at App. G-2, G-3, G-4, G-5.

100. *Ralston Purina Calls It Quits for Smoking Employees at All Sites*, 6 Empl. Rel. Weekly (BNA) 847 (1988).

101. See Barrus, *Smokers', Nonsmokers' Rights Collide in the Work Environment*, Occup. Health & Safety, Feb. 1985, at 31; Malcolm, *Mounting Drive on Smoking Stirs Tensions in Workplace*, N.Y. Times, Feb. 20, 1987, at A1, col. 1.

102. Health Insurance Association of America, Survey of Health Promotion Insurance Underwriting Practices (1986).

103. *Non-Smoking Discount Offered*, Am. Med. News, Jan. 16, 1984, at 29 (Blue Cross and Blue Shield of Minn., individual policy).

104. Kristein, *How Much Can Business Expect to Profit From Smoking Cessation?*, 12 Preventive Med. 358, 361 (1983).

105. *See generally*, Hendrix & Taylor, A *Multivariate Analysis of the Relationship Between Cigarette Smoking and Absence From Work*, 1 Am. J. Health Promotion, Fall 1987, at 5; Van Tuinen & Land, *Smoking and Excess Sick Leave in a Department of Health*, 28 J. Occup. Med. 33 (1986).

106. Kristein, *supra* note 104.

107. *See* Rothstein, *Refusing to Employ Smokers: Good Public Health or Bad Public Policy?*, 62 Notre Dame L. Rev. 940 (1987).

108. 816 F.2d 539 (10th Cir. 1987).

109. The basis for this requirement is to maintain a healthy work force and to reduce workers' compensation costs. Telephone interview with Diane Davis Huckins, Assistant Municipal Counselor for City of Oklahoma City, Jan. 26, 1987. It is not clear why the Oklahoma City restriction applied only to the first year of employment.

110. *See* Weiss, *Watch Out: Urine Trouble*, Harper's, June, 1986, at 56.

111. 'No Smoking' Sweeps America, Bus. Week, July 27, 1987, at 40, 42.

112. Certain components of cigarette smoke and their metabolites are measureable in the blood, urine, and saliva of smokers. The most tobacco-specific substance for which commercial tests are available is cotinine, the primary metabolite of nicotine. Cotinine, which has a half-life of 20 to 30 hours, appears in elevated levels from continued exposure, and its presence correlates with changes in smoking habits and with the nicotine content in the cigarettes smoked. A urinalysis for cotinine using gas chromotography costs around $25 and appears to be the most popular technique. Other methods are thin layer chromotography and radioimmunoassay techniques. *See generally* Environmental Tobacco Smoke, *supra* note 63, at §137–45; Passive Smoking, *supra* note 65, at §12–14;

Haley & Hoffmann, *Analysis for Nicotine and Cotinine in Hair to Determine Cigarette Smoker Status*, 31 Clinical Chem. 1598 (1985); Jarvis, Tunstall-Pedoe, Feyerabend, et al., *Comparison of Tests Used to Distinguish Smokers From Nonsmokers*, 77 Am. J. Pub. Health 1435 (1987); Matsukura, et al., *Effects of Environmental Tobacco Smoke on Urinary Cotinine Excretion in Nonsmokers*, 311 New Eng. J. Med. 828 (1984).

113. *Pre-Job Urinalysis Used to Screen Out Smokers, Expert Says*, Houston Chronicle, Aug. 29, 1986, at 15, col. 1.

114. Fenton, Schaffer, Chen, et al., *A Comparison of Enzyme Emmunoassay and Gas Chromatography/Mass Spectrometry in Forensic Toxicology*, 25 J. Forensic Sci. 314 (1980).

115. False positive rates vary based on the substance tested for and the test procedure used. The EMIT test false positive rates are: cocaine–10%; opiates–5.6%; barbiturates–5.1%; amphetamines–12.5%; and marijuana–19%. *Id.* The average is about 10%, for a specificity of 90%.

116. About 5% to 10% of applicants at major corporations test positively for one or more drugs. The prevalence for any single substance may well be lower than the assumed 5%. A lower prevalence would result in an even lower predictive value (positive). For example, with a 1% prevalence, the predictive value (positive) of an unconfirmed EMIT test would be 9%.

117. Office of Technology Assessment, U.S. Congress, Scientific Validity of Polygraph Testing 97 (1983). These figures vary widely depending on the type of study, questioning techniques, examiner, and subject.

118. *Id.* at 98–99.

119. *Id.*

120. R. Galen & S. Gambino, Beyond Normality: The Predictive Value and Efficiency of Medical Diagnosis 18 (1975).

121. *Chest X-Ray Examinations in Occupational Medicine*, 25 J. Occup. Med. 773 (1983).

122. *See* Halperin, Ratcliffe, Frazier, et al., *Medical Screening in the Workplace: Proposed Principles*, 28 J. Occup. Med. 547, 550 (1986).

Chapter 4

1. Schulte, *Simultaneous Assessment of Genetic and Occupational Risk Factors*, 29 J. Occup. Med. 884, 889 (1987), *citing* Chetwynd, *Toxic Jaundice in Munition Workers*, 10 Proc. Royal Soc'y Med. 6 (1917).

2. J.B.S. Haldane, Heredity and Politics 179–80 (1938).

3. E. Calabrese, Ecogenetics: Genetic Variation in Susceptibility to Environmental Agents 6 (1984).

4. Stokinger & Mountain, *Test for Hypersusceptibility to Hemolytic Chemicals*, 6 Archives Envtl. Health 495 (1963).

5. Stokinger & Scheel, *Hypersusceptibility and Genetic Problems in Occupational Medicine—A Consensus Report*, 15 J. Occup. Med. 564 (1973).

6. *Id.* at 572.

7. *Id.*

8. *Id.*

9. Reinhardt, *Chemical Hypersusceptibility*, 20 J. Occup. Med. 319, 320 (1978).

10. Severo, *Genetic Tests by Industry Raise Questions on Rights of Workers*, N.Y. Times, Feb. 3, 1980, at 1; Severo, *Screening of Blacks by Du Pont Sharpens Debate on Gene Tests*, N.Y. Times, Feb. 4, 1980, at 1; Severo, *Dispute Arises Over Dow Studies on Genetic Damage in Workers*, N.Y. Times, Feb. 5, 1980, at 1; Severo, *Federal Mandate for Gene Tests Disturbs U.S. Job Safety Official*, N.Y. Times, Feb. 6, 1980, at 1.

11. Genetic Screening and the Handling of High-Risk Groups in the Workplace: Hearings Before the Subcommittee on Investigations and Oversight, House Committee on Science and Technology, 97th Cong., 1st Sess. (Oct. 14, 15, 1981); Genetic Screening of Workers: Hearings Before the Subcommittee on Investigations and Oversight, House Committee on Science and Technology, 97th Cong., 2d Sess. (June 22, 1982).

12. United States Congress, Office of Technology Assessment, The Role of Genetic Testing in the Prevention of Occupational Disease 33 (1983).

13. *Id.* at 9–10.

14. For a further discussion, see M. Rothstein, Medical Screening of Workers 52–61 (1984).

15. Hunt, *The Total Gene Screen*, N.Y. Times Mag., Jan. 19, 1986, at 33, 56; Zoler, *Genetic Tests Creating a Deluge of Dilemmas*, Med. World News, Sept. 22, 1986, at 34, 52.

16. Bureau of National Affairs, Recruiting and Selection Procedures 17 (1988) (Table 7).

17. *See* Gusella, Wexler, Conneally, et al., *A Polymorphic DNA Marker Genetically Linked to Huntington's Disease*, 306 Nature 234 (1983).

18. Much of this discussion has been adapted from Office of Technology Assessment, U.S. Congress, Tests for Human Genetic Disorders ch. 3 (1987).

19. Meissen, Myers, Mastromauro, et al., *Predictive Testing for Huntington's Disease with Use of a Linked DNA Marker*, 318 New Eng. J. Med. 535 (1988).

20. Barnes, *Defect in Alzheimer's Is on Chromosome 21*, 235 Science 846 (1987).

21. Wiggs, Janey, Nordenskjold, et al., *Prediction of the Risk of Hereditary Retinoblastoma Using DNA Polymorphisms Within the Retinoblastoma Gene*, 318 New Eng. J. Med. 151 (1988).

22. Brown & Goldstein, *A Receptor-Mediated Pathway for Cholesterol Homeostasis*, 232 Science 34 (1986).

23. Reeders, Breuning, Davies, et al., *A Highly Polymorphic DNA Marker Linked to Adult Polycystic Kidney Disease on Chromosome 16*, 317 Nature 542 (1985); Romeo, Devoto, Costa, et al., *A Second Genetic Locus for Autosomal Dominant Polycystic Kidney Disease*, 2 Lancet 8 (1988).

24. Caskey, *Disease Diagnosis by Recombinant DNA Methods*, 236 Science 1223 (1987).

25. Monaco, Neve, Colletti-Fenner, et al., *Isolation of Candidate cDNA for Portions of the Duchenne Muscular Dystrophy Gene*, 323 Nature 646 (1986).

26. Estivill, Farrall, Scambler, et al., *A Candidate for the Cystic Fibrosis Locus Isolated by Selection for Methylation-Free Islands*, 326 Nature 840 (1987).

27. Wertelecki, Rouleau, Superneau, et al., *Neurofibromatosis 2: Clinical and DNA Linkage Studies of a Large Kindred*, 319 New Eng. J. Med. 278 (1988).

28. Mendlewicz, Simon, Sevy, et al., *Polymorphic DNA Marker on X Chromosome and Manic Depression*, 1 Lancet 1230 (1987).

29. Merz, *With Current Gene Markers, Presymptomatic Diagnosis of Heritable Diseases Is Still a Family Affair*, 258 J.A.M.A. 1132 (1987).

30. Hood, *Biotechnology and Medicine of the Future*, 259 J.A.M.A. 1837, 1841 (1988).

31. *New Genetic Linkage Map Is First to Span Entire Human Genome*, Med. World News, Nov. 9, 1987, at 77.

32. *Id.*

33. *See, e.g.*, Boffey, *Rapid Advances Point to the Mapping of All Human Genes*, N.Y. Times, July 15, 1986, at 17, col. 1; Merz, *Mapping the Human Genome Raises Question: Which Road to Take?*, 258 J.A.M.A. 1131 (1987); Roberts, *Academy Backs Genome Project*, 239 Science 725 (1988).

34. Roberts, *supra* note 33, at 726. *See generally* Office of Technology Assessment, U.S. Congress, Mapping Our Genes (1988).

35. Rowley, *Genetic Screening: Marvel or Menace?*, 225 Science 138 (1984).

36. Zoler, *Genetic Testing Projected to Double by Early 1990s*, Med. World News, Apr. 11, 1988, at 58.

37. Zoler, *supra* note 15, at 49–50.

38. Blakeslee, *Genetic Discoveries Raise Painful Questions*, N.Y. Times, Apr. 21, 1987, at 19, col. 5, 23, col. 1.

39. Zoler, *supra* note 15, at 48.

40. Young, *DNA Probes*, 258 J.A.M.A. 2404, 2406 (1987).

41. *The Hereditability of Heart Disease*, 259 J.A.M.A. 3319 (1988), *reprinted from* 10 J.A.M.A. 721 (1888).

42. Kolata, *Genetic Screening Raises Questions for Employers and Insurers*, 232 Science 317, 319 (1986).

43. Fla. Stat. Ann. §448.075 (West 1981).

44. La. Rev. Stat. Ann. §§23:1001 to :1005 (West 1985).

45. N.C. Gen. Stat. §95-28.1 (1985).

46. N.J. Stat. Ann. §10:5-5(x)-(cc) to :5-12 (West 1976 & Supp. 1988).

47. 42 U.S.C. §2000e (1982).

48. Office of Technology Assessment, U.S. Congress, The Role of Genetic Testing in the Prevention of Occupational Disease 124 (1983).

49. Blakeslee, *supra* note 38.

50. Kolata, *supra* note 42.

Chapter 5

1. *See* Gottlieb, Schroff, Schanker, et al., *Pneumocystis Carinii Pneumonia and Mucosal Candidiasis in Previously Healthy Homosexual Men*, 305 New Eng. J. Med. 1425 (1981); Masur, Michelis, Greene, et al., *An Outbreak of Community-Acquired Pneumocystis Carinii Pneumonia: Initial Manifestation of Cellular Immune Dysfunction*, 305 New Eng. J. Med. 1431 (1981).

2. Institute of Medicine, National Academy of Sciences, Confronting AIDS 8 (1986).
3. The discussion of AIDS etiology has been adapted from Green, *The Transmission of AIDS*, in AIDS and the Law (H. Dalton & S. Burris, eds. 1987).
4. *See Revision of the CDC Surveillance Case Definition for Acquired Immunodeficiency Syndrome*, 36 Morbidity & Mortality Weekly Rep. 3S (1987).
5. *See, e.g.*, Fischl, Dickinson, Scott, et al., *Evaluation of Heterosexual Partners, Children, and Household Contacts of Adults With AIDS*, 257 J.A.M.A. 640 (1987); Lifson, *Do Alternate Modes for Transmission of Human Immunodeficiency Virus Exist?*, 259 J.A.M.A. 1353 (1988).
6. *Update: Acquired Immunodeficiency Syndrome—United States*, 35 Morbidity & Mortality Weekly Rep. 757, 758 (1986). *See also* Curran, Jaffe, Hardy, et al., *Epidemiology of HIV Infection and AIDS in the United States*, 239 Science 610 (1988).
7. *See, e.g.*, Board of Trustees, American Medical Association, *Prevention and Control of Acquired Immunodeficiency Syndrome*, 258 J.A.M.A. 2097 (1987).
8. For a discussion of HIV testing, see Rothstein, *Screening Workers for AIDS*, in AIDS and the Law (H. Dalton & S. Burris, eds. 1987).
9. For a technical discussion of how the ELISA test works, see Council on Scientific Affairs, American Medical Association, *Status Report on the Acquired Immunodeficiency Syndrome—Human T-Cell Lymphotropic Virus Type III Testing*, 254 J.A.M.A. 1342 (1985); Schwartz, Dans & Kinosian, *Human Immunodeficiency Virus Test Evaluation, Performance, and Use*, 259 J.A.M.A. 2574 (1988); *Update: Serologic Testing for Antibody to Human Immunodeficiency Virus*, 36 Morbidity & Mortality Weekly Rep. 833 (1988).
10. Levine & Bayer, *Screening Blood: Public Health and Medical Uncertainty*, Hastings Center Rep., Aug. 1985, at 8, 9.
11. *Id.*; Council on Scientific Affairs, *supra* note 9, at 1343; *see Puzzling Western Blot Results Worry Nation's Blood Bankers*, Med. World News, Dec. 22, 1986, at 69.
12. *See* Consortium for Retrovirus Serology Standardization, *Serological Diagnosis of Human Immunodeficiency Virus Infection by Western Blot Testing*, 260 J.A.M.A. 674 (1988).
13. *See Acquired Immunodeficiency Syndrome (AIDS) Update—United States*, 32 Morbidity & Mortality Weekly Rep. 309 (1983) (AIDS diagnosis requires underlying immunodeficiency and presence of unexplained opportunistic infection or Kaposi's sarcoma in patient under 60 years of age); *AIDS Antibody Screening Test*, 57 Analytical Chem. 773A (1985) ("Because the ELISA screening test detects only antibodies to the AIDS virus, it is not a test for AIDS virus and is not intended to diagnose AIDS").
14. Curran, Morgan, Hardy, et al., *The Epidemiology of AIDS: Current Status and Future Prospects*, 229 Science 1352, 1354 (1985); *see also* Marlink, et al., 315 New Eng. J. Med. 1549 (1986) (letter) (low sensitivity of ELISA testing in early HIV infection).
15. Leeson, *HTLV-III Antibody Tests and Health Education*, 1 Lancet 911 (1986).
16. *See, e.g.*, Lester, *Prejudice Toward AIDS Patients Versus Other Terminally Ill Patients* (letter and table), 78 Am. J. Pub. Health 854 (1988). *See*

generally D. Black, The Plague Years (1985); R. Shilts, And the Band Played On (1987).

17. *Summary: Recommendations for Preventing Transmission of Infection With Human T-Lymphotropic Virus Type II/Lymphadenopathy-Associated Virus in the Workplace*, 34 Morbidity & Mortality Weekly Rep. 681 (1985).

18. *State Legislatures Are Cautious in Addressing AIDS Issues, Study Says*, 5 Empl. Rels. Weekly (BNA) 1597 (1987) (citing study by George Washington University's Intergovernmental Health Policy Project).

19. Cal. Health & Safety Code §§199.21(f), −.38 (West Supp. 1988).

20. Del. H.B. 136 (1988).

21. Fla. Stat. §381.606(5) (1986).

22. Iowa Code Ann. §§601A.2 (11), 601A.6(1)(d) (West 1988).

23. Mass. Gen. Laws Ann. ch. 111, §70f (Supp. 1988).

24. R.I. Pub. L. 88-405 (1988).

25. Vermont H. 239 (1988).

26. Wash. Rev. Code §49.60 (1988).

27. Wis. Stat. Ann. §103.15(2)(a), (2)(b), (3) (West Supp. 1988).

28. Tex. Rev. Stat. Ann. art. 4419b-1, §9.02 (1988).

29. Austin Ord. No. 861211-V (Dec. 11, 1986).

30. Los Angeles Code art. 5.8, §§45.80–45.93 (1985).

31. Phila. Exec. Order No. 4-86 (Apr. 15, 1986).

32. San Francisco Police Code §§3801–3816 (1985).

33. 480 U.S. 273 (1987).

34. *Arline v. School Board*, 772 F.2d 759 (11th Cir. 1985).

35. 480 U.S. at 282 n.7.

36. *See generally* Leonard, *AIDS in the Workplace*, in AIDS and the Law (H. Dalton & S. Burris, eds. 1987); Comment, *After School Board of Nassau County v. Arline: Employees With AIDS and the Concerns of the "Worried Well*," 37 Am. U. L. Rev. 867 (1988); Note, *Asymptomatic Infection with the AIDS Virus as a Handicap Under the Rehabilitation Act of 1973*, 88 Colum. L. Rev. 563 (1988).

37. 480 U.S. at 284–285 (footnotes omitted).

38. *See id.* at 287 n. 16.

39. *Id.* at 288.

40. *Arline v. School Board*, 692 F. Supp. 1286 (M.D. Fla. 1988).

41. 840 F.2d 701 (9th Cir. 1988).

42. *See also Glover v. Eastern Neb. Commun. Office of Retardation*, 686 F. Supp. 243 (D. Neb. 1988) (enjoining mandatory HIV testing of employees of agency providing services to the mentally retarded).

43. Pub. L. 100-259, 100th Cong., 2d Sess. (1988).

44. Section 9, Pub. L. 100-259, 100th Cong., 2d Sess. (1988), amending 29 U.S.C. §706(7)(B) (1982).

45. 134 Cong. Rec. H1065 (daily ed. Mar. 22, 1988) (remarks of Sen. Harkin).

46. *See, e.g., Cronan v. New Eng. Tel. Co.*, 41 FEP Cases 1273 (Mass. Super. Ct. 1986); *Raytheon Co. v. Fair Empl. & Housing Comm'n*, 46 FEP Cases 1089 (Cal. Super. Ct. 1988).

47. Tenn. Code Ann. §8-50-103(c) (Supp. 1987).

48. Ricklefs, *Victims of AIDS-Related Discrimination Are Fighting Back—and Getting Results*, Wall St. J., July 15, 1988, at 17, col. 3.

49. *Id.*
50. 521 N.E.2d 350 (Ind. App. 1988).
51. *Id.* at 352.
52. Hardy, Rauch, Echenberg, et al., *The Economic Impact of the First 10,000 Cases of Acquired Immunodeficiency Syndrome in the United States*, 255 J.A.M.A. 209 (1986).
53. Andrulis, Beers, Bentley, et al., *The Provision and Financing of Medical Care for AIDS Patients in U.S. Public and Private Teaching Hospitals*, 258 J.A.M.A. 1343 (1987).
54. Seage, Landers, Barry, et al., *Medical Care Costs of AIDS in Massachusetts*, 256 J.A.M.A. 3107 (1986).
55. *See* Chase, *AIDS Treatments in 1991 May Cost About $4.5 Billion*, Wall St. J., May 26, 1988, at 14, col. 1.
56. Bloom & Carliner, *The Economic Impact of AIDS in the United States*, 239 Science 604 (1988). *See* Scitovsky, *The Economic Impact of AIDS in the United States*, 7 Health Affairs 32 (Fall 1988).
57. For a discussion of different approaches to this problem, see Epstein, *AIDS and Employee Testing*, 1988 U. Chi. Legal F. 33; Liebman, *Too Much Information: Predictions of Employee Disease and the Fringe Benefit System*, 1988 U. Chi. Legal F. 57; Rothstein, *Medical Screening and Employment Law: A Note of Caution and Some Observations*, 1988 U. Chi. Legal F. 1.
58. *Employers' Share of the Cost of AIDS and Related Conditions*, Med. Benefits, Oct. 15, 1988, at 6 (based on Coolfont Report).
59. Office of Technology Assessment, U.S. Congress, Medical Testing and Health Insurance 108–116 (1988). *Compare* Clifford & Iuculano, *AIDS and Insurance: The Rationale for AIDS-Related Testing*, 100 Harv. L. Rev. 1806 (1987) *with* Schatz, *The AIDS Insurance Crisis: Underwriting or Overreaching?*, 100 Harv. L. Rev. 1782 (1987).
60. *See* Weiss & Thier, *HIV Testing is the Answer—What's the Question*, 319 New Eng. J. Med. 1010 (1988).
61. Committee Report, *AIDS in the Workplace: Guidelines*, 30 J. Occup. Med. 578 (1988).
62. Citizens Commission on AIDS for New York City and Northern New Jersey, Responding to AIDS: Ten Principles for the Workplace 3–5 (1988).
63. *See* Davidson, *Head of Reagan's AIDS Panel Urges President to Sign Order to Prohibit Bias*, Wall St. J. June 3, 1988, at 32, col. 5.
64. *See* Davidson, *Science Panel's Report on AIDS Urges Passage of Law Blocking Discrimination*, Wall St. J., June 2, 1988, at 22, col. 3.
65. *See AMA House of Delegates Adopts Comprehensive Measures on AIDS*, 258 J.A.M.A. 425 (1987).
66. Davidson, *supra* note 63. *See* Blendon & Donelon, *Discrimination Against People With AIDS*, 319 New Eng. J. Med. 1022 (1988).

Chapter 6

1. Some of the discussion in this chapter has been adapted from Rothstein, *Drug Testing in the Workplace: The Challenge to Employment Relations and Employment Law*, 63 Chi.-Kent L. Rev. 683 (1987). *See also Survey of the Law of Employee Drug Testing*, 42 U. Miami L. Rev. 553 (1988).

2. Press Office, National Institute on Drug Abuse, *Highlights of the 1985 National Household Survey on Drug Abuse*, NIDA Capsules (Nov. 1986 rev.) [hereinafter NIDA Highlights].

3. *Id.*

4. Smith & Silberman, *Treatment Resources for Chemical Dependency*, 1 Seminars in Occup. Med. 265 (1986) (citing the National Institute on Alcohol Abuse and Alcoholism (NIAAA), *Fifth Special Report to Congress on Alcohol and Health* (1984)).

5. NIDA Highlights, *supra* note 2.

6. Smith & Silberman, *supra* note 4 (citing unpublished NIAAA Report submitted to Congress).

7. Ross & Walsh, *Treatment for Chemical Dependency and Mental Illness: The Payer's Perspective*, 1 Seminars in Occup. Med. 277 (1986).

8. *See, e.g.*, Weisman, *I Was a Drug-Hype Junkie*, New Republic, Oct. 6, 1986, at 14.

9. *See* Barnes, *Drugs: Running the Numbers*, 240 Science 1729 (1988).

10. *See* Brinkley, *Drug Use Held Mostly Stable or Lower*, N.Y. Times, Oct. 10, 1986, at 10, col. 1 (quoting Dr. Charles R. Shuster, Director of NIDA).

11. *See* Kerr, *Rich vs. Poor: Drug Patterns Are Diverging*, N.Y. Times, Aug. 30, 1987, at 1, col. 2, 17, col. 1.

12. *See* Kerr, *The American Drug Problem Takes on Two Faces*, N.Y. Times, July 10, 1988, at E5, col. 1.

13. President's Commission on Organized Crime, America's Habit: Drug Abuse, Drug Trafficking, and Organized Crime 67 (1986) [hereinafter President's Commission]. For example, one synthetic drug, 3-methyl fentanyl is up to 1,000 times more potent than morphine. *Id.*

14. *Id.* at 60.

15. *See* Tolbert, *Health Professionals Should Monitor Workers' Over-the-Counter Drug Use*, Occup. Health & Safety, Dec. 1987, at 52.

16. *See* Russo & Sparadeo, *Substance Abuse and Impairment in the Workplace: A Labor Perspective*, 1 Seminars in Occup. Med. 301 (1986).

17. L. Dogoloff & R. Angarola, Urine Testing in the Workplace 8 (1985).

18. *Id.* at 237–38.

19. *See, e.g.*, *CEOs Call Drug Problem Worse But Applaud Company Action*, 3 Nat'l Rep. on Substance Abuse (BNA), Jan. 4, 1989, at 3; Freudenheim, *Workers' Substance Abuse Is Increasing Survey Says*, N.Y. Times, Dec. 12, 1988, at 25, col. 1.

20. Dogoloff, *Drug Abuse in the Workplace*, 1 Occup. Med.: State of the Art Revs. 643 (1986) (67 percent); Imwinkelried, *Some Preliminary Thoughts on the Wisdom of Governmental Prohibition or Regulation of Employee Urinalysis Testing*, 11 Nova L. Rev. 563, 565 (1987) (65 percent); *Alcohol, Drug Factor in Accidents Discussed, Disputed at Montreal Session*, 17 Occup. Safety & Health Rep. (BNA) 93 (1987) (50%–65%); [hereinafter *Montreal Session*].

21. P. Bensinger, Drugs in the Workplace: Employers Rights and Responsibilities 1 (1984).

22. Dogoloff, *supra* note 20, at 645 (2.5 times); Imwinkelreid, *supra* note 20, at 565 (16 times).

23. Walsh & Gust, *Drug Abuse in the Workplace: Issues, Policy Decisions, and Corporate Response*, 1 Seminars in Occup. Med. 237 (1986) (citing study by Kandel & Yamaguchi).

24. BNA Special Report, Alcohol and Drugs in the Workplace: Costs, Controls, and Controversies 7 (1986) [hereinafter BNA Special Report].
25. *Id.* at 7 (quoting P. Bensinger).
26. *See id.* at 9 (citing information provided by the Federal Railroad Administration).
27. *Id.* at 8.
28. Montreal Session, *supra* note 20, at 93-94.
29. *Id. See also Few Sound Studies Link Drug, Alcohol Abuse With Workplace Accident Rates, Physician Says*, 17 Occup. Safety & Health Rep. (BNA) 825 (1987) (quoting Dr. Bob Brewer of the Rush Occupational Health Network).
30. *Study: $50 Billion Wasted Annually From Abuse of Drugs and Alcohol*, 4 Employee Rels. Weekly (BNA) 1554 (1986) (citing a study by the Comprehensive Care Corp.).
31. BNA Special Report, *supra* note 24, at 7.
32. *Gariup Constr. Co. v. Foster*, 519 N.E.2d 1224 (Ind. 1988); *Otis Eng'g Corp. v. Clark*, 668 S.W.2d 307 (Tex. 1983).
33. 305 Or. 439, 753 P.2d 404 (1988).
34. *See* Morgan, *The "Scientific" Justification for Urine Drug Testing*, 36 Kan. L. Rev. 683 (1988).
35. *Workplace Next Battleground in Drug Crusade, Reagan Tells Meeting*, 6 Empl. Rel. Weekly (BNA) 205 (1988) (reporting speech at Duke University, Feb. 8, 1988).
36. *Reagan Undergoes Urinary Test and Reports "Everything's Fine,"* N.Y. Times, Aug. 10, 1986, at 24, col. 1.
37. Sims, *Boom in Drug Tests Expected*, N.Y. Times, Sept. 8, 1986, at 1, col. 1.
38. McBay, *Efficient Drug Testing: Addressing the Basic Issues*, 11 Nova L. Rev. 647, 648 (1987).
39. President's Commission, *supra* note 13, at 452.
40. Exec. Order 12,564, 51 Fed. Reg. 32,889 (1986).
41. *See* Weinraub, *Reagan Aides Back Testing for Drugs in U.S. Employees*, N.Y. Times, Sept. 11, 1986, at A1, col. 5.
42. Section 503 of Pub. L. 100-71, Supplemental Appropriations Act for 1987.
43. *See Congress Okays Testing Regulations; Signature by President Is Expected*, 1 Nat'l Rep. on Substance Abuse (BNA), July 8, 1987, at 1.
44. 52 Fed. Reg. 30,638 (1987).
45. *Id.* at 30,639. The Controlled Substances Act, Pub. L. 99-646 (1986), (codified in scattered sections of 18 and 21 U.S.C.).
46. Schroeder, *On Beyond Drug Testing: Employer Monitoring and the Quest for the Perfect Worker*, 36 Kan. L. Rev. 869, 870 (1988).
47. Chapman, *The Ruckus Over Medical Testing*, Fortune, Aug. 19, 1985, at 57, 58 (increase in testing from 1982 to 1985); Fowler, *Drug Testing Common for Job Seekers*, N.Y. Times, Jan. 19, 1988, at 47, col. 1 (48% of 252 *Fortune* 500 companies test applicants).
48. *Drug Testing Popular*, Occup. Health & Safety, Aug. 1987, at 12 (based on survey by Business and Legal Reports).
49. *See Statements on Drug/Alcohol Abuse in the Workplace Before House Labor Subcommittee on Health and Safety*, Daily Lab. Rep. (BNA), Dec. 15, 1985, at D-2.

50. Godefroi & McCunney, *Drug Screening Practices in Small Businesses: A Survey* (letter), 30 J. Occup. Med. 300, 302 (1988).
51. *Survey Shows Little Use of Random Test Programs*, 1 Nat'l Rep. on Substance Abuse (BNA), Sept. 16, 1987, at 2 (citing study by Executive Knowledgeworks).
52. *Teleconference on Drug Testing*, U.S.A. Today, Feb. 5, 1987, at 1, col. 1.
53. Marshall, *Testing Urine for Drugs*, 241 Science 150 (1988).
54. *Testing for Drug Use: Handle With Care*, Bus. Week, Mar. 28, 1988, at 65.
55. *See* Council on Scientific Affairs, American Medical Association, *Scientic Issues in Drug Testing* 257 J.A.M.A. 3110, 3111 (1987); Miike & Hewitt, *Accuracy and Reliability of Urine Drug Tests*, 36 Kan. L. Rev. 641 (1988); Schnoll & Lewis, *Drug Screening in the Workplace: Pros and Cons*, 1 Seminars in Occup. Med. 243, 245 (1986).
56. For a further discussion of these other drug tests, see R. Decresce & M. Lifshitz, Drug Testing in the Workplace (1989); Dubowski, *Drug-Use Testing: Scientific Perspectives*, 11 Nova L. Rev. 415, 428–33 (1987).
57. *Id. See also* L. Dogoloff & R. Angarola, *supra* note 17, at 30; Denenberg & Denenberg, *Drug Testing From the Arbitrator's Perspective*, 11 Nova L. Rev. 371, 402 (1987).
58. Testimony of Lawrence Miike, Office of Technology Assessment, United States Congress, before the Subcommittee on Human Resources of the House Post Office and Civil Service Committee, *Accuracy and Reliability of Urine Drug Tests*, Sept. 16, 1986, at 1-2, 19; Dubowski, *supra* note 56, at 436–37, 540 (citing the NIDA Draft Standards for Accreditation of Laboratories Engaged in Drug Testing, Jan. 1987).
59. Dubowski, *supra* note 56, at 437.
60. For a discussion of color or spot tests, see Council on Scientific Affairs, *supra* note 55, at 3112; Schnoll & Lewis, *supra* note 55, at 246.
61. For a discussion of thin layer chromatography, see Council on Scientific Affairs, *supra* note 55, at 3112; Miike, *supra* note 58, at 3; Schnoll & Lewis, *supra* note 58, at 246.
62. For a discussion of RIA, see Council on Scientific Affairs, *supra* note 55, at 3112; Schnoll & Lewis, *supra* note 55, at 248.
63. For a discussion of FPIA, see Council on Scientific Affairs, *supra* note 55 at 3113; Dubowski, *supra* note 56, at 460–62.
64. For a discussion of HPLC, see Council on Scientific Affairs, *supra* note 55, at 3114; Dubowski, *supra* note 56, at 475–77; Schnoll & Lewis, *supra* note 55, at 249.
65. Hoyt, Finnigan, Nee, et al., *Drug Testing in the Workplace—Are Methods Legally Defensible?*, 258 J.A.M.A. 504, 508 (1987).
66. *Id. See also* Hudner, *Urine Testing for Drugs*, 11 Nova L. Rev. 553, 555 (1987); McBay, *Efficient Drug Testing: Addressing the Basic Issues*, 11 Nova L. Rev. 647, 648 (1987); Morikawa, Hurtgen, Connor, et al., *Implementation of Drug and Alcohol Testing in the Unionized Workplace*, 11 Nova L. Rev. 653, 656 (1987); Schroeder & Nelson, *Drug Testing in the Federal Government*, 11 Nova L. Rev. 685, 688–89 (1987).
67. Council on Scientific Affairs, *supra* note 55, at 3111; Schnoll & Lewis, *supra* note 55, at 246.

68. Council on Scientific Affairs, *supra* note 54, at 3111; McBay, *supra* note 66, at 649.

69. Kerns & Schnoll, *Effects of Drugs on Occupational Performance*, 1 Seminars in Occup. Med. 229, 230 (1986); Walsh & Gust, *supra* note 23, at 238–39.

70. Kerns & Schnoll, *supra* note 69, at 229–30; Walsh & Gust, *supra* note 23, at 238.

71. Professor Ronald K. Seigel of UCLA Medical School, forensic psychopharmacologist, *quoted in* Deneberg & Deneberg, *supra* note 57, at 399.

72. *See* Council on Scientific Affairs, *supra* note 55, at 3113; Morgan, *Problems of Mass Urine Screening for Misused Drugs*, 16 J. Psychoactive Drugs 305 (1984).

73. *See* Marshall, *supra* note 53, at 152.

74. *See* Zeidenberg, Bourdon & Nahas, *Marijuana Intoxication by Passive Inhalation: Documentation by Detection of Urinary Metabolites*, 134 Am. J. Psychiatry 76 (1977); *Passive Inhalation of Marijuana Smoke*, 250 J.A.M.A. 898 (1983) (letter).

75. *Id.*

76. *See, e.g.*, Zeese, *Drug Hysteria Causing Use of Useless Urine Tests*, 11 Nova L. Rev. 815, 819 (1987).

77. *See* Dubowski, *supra* note 56, at 540; Sonnenstuhl, Trice, Staudenmeir, et al., *Employee Assistance and Drug Testing: Fairness and Injustice in the Workplace*, 11 Nova L. Rev. 709, 719 (1987). *See generally* Note, *Drug Testing in the Workplace: The Need for Quality Assurance Legislation*, 48 Ohio St. L.J. 877 (1987).

78. 384 U.S. 757 (1966).

79. *See, e.g..*, *Division 241, Amalgamated Transit Union v. Suscy*, 538 F.2d 1264 (7th Cir.), *cert. denied*, 429 U.S. 1029 (1976); *Allen v. City of Marietta*, 601 F. Supp. 482 (N.D. Ga. 1985); *Ewing v. State*, 160 Ind. App. 138, 310 N.E.2d 571 (1974).

80. *Katz v. United States*, 389 U.S. 347, 351 (1967); *McDonell v. Hunter*, 809 F.2d 1302, 1305 (8th Cir. 1987); *National Fed'n of Fed. Employees v. Weinberger*, 818 F.2d 935, 942–43 (D.C. Cir. 1987).

81. *Allen v. City of Marietta*, 601 F. Supp. 482, 491 (N.D. Ga. 1985).

82. *Id.*

83. *Whalen v. Roe*, 429 U.S. 589, 599–600 (1977).

84. *Amalgamated Transit Union, Local 1277 v. Sunline Transit Agency*, 663 F. Supp. 1560, 1572 (C.D. Cal. 1987). *See also Shoemaker v. Handel*, 795 F.2d 1136 (3d Cir. 1986).

85. *Jones v. McKenzie*, 833 F.2d 335 (D.C. Cir. 1987).

86. *Banks v. FAA*, 687 F.2d 92 (5th Cir. 1982).

87. *Everett v. Napper*, 825 F.2d 341 (11th Cir. 1987). *See also Cleveland Bd. of Educ. v. Loudermill*, 470 U.S. 532 (1985).

88. *See, e.g.*, *Copeland v. Philadelphia Police Dep't*, 840 F.2d 1139 (3d Cir. 1988); *Lavery v. Department of Highway Safety*, 523 So. 2d 696 (Fla. 1988).

89. *See, e.g.*, *Lovvorn v. City of Chattanooga*, 846 F.2d 1539 (6th Cir. 1988); *City of East Point v. Smith*, 365 S.E.2d 432 (Ga. 1988).

90. *McDonell v. Hunter*, 809 F.2d 1302 (8th Cir. 1987); *Taylor v. O'Grady*, 669 F. Supp. 1422 (N.D. Ill. 1987).

91. *National Fed'n of Fed. Employees v. Carlucci*, 680 F. Supp. 416 (D.D.C. 1988).
92. *Rushton v. Nebraska Pub. Power Dist.*, 844 F.2d 562 (8th Cir. 1988).
93. *Transport Workers Union v. SEPTA*, 678 F. Supp. 543 (E.D. Pa. 1988); *Fiorenza v. Gunn*, 140 A.D.2d 295, 527 N.Y.S.2d 806 (App. Div. 1988).
94. *Jones v. McKenzie*, 833 F.2d 335 (D.C. Cir. 1987).
95. *Patchogue-Medford Congress of Teachers v. Patchogue–Medford Union Free School Dist.*, 70 N.Y.2d 57, 510 N.E.2d 325, 517 N.Y.S.2d 456 (1987).
96. *Shoemaker v. Handel*, 795 F.2d 1136 (3d Cir. 1986).
97. *National Treasury Employees Union v. Von Raab*, 109 S.Ct. ___ (1989).
98. *Skinner v. Railway Labor Exec. Ass'n*, 109 S.Ct. ___ (1989).
99. Ariz. Const. art. II, §8; Cal. Const. art. I, §1; Hawaii. Const. art. I, §5; Ill. Const. art. I, §6; La. Const. art. I, §5; Mo. Const. art. I, §§1–4; Wash. Const. art. I, §7.
100. *See, e.g., Wilkinson v. Times Mirror Books*, No. 636361-3 (Alameda County, Cal. Super. Ct., June 8, 1988), *cited in* 2 Nat'l Rep. on Substance Abuse (BNA), June 22, 1988, at 6.
101. *Governor, Staff Covered by Drug Testing Measure*, 2 Nat'l Rep. on Substance Abuse (BNA), May 11, 1988, at 7.
102. Senate Bill No. 643 (1988).
103. H.B. 1618 (1988).
104. Utah Code Ann. §§34-38-1 to –15 (1987).
105. Pub. Act. No. 87-551 (1987).
106. Iowa H.F. 469 (1987).
107. Minn. Stat. Ann. §§181.93 to –.995 (West 1987).
108. Mont. Code Ann. §39-2-304 (1987).
109. Neb. Legis. Bill No. 582 (1988).
110. R.I. Gen. Laws. §§28-6.5-1 to –2 (1987).
111. Vt. Stat. Ann. tit. 21, Ch. 5, §§511–520 (1987).
112. San Francisco Police Code art. 33A, §§3300 A.1 to –.11 (1985).
113. 29 U.S.C. §§701–796 (Supp. 1988).
114. *Id.* §706(7)(B).
115. *See* 124 Cong. Rec. 14,507 (daily ed. May 18, 1978) (remarks of Rep. Hyde).
116. 29 U.S.C. §706(7)(B)(1982).
117. 480 U.S. 273 (1987).
118. *Id.* at 285 n. 14.
119. *See* 124 Cong. Rec. S19,002 (daily ed. Oct. 14, 1978) (remarks of Sen. Williams).
120. 683 F. Supp. 758 (D. Kan. 1988).
121. 803 F.2d 67 (2d Cir. 1986). *Accord, Copeland v. Philadelphia Police Dep't*, 840 F.2d 1139 (3d Cir. 1988).
122. 9 FEP Cases 225 (E.D. Mich. 1985).
123. 29 C.F.R. §1613.702(c) (1987).
124. 680 F. Supp. 590 (S.D.N.Y. 1988).
125. *Id.* at 597.

126. S. Rep. No. 318, 93d Cong., 1st Sess., *reprinted in* 1973 U.S. Code Cong. & Admin. News 2078, 2092.
127. For a table listing the various state laws, see Rothstein, *supra* note 1, at 719–20.
128. *See* Ellenberger, *AFL-CIO Urges Privacy Protection, Treatment in Drug Abuse Testing*, Bus. & Health, Oct. 1987, at 58.
129. Council on Scientific Affairs, American Medical Association, *Issues in Employee Drug Testing*, 258 J.A.M.A. 2089 (1987).
130. *Id.* at 2095.
131. Neal, *Mandatory Drug Testing*, A.B.A.J., Oct. 1, 1988, at 58, 63.
132. Mohr, *Drug Test Policy Caught in Snags*, N.Y. Times, Dec. 18, 1988, at 17, col. 1.
133. R. Decresce & M. Lifshitz *supra* note 56, at 8.
134. *See* Bureau of National Affairs, Alcohol and Drugs in the Workplace 15 (1986) (cocaine hotline survey showed 83 percent of callers used some drug on the job); Note, *Employee Drug Testing—Issues Facing Private Sector Employees*, 65 N.C.L. Rev. 832 (1987) (citing National Institute of Drug Abuse survey showing 10%-23% of all workers use drugs at work; 90% of cocaine users use it during work hours).
135. *See, e.g., Bowen Expresses Pessimism in Administration Drug War*, 2 Nat'l Rep. on Substance Abuse (BNA), May 11, 1988, at 4,5.
136. *See In re Meese*, No. 87-1 (D.C. Cir., July 5, 1988) (Report of the Independent Counsel), at 27–29.
137. *Your Boss Is Not a Cop*, New Republic, June 6, 1988, at 7-8.
138. American Occupational Medical Association, *Drug Screening in the Workplace: Ethical Guidelines*, 28 J. Occup. Med. 1240 (1986).
139. Lewis & Cooper, *Alcohol, Other Drugs, and Fatal Work-Related Injuries*, 31 J. Occup. Med. 23 (1989).
140. *Drugs a Serious Problem, Subcontractors Group Told*, 2 Nat'l Rep. on Substance Abuse (BNA), Apr. 13, 1988, at 7.
141. Nelson, *Drug Abusers on the Job*, 23 J. Occup. Med. 403 (1981).
142. *See* McLatchie, Grey, Johns, et al., *A Component Analysis of an Alcohol and Drug Program: Employee Education*, 23 J. Occup. Med. 477 (1981).
143. Masi, *Employee Assistance Programs*, 1 Occup. Med.: State of the Art Revs. 653 (1986).
144. Bureau of National Affairs, *supra* note 134, at 39.
145. *Id.* at 40.

Chapter 7

1. E. Berkowitz, Disabled Policy 212 (1987) (footnote omitted).
2. 29 U.S.C. §791 (1988).
3. *Id.* §793.
4. 45 C.F R. §84.3(j)(2)(ii) (1988) (§504 regulation).
5. *Compare Beam v. Sun Shipbuilding & Dry Dock Co.*, 679 F.2d 1077 (3d Cir. 1982) *and Simpson v. Reynolds Metals Co.*, 629 F.2d 1226 (7th Cir. 1980) (no private right of action) *with Philip Morris, Inc. v. Block*, 755 F.2d 368 (4th Cir. 1985) *and California Ass'n of Physically Handicapped, Inc. v. FCC*, 721 F.2d 667 (9th Cir.) *cert. denied*, 469 U.S. 832 (1983) (permitting a private right of action).

6. 29 U.S.C. §794 (1988).
7. 45 C.F.R. §85.5 (1988).
8. *See e.g.*, *Rogers v. Frito-Lay, Inc.*, 611 F.2d 1074 (5th Cir.), *cert. denied*, 449 U.S. 886 (1980). *See generally* L. Rothstein, Rights of Physically Handicapped Persons §3.18 (1983).
9. Section 103(d)(2)(B) of the Rehabilitation Act Amendments of 1986, 100 Stat. 1807, 1810.
10. H. Rep. No. 571, 99th Cong., 2d Sess. 17, *reprinted in* 1986 U.S. Code Cong. & Admin. News 3471, 3487.
11. *See, e.g.*, Note, *Defining "Handicap" for Purposes of Employment Discrimination*, 30 Ariz. L. Rev. 633, 659–70 (1988) (collecting state definitions).
12. 45 C.F.R. 84.14 (1988).
13. *See, e.g.*, Cal. Fair Empl. Practice Regs. §7294.0 (1988).
14. 19 FEP Cases 1624 (U.S. Dep't of Labor 1979).
15. *Id.* at 1631 (footnote omitted).
16. *E.E. Black, Ltd. v. Marshall*, 497 F. Supp. 1088 (D. Hawaii 1980).
17. *E.E. Black, Ltd. v. Donovan*, 26 FEP Cases 1183 (D. Hawaii 1981).
18. Cal. Fair Empl. Practice Regs. §7293.8(d) (1988).
19. *See, e.g.*, *Sterling Transit Co. v. Fair Empl. Practice Comm'n*, 121 Cal. App. 3d 791, 175 Cal. Rptr. 548 (1981).
20. 80 Or. App. 464, 722 P.2d 1282 (1986), *rev. denied*, 302 Or. 460, 730 P.2d 1250 (1986).
21. 722 P.2d at 1284 (emphasis in original).
22. 497 F. Supp. at 1104.
23. *School Dist. v. Friedman*, 96 Pa. Commw. 267, 507 A.2d 882 (1986).
24. *Leggett v. First Interstate Bank*, 86 Or. App. 523, 739 P.2d 1083 (1987).
25. *American Motors Corp. v. Labor & Indus. Rev. Comm'n*, 119 Wis. 2d 706, 350 N.W.2d 120 (1984).
26. *Rezza v. United States Dep't of Justice*, 698 F. Supp. 586 (E.D. Pa. 1988).
27. *de la Torres v. Bolger*, 781 F.2d 1134 (5th Cir. 1986).
28. 794 F.2d 931 (4th Cir. 1986).
29. *Id.* at 934.
30. *Id.* at 933.
31. 745 S.W.2d 314 (Tex. 1987).
32. *Id.* at 317.
33. *Bayport-Blue Pt. School Dist. v. State Div. of Human Rights*, 131 A.D.2d 849, 517 N.Y.S.2d 209 (App. Div. 1987).
34. *See* Rothstein, *Legal Issues in the Medical Assessment of Physical Impairment by Third-Party Physicians*, 5 J. Legal Med. 503, 516–17 (1984).
35. 425 Mich. 313, 389 N.W.2d 686 (1986).
36. 410 N.W.2d 250 (Iowa 1987).
37. 147 Mich. App. 573, 382 N.W.2d 823 (1985).
38. 617 F. Supp. 156 (D.D.C. 1985).
39. 76 Or. App. 617, 711 P.2d 139 (1985).
40. 110 N.J. 363, 541 A.2d 682 (1988).
41. 541 A.2d at 689.
42. 358 N.W.2d 432 (Minn. App. 1984).
43. 70 N.Y.2d 100, 510 N.E.2d 799, 517 N.Y.S.2d 715 (1987).
44. 70 N.Y.2d at 107, 510 N.E.2d at 802, 517 N.Y.S.2d at 718.

45. 47 FEP Cases 179 (Me. 1986).

46. *Id.* at 182 (quoting lower court opinion).

47. 373 N.W.2d 377 (Minn. App. 1985).

48. 567 F. Supp. 369 (E.D. Pa. 1983), *aff'd*, 732 F.2d 146 (3d Cir. 1984), *cert. denied*, 469 U.S. 1188 (1985).

49. *See Dean v. Municipality of Metropolitan Seattle-Metro*, 104 Wash. 2d 627, 708 P.2d 393 (1985).

50. *See Jenks v. Avco Corp.*, 340 Pa. Super. 542, 490 A.2d 912 (1985).

51. *See Harrison v. Marsh*, 691 F. Supp. 1223 (W.D. Mo. 1988).

52. *See Bento v. ITO Corp.*, 599 F. Supp. 731 (D.R.I. 1984).

53. *See Jasany v. United States Postal Serv.*, 755 F.2d 1244 (6th Cir. 1985); *Rancour v. Detroit Edison Co.*, 47 FEP Cases 1284 (Mich. App. 1986).

54. *See Treadwell v. Alexander*, 707 F.2d 473 (11th Cir. 1983); *Bowerman v. Malloy Lithographing, Inc.*, 430 N.W.2d 742 (Mich. App. 1988).

55. 694 F.2d 666 (11th Cir. 1983).

56. 549 F. Supp. 85 (W.D. Wash. 1982).

57. *Id.* at 87.

58. 480 U.S. 273 (1987).

59. *Id.* at 289 n. 19. *See Coley v. Secretary of the Army*, 689 F. Supp. 519 (D. Md. 1987).

60. 662 F.2d 292 (5th Cir. 1981).

61. *Id.* at 308.

62. *See, e.g., Dothard v. Rawlinson*, 433 U.S. 321 (1977).

63. *See, e.g., Washington v. Davis*, 426 U.S. 229 (1976).

64. *See, e.g., Green v. Missouri Pac. R.R.*, 523 F.2d 1290 (8th Cir. 1975).

65. *See, e.g., Wallace v. Delron Corp.*, 494 F.2d 674 (8th Cir. 1974).

66. 473 N.E.2d 325 (Ohio C.P. 1981).

67. *Id.* at 328.

68. 687 F. Supp. 1115 (E.D. Mich. 1988).

69. *Id.* at 1121, *quoting* Wegner, *The Antidiscrimination Model Reconsidered: Ensuring Equal Opportunity Without Respect to Handicap Under §504 of the Rehabilitation Act of 1973*, 59 Cornell L. Rev. 401, 490 (1984).

70. 128 Mich. App. 435, 340 N.W.2d 117 (1983).

71. 340 N.W.2d at 118. *See also State ex rel. Khalifa v. Hennepin County*, 420 N.W.2d 634 (Minn. App. 1988).

72. *Mass Transit Admin. v. Maryland Comm'n on Human Rels.*, 68 Md. App. 703, 515 A.2d 781 (Ct. Spec. App. 1986).

73. *Lewis v. Metropolitan Transit Comm'n*, 320 N.W.2d 426 (Minn. 1982).

74. *Boynton Cab Co. v. Department of Indus., Labor & Human Rels.*, 96 Wis. 2d 396, 291 N.W.2d 850 (1980).

75. 110 N.J. 363, 541 A.2d 682 (1988).

76. 224 Neb. 731, 401 N.W.2d 461 (1987).

77. *See, e.g., Baltimore & O.R.R. v. Bowen*, 60 Md. App. 299, 482 A.2d 921 (Ct. Spec. App. 1984); *Bucyrus-Erie Co. v. Department of Indus., Labor & Human Rels.*, 90 Wis. 2d 408, 280 N.W.2d 142 (1979). *Cf. In re Montgomery Ward & Co.*, 280 Or. 163, 570 P.2d 76 (1977) ("high probability").

78. *See, e.g., Allen v. Southeastern Mich. Transp. Auth.*, 132 Mich. App. 533, 349 N.W.2d 204 (1984) (bus driver with arthritis); *Boynton Cab Co. v.*

Department of Indus., Labor & Human Rels., 96 Wis. 2d 396, 291 N.W.2d 850 (1980) (taxi driver with one arm).

79. 471 A.2d 288 (Me. 1984)
80. *Id.* at 292.
81. 748 S.W.2d 390 (Mo. App. 1988).
82. *Id.* at 398.
83. 14 FEP Cases 344 (Wis. Cir. Ct. 1976).
84. Pa. Stat. Ann. tit. 43, §954(p) (Purdon Supp. 1988).
85. 65 N.Y.2d 213, 480 N.E.2d 695, 491 N.Y.S.2d 106 (1985).
86. 65 N.Y.2d at 218, 480 N.E.2d at 698, 491 N.Y.S.2d at 109.
87. 29 U.S.C. §706(8)(B)(1988).
88. 42 U.S.C. §290dd-1(a)(1988).
89. *Compare Clowes v. Terminix, Int'l, Inc.*, 109 N.J. 575, 538 A.2d 794 (1988) (covered) *with Welsh v. Municipality of Anchorage*, 676 P.2d 602 (Alaska 1984) (not covered). For a compilation of state coverage, see Rothstein, *Drug Testing in the Workplace: The Challenge to Employment Relations and Employment Law*, 63 Chi.-Kent L. Rev. 683, 719–20 (1987).
90. *Compare Clowes v. Terminix, Int'l, Inc.*, 109 N.J. 575, 538 A.2d 794 (1988) (must be introduced) *with Consolidated Freightways, Inc. v. Cedar Rapids Civil Rights Comm'n*, 366 N.W.2d 522 (Iowa 1985) (need not be introduced).
91. 598 F. Supp. 126 (D.D.C. 1984), *aff'd mem. sub nom. Whitlock v. Brock*, 790 F.2d 964 (D.C. Cir. 1986). *Accord Callicotte v. Carlucci*, 698 F. Supp. 944 (D.D.C. 1988).
92. *Consolidated Freightways, Inc. v. Cedar Rapids Civil Rights Comm'n*, 366 N.W.2d 522 (Iowa 1985); *Hazlett v. Martin Chevrolet, Inc.*, 25 Ohio St. 3d 279, 496 N.E.2d 478 (1986).
93. *Crew v. Office of Personnel Management*, 834 F.2d 140 (8th Cir. 1987); *Lemere v. Burnley*, 683 F. Supp. 275 (D.D.C. 1988).
94. 363 N.W.2d 94 (Minn. App. 1985).
95. *Robinson v. Devine*, 37 FEP Cases 728 (D.D.C. 1985); *Salazar v. Ohio Civil Rights Comm'n*, 39 Ohio App. 3d 26, 528 N.E.2d 1303 (1987); *Brady v. Daily World*, 105 Wash. 2d 770, 718 P.2d 785 (1986); *Squires v. Labor & Indus. Rev. Comm'n*, 30 FEP Cases 398 (Wis. Ct. App. 1980).
96. *Gruening v. Pinotti*, 392 N.W.2d 670 (Minn. App. 1986).
97. *Richardson v. United States Postal Serv.*, 613 F. Supp. 1213 (D.D.C. 1985).
98. *Smith v. Ortiz*, 136 Misc. 2d 110, 517 N.Y.S.2d 352 (Sup. Ct. 1987).
99. *Hubbard v. United Press, Int'l*, 31 FEP Cases 139 (Minn. 1983); *Clowes v. Terminix Int'l, Inc.*, 109 N.J. 575, 538 A.2d 794 (1988).
100. 138 Ill. App. 3d 71, 485 N.E.2d 33 (1985).
101. *See, e.g., Longoria v. Harris*, 554 F. Supp. 102 (S.D. Tex. 1982); *Coleman v. Casey County Bd. of Educ.*, 510 F. Supp. 301 (W.D. Ky. 1980); *Melvin v. City of West Frankfort*, 93 Ill. App. 3d 425, 417 N.E.2d 260 (1981).
102. 96 Wis. 2d 396, 291 N.W.2d 850 (1980). *Accord Ranger Div., Ryder Truck Lines, Inc. v. Bayne*, 333 N.W.2d 891 (Neb. 1983).
103. 748 S.W.2d 390 (Mo. App. 1988).
104. *See, e.g., Guinn v. Bolger*, 598 F. Supp. 196 (D.D.C. 1984).
105. *J.C. Penney Co. v. Department of Indus., Labor, & Human Rels.*, 12 FEP Cases 1109 (Wis. Cir. Ct. 1976).

106. *Green v. Union Pac. R.R.*, 548 F. Supp. 3 (W.D. Wash. 1981).
107. *Allen v. Southeastern Mich. Transp. Auth.*, 132 Mich. App. 533, 349 N.W.2d 204 (1984).
108. *Davis v. United States Postal Serv.*, 675 F. Supp. 225 (M.D. Pa. 1987).
109. See Chapter 3 under the heading "The Limits of Predictive Screening."
110. *City of New York v. State Div. of Human Rights (Granelle)*, 70 N.Y.2d 100, 510 N.E.2d 799, 517 N.Y.S.2d 715 (1987); *Pacific Motor Trucking Co. v. Bureau of Labor & Indus.*, 64 Or. App. 361, 668 P.2d 446 (1983); *Western Weighing Bureau v. Wisconsin Dep't of Indus., Labor & Human Rels.*, 21 FEP Cases 1733 (Wis. Cir. Ct. 1977).
111. *Salt Lake City Corp. v. Confer*, 674 P.2d 632 (Utah 1983).
112. *Action Indus., Inc. v. Commonwealth*, 102 Pa. Commw. 382, 518 A.2d 610 (1986). *But see Dauten v. County of Muskegon*, 128 Mich. App. 435, 340 N.W.2d 117 (1983) (upholding refusal to hire lifeguard with scoliosis).
113. *Anderson v. Exxon Co.*, 89 N.J. 483, 446 A.2d 486 (1982).
114. *Baltimore & O.R.R. v. Bowen*, 60 Md. App. 299, 482 A.2d 921 (Md. Ct. Spec. App. 1984).
115. 139 Wis. 2d 740, 407 N.W.2d 510 (1987).
116. *Frank v. American Freight System, Inc.*, 398 N.W.2d 797 (Iowa 1987).
117. *Gomez-Bethke v. Metropolitan Airport Comm'n*, 358 N.W.2d 432 (Minn. App. 1984).
118. *Department of Civil Rights v. A & C Carriers*, 157 Mich. App. 534, 403 N.W.2d 586 (1987).
119. *School Bd. v. Rateau*, 449 So. 2d 839 (Fla. Dist. Ct. App. 1984).
120. *Silk v. Huck Installation & Equip. Div.*, 109 A.D.2d 930, 486 N.Y.S.2d 406 (App. Div. 1985).
121. *Dugger v. Delta Airlines, Inc.*, 173 Ga. App. 16, 325 S.E.2d 394 (1984), *cert. denied*, 471 U.S. 1103 (1985). *Accord Andrews v. Consolidated Rail Corp.*, 831 F.2d 678 (7th Cir. 1987) (spondylolisthesis).
122. *Carr v. General Motors Corp.*, 425 Mich. 313, 389 N.W.2d 686 (1986).
123. *Diaz v. United States Postal Serv.*, 658 F. Supp. 484 (E.D. Cal. 1987).
124. *Providence Journal Co. v. Mason*, 116 R.I. 614, 359 A.2d 682 (1976).
125. *Brown v. Hy-Vee Food Stores, Inc.*, 407 N.W.2d 598 (Iowa 1987).
126. 121 Cal. App. 3d 791, 175 Cal. Rptr. 548 (1981).
127. *Perez v. Philadelphia Housing Auth.*, 677 F. Supp. 357 (E.D. Pa. 1987), *aff'd*, 841 F.2d 1120 (3d Cir. 1988).
128. *Sommers v. Iowa Civil Rights Comm'n*, 337 N.W.2d 470 (Iowa 1983).
129. See *Blackwell v. Department of Treasury*, 656 F. Supp. 713 (D.D.C. 1986), *opinion vacated judgment aff'd*, 830 F.2d 1183 (D.C. Cir. 1987).
130. Cal. Gov't Code §12926(f) (West 1987). *See Fisher v. Superior Court*, 177 Cal. App. 3d 779, 223 Cal. Rptr. 203 (1986).
131. Vt. Stat. Ann. tit. 21, §495d(7)(C) (Supp. 1985).
132. *Harrison v. Marsh*, 691 F. Supp. 1223 (W.D. Mo. 1988).
133. H.R. 1546, 100th Cong., 1st Sess. (1987). *See generally* Canfield, *Cancer Patients' Prognosis: How Terminal Are Their Employment Prospects?*, 38 Syracuse L. Rev. 801 (1987); Hoffman, *Employment Discrimination Based on Cancer History: The Need for Federal Legislation*, 59 Temple L.Q. 1 (1986).
134. See *Katradio v. Dav-El*, 846 F.2d 1482 (D.C. Cir. 1988) (colon cancer did not substantially limit major life activities); *Shaw v. W.M. Wrigley, Jr.*,

Co., 183 Ga. App. 699, 359 S.E.2d 723 (1987) (personality conflicts and not breast cancer caused discharge); *Lyons v. Heritage House Restaurants, Inc..*, 89 Ill. App. 2d 163, 432 N.E.2d 270 (1982) (uterine cancer not a handicap under then-existing law).

135. 14 FEP Cases 344 (Wis. Cir. Ct. 1976).
136. *Accord, Goldsmith v. New York Psychoanalytic Inst.*, 73 A.D.2d 16, 425 N.Y.S.2d 561 (1980) (Hodgkin's disease).
137. Emmett, *Dermatological Screening*, 28 J. Occup. Med. 1045 (1986); Lammintausta & Mailbach, *Dermatologic Considerations in Worker Fitness Evaluations*, 3 Occup. Med.: State of the Art Revs. 341 (1988).
138. 63 A.D.2d 170, 406 N.Y.S.2d 912 (1978), *aff'd*, 425 N.Y.S.2d 74 (1980).
139. 115 Mich. App. 98, 320 N.W.2d 306 (1982).
140. *Hines v. Grand Trunk W. R.R.*, 151 Mich. App. 585, 391 N.W.2d 750 (1985).
141. *Davis v. Meese*, 692 F. Supp. 505 (E.D. Pa. 1988).
142. *Jackson v. State*, 544 A.2d 291 (Me. 1988).
143. 694 F.2d 619 (9th Cir. 1982).
144. *Id.* at 623 n.3.
145. *Agnello v. Adolph Coors Co.*, 689 P.2d 1162 (Colo. App. 1984).
146. *Pannell v. Wanke Panel Co.*, 618 F. Supp. 41 (D. Or. 1985); *Spicer v. Martin Brower Co.*, 177 Ga. App. 197, 338 S.E.2d 773 (1985).
147. *See, e.g., Reynolds v. Brock*, 815 F.2d 571 (9th Cir. 1987).
148. *See, e.g., Jansen v. Food Circus Supermarkets, Inc.*, 110 N.J. 363, 541 A.2d 682 (1988).
149. *See Silverstein v. Sisters of Charity*, 43 Colo. App. 446, 614 P.2d 891 (1979) (unlawful for hospital to deny all epileptics direct patient care positions).
150. 633 F. Supp. 927 (S.D. Fla. 1986).
151. *Id.* at 935.
152. *Mantolete v. Bolger*, 767 F.2d 1416 (9th Cir. 1985); *Higgins v. Maine Cent. R.R.*, 471 A.2d 288 (Me. 1984).
153. *Chicago, M. St. P. & Pac. R.R. v. Department of Indus., Labor & Human Rels.*, 62 Wis. 2d 392, 215 N.W.2d 443 (1974).
154. *See, e.g., Salmon Pineiro v. Lehman*, 653 F. Supp. 483 (D.P.R. 1987); *Lewis v. Remmele Eng'g, Inc.*, 314 N.W. 2d 1 (Minn. 1981).
155. 318 N.W.2d 162 (Iowa 1982).
156. *Rice v. Schuyler County Civil Serv. Comm'n*, 137 A.D.2d 359, 528 N.Y.S.2d 944 (1988).
157. *Consolidation Coal Co. v. Ohio Civil Rights Comm'n*, 473 N.E.2d 325 (Ohio C.P. 1981).
158. *Crane v. Dole*, 617 F. Supp. 156 (D.D.C. 1985).
159. *Strathie v. Department of Transp.*, 716 F.2d 227 (3d Cir. 1983); *Packard v. Gordon*, 148 Vt. 579, 537 A.2d 140 (1987). *See Milan v. Illinois Human Rights Comm'n*, 169 Ill. App. 3d 979, 523 N.E.2d 1155 (1988).
160. *See* Temte, *Cardiovascular Conditions and Worker Fitness and Risk*, 3 Occup. Med.: State of the Art Revs. 241 (1988).
161. See Figure 1-1 in Chapter 1.
162. *See Walker v. Attorney General*, 572 F. Supp. 100 (D.D.C. 1983) (upholding defendant when plaintiff's own physician made erroneous diagnosis of coronary artery disease).

163. *Carty v. Carlin*, 623 F. Supp. 1181 (D. Md. 1985).
164. *Bey v. Bolger*, 540 F. Supp. 910 (E.D. Pa. 1982).
165. *Treadwell v. Alexander*, 707 F.2d 473 (11th Cir. 1983).
166. *Bailey v. Tisch*, 683 F. Supp. 652 (S.D. Ohio 1988).
167. *Miller v. Ravitch*, 130 A.D.2d 579, 515 N.Y.S.2d 518 (App. Div. 1987).
168. *Sitler v. New York State Div. of Human Rights*, 133 A.D.2d 938, 520 N.Y.S.2d 653 (App. Div. 1987).
169. *Kendall Mfg. Co. v. Illinois Human Rights Comm'n*, 152 Ill. App. 3d 695, 504 N.E.2d 805, *cert. denied*, 511 N.E.2d 429 (Ill. 1987).
170. *Bento v. ITO Corp.*, 599 F. Supp. 731 (D.R.I. 1984).
171. 458 A.2d 1225 (Me. 1983).
172. *See also Montgomery Ward & Co. v. Bureau of Labor*, 280 Or. 163, 570 P.2d 76 (1977).
173. 675 F. Supp. 225 (M.D. Pa. 1987).
174. *Missouri Comm'n on Human Rights v. Southwestern Bell Tel. Co.*, 699 S.W.2d 75 (Mo. App. 1985).
175. *Greene v. Union Pac. R.R.*, 548 F. Supp. 3 (W.D. Wash. 1981).
176. *Jurgella v. Danielson*, 46 FEP Cases 1182 (Ariz. App. 1988); *Devaux v. State*, 68 Or. App. 322, 681 P.2d 156 (1984).
177. 68 Md. App. 703, 515 A.2d 781 (1986).
178. 32 Cal. 3d 603, 651 P.2d 1151, 186 Cal. Rptr. 345 (1982).
179. 480 U.S. 273 (1987).
180. 694 F.2d 666 (11th Cir. 1983). *See also Fitzgerald v. Green Valley Area Educ. Agency*, 589 F. Supp. 1130 (S.D. Iowa 1984) (dyslexia, epilepsy, cerebral palsy).
181. 107 A.D.2d 153, 485 N.Y.S.2d 907 (App. Div. 1985).
182. *Rhone v. United States Dep't of the Army*, 665 F. Supp. 734 (E.D. Mo. 1987); *Dean v. Municipality of Metro. Seattle–Metro*, 104 Wash. 2d 627, 708 P.2d 393 (1985).
183. 131 A.D.2d 849, 517 N.Y.S.2d 209 (App. Div. 1987).
184. 517 N.Y.S.2d at 211. *See Recanzone v. Washoe County School Dist.*, 696 F. Supp. 1372 (D. Nev. 1988) (school teacher with multiple sclerosis and viral myelitis).
185. 849 F.2d 1048 (7th Cir. 1988).
186. *Board of Educ. v. State Div. of Human Rights*, 130 A.D.2d 614, 515 N.Y.S.2d 543 (App. Div. 1987).
187. *Deerson v. Metal-Matic, Inc.*, 423 N.W.2d 393 (Minn. App. 1988).
188. 589 F. Supp. 1130 (S.D. Iowa 1984).
189. *Id.* at 1136.
190. *See Holland v. Boeing Co.*, 18 FEP Cases 37 (Wash. 1978) (cerebral palsy is a handicap). *But cf. Pridemore v. Legal Aid Soc'y*, 625 F. Supp. 1171 (S.D. Ohio 1985) (borderline cerebral palsy, which does not interfere with major life activity, is not a handicap). *See also Rosiak v. United States Dep't of the Army*, 679 F. Supp. 444 (M.D. Pa. 1987), *aff'd*, 845 F.2d 1014 (3d Cir. 1988) (carpenter with neurological symptoms of allergy to contact cement not otherwise qualified); *Bruegging v. Burke*, 696 F. Supp. 674 (D.D.C. 1987) (Federal Register employee with cerebral palsy not otherwise qualified for promotion).
191. *See, e.g., Krein v. Marian Manor Nursing Home*, 415 N.W.2d 793 (N.D. 1987).

192. *Missouri Comm'n on Human Rights v. Southwestern Bell Tel. Co.*, 699 S.W.2d 75 (Mo. App. 1985).
193. *Philadelphia Elec. Co. v. Commonwealth*, 68 Pa. Commw. 212, 448 A.2d 701 (1982).
194. *Greene v. Union Pac. R.R.*, 548 F. Supp. 3 (W.D. Wash. 1981).
195. *Velger v. Williams*, 118 A.D.2d 1037, 500 N.Y.S.2d 411 (App. (Div. 1986).
196. *See, e.g., Devaux v. State*, 68 Or. App. 327, 681 P.2d 158 (1984).
197. 65 N.Y.2d 213, 480 N.E.2d 695, 491 N.Y.S.2d 106 (1985).
198. 65 N.Y.2d at 216, 480 N.E.2d at 698, 491 N.Y.S.2d at 109.
199. *State ex rel. Khalifa v. Hennepin County*, 420 N.W.2d 634 (Minn App. 1988).
200. *Colorado Civil Rights Comm'n v. North Washington Fire Protection Dist.*, 754 P.2d 393 (Colo. App. 1987).
201. *Elstner v. Southwestern Bell Tel. Co.*, 659 F. Supp. 1328 (S.D. Tex. 1987).
202. *Caterpillar, Inc. v. Human Rights Comm'n*, 154 Ill. App. 3d 424, 506 N.E.2d 1029 (1987).
203. *Alderson v. Postmaster General*, 598 F. Supp. 49 (W.D. Okla. 1984).
204. *Maine Human Rights Comm'n v. Canadian Pac., Ltd.*, 458 A.2d 1225 (Me. 1983).
205. *Brown v. City of Portland*, 80 Or. App. 464, 722 P.2d 1282, *review denied*, 302 Or. 460, 730 P.2d 1250 (1986).
206. *Reese v. Sears, Roebuck & Co.*, 107 Wash. 2d 563, 731 P.2d 497 (1987).
207. *Franklin v. United States Postal Serv.*, 687 F. Supp. 1214 (S.D. Ohio 1988); *Swann v. Walters*, 620 F. Supp. 741 (D.D.C. 1984); *Tatum v. Labor & Indus. Rev. Comm'n*, 132 Wis. 2d 411, 392 N.W.2d 840 (Wis. App. 1986).
208. *Gardner v. Morris*, 752 F.2d 1271 (8th Cir. 1985); *Matzo v. Postmaster General*, 685 F. Supp. 260 (D.D.C. 1987).
209. *Anastasi v. Civil Serv. Comm'n*, 88 Pa. Commw. 6, 488 A.2d 384 (1985).
210. *Forrisi v. Bowen*, 794 F.2d 931 (4th Cir. 1986).
211. *Leggett v. First Interstate Bank*, 86 Or. App. 523, 739 P.2d 1083 (1987).
212. 144 Ill. App. 3d 860, 494 N.E.2d 619 (1986).
213. *School Dist. v. Friedman*, 96 Pa. Commw. 267, 507 A.2d 882 (1986).
214. 46 FEP Cases 1366 (E.D. Pa. 1988).
215. 512 Pa. 534, 517 A.2d 1253 (1986).
216. 116 A.D.2d 141, 500 N.Y.S.2d 246 (App. Div. 1986).
217. *Advocates for Handicapped v. Sears, Roebuck & Co.*, 67 Ill. App. 3d 512, 385 N.E.2d 39 (1978); *cert. denied*, 444 U.S. 981 (1979).
218. *Carter v. Tisch*, 822 F.2d 465 (4th Cir. 1987); *Ackerman v. Western Elec. Co.*, 643 F. Supp. 836 (N.D. Cal. 1986); *Chicago M., St. P. & Pac. R.R. v. Department of Indus., Labor & Human Rels.*, 8 FEP Cases 937 (Wis. Cir. Ct. 1971), *aff'd as modified*, 62 Wis. 2d 392, 215 N.W.2d 443 (1974).
219. *Reese v. Sears, Roebuck & Co.*, 107 Wash. 2d 563, 731 P.2d 497 (1987).
220. *Fynes v. Weinberger*, 677 F. Supp. 315 (E.D. Pa. 1985).
221. *Vickers v. Veterans Admin.*, 549 F. Supp. 85 (W.D. Wash. 1982).
222. *Rogers v. Campbell Foundry Co.*, 185 N.J. Super. 109, 447 A.2d 589 (App. Div. 1982).
223. *Probasco v. Iowa Civil Rights Comm'n*, 420 N.W.2d 432 (Iowa 1988).
224. *Reese v. Sears, Roebuck & Co.*, 107 Wash. 2d 563, 731 P.2d 497 (1987).
225. *Vickers v. Veterans Admin.*, 549 F. Supp. 85 (W.D. Wash. 1982).

226. *Carter v. Tisch*, 822 F.2d 465 (4th Cir. 1987).
227. 119 Wis. 2d 706, 350 N.W.2d 120 (1984).
228. 608 F. Supp. 739 (C.D. Cal. 1984).
229. 660 F. Supp. 1418 (D. Conn. 1987).
230. 760 F.2d 859 (8th Cir. 1985).
231. 106 Wash. 2d 560, 720 P.2d 793 (1986).
232. *But see Connecticut Inst. for Blind v. Connecticut Comm'n on Human Rights*, 176 Conn. 88, 405 A.2d 618 (1978) (school for blind could not refuse to hire teacher's aide with impaired vision).
233. 556 F.2d 184 (3d Cir. 1977), *cert. denied*, 450 U.S. 923 (1981).
234. 567 F. Supp. 369 (E.D. Pa. 1983), *aff'd*, 732 F.2d 146 (3d Cir. 1984), *cert. denied*, 469 U.S. 1188 (1985).
235. 840 F.2d 63 (D.C. Cir. 1988).
236. *Colorado Civil Rights Comm'n v. Conagra Flour Milling Co.*, 736 P.2d 842 (Colo. App. 1987).
237. *Rhone v. United States Dep't of the Army*, 665 F. Supp. 734 (E.D. Mo. 1987); *Dean v. Municipality of Metro. Seattle–Metro*, 104 Wash. 2d 627, 708 P.2d 393 (1985).
238. *Halsey v. Coca-Cola Bottling Co.*, 410 N.W.2d 250 (Iowa 1987).
239. *Lewis v. Metropolitan Transit Comm'n*, 320 N.W.2d 426 (Minn. 1982). *See Harris v. Borman's, Inc.*, 428 N.W.2d 790 (Mich. App. 1988) (bakery clerk with congenital nystagmus not otherwise qualified).
240. *City of Belleville v. Human Rights Comm'n*, 167 Ill. App. 3d 834, 522 N.E.2d 268 (1988).
241. *Brown County v. Labor & Indus. Review Comm'n*, 124 Wis. 2d 560, 369 N.W.2d 735 (1985).
242. *Padilla v. City of Topeka*, 238 Kan. 218, 708 P.2d 543 (1985).
243. *City of Columbus v. Ohio Civil Rights Comm'n*, 23 Ohio App. 3d 178, 492 N.E.2d 482 (1985).
244. *In re Gargano*, 754 P.2d 393 (Colo. App. 1987).
245. *Burgess v. Joseph Schlitz Brewing Co.*, 298 N.C. 520, 259 S.E.2d 248 (Ct. App. 1979).
246. *Quinn v. Southern Pac. Transp. Co.*, 76 Or. App. 617, 711 P.2d 139 (1985).
247. *Jasany v. United States Postal Serv.*, 755 F.2d 1244 (6th Cir. 1985).
248. 781 F.2d 1134 (5th Cir. 1986).
249. *Id.* at 1138.

Chapter 8

1. L. Tribe, American Constitutional Law 1688 (2d ed. 1988).
2. 704 F.2d 661 (2d Cir. 1983), *vacated and remanded on other grounds*, 465 U.S. 1016 (1984).
3. *But cf. Garrett v. Los Angeles City Unified School Dist.*, 116 Cal. App. 3d 472, 172 Cal. Rptr. 170 (1981) (no due process violation to refuse to hire pregnant elementary school teacher who objected to chest x-ray).
4. 816 F.2d 539 (10th Cir. 1987).
5. *See, e.g., Kelley v. Johnson*, 425 U.S. 238 (1976) (upholding hair-length regulation for police).

6. *See, e.g., Pettit v. State Bd. of Educ.*, 10 Cal. 3d 29, 513 P.2d 889, 109 Cal. Rptr. 665 (1973) (upholding discharge of 48 year-old elementary school teacher who, with her husband, were members of a "swingers" club and had pleaded guilty to the misdemeanor of "outraging public decency"); *Broderick v. Police Comm'r*, 368 Mass. 33, 330 N.E.2d 199 (1975), *cert. denied*, 423 U.S. 1048 (1976) (requiring completion of questionnaire inquiring into police officers' activities following weekend of hooliganism).

7. *See, e.g., Andrews v. Drew Mun. Separate School Dist.*, 507 F.2d 611 (5th Cir. 1975), *cert. dismissed*, 425 U.S. 559 (1976) (prohibiting refusal to rehire unwed mother as school teacher); *Murray v. Jamison*, 333 F. Supp. 1379 (W.D.N.C. 1971) (unconstitutional to discharge building inspection dispatcher because he was the Grand Dragon of the Ku Klux Klan of North Carolina).

8. Alas. Const. art. 1, §22; Ariz. Const. art. 2, §8; Cal. Const. art. 1, §1; Haw. Const. art. I, §5; Ill. Const. art. 1, §6; La. Const. art. 1, §5; Mont. Const. art. 2, §10.

9. Cal. Const. art. 1, §1.

10. *See e.g., Price v. Pacific Ref. Co.*, No. 292000 (Contra Costa, Cal. Super. Ct., Feb. 10, 1987).

11. *See Adair v. United States*, 208 U.S. 161, 172–75 (1908) (union membership). *See also Coppage v. Kansas*, 236 U.S. 1, 11 (1915) (union membership; employer's "liberty of contract" a constitutional right).

12. *See Dillon v. Great Atl. & Pac. Tea Co.*, 43 Md. App. 161, 403 A.2d 406, 407–08 (Ct. Spec. App. 1979).

13. *Odell v. Humble Oil & Ref. Co.*, 201 F.2d 123 (10th Cir.), *cert. denied*, 345 U.S. 941 (1953); *Hinrichs v. Tranquilaire Hosp.*, 352 So. 2d 1130 (Ala. 1977); *Forrer v. Sears, Roebuck & Co.*, 36 Wis. 2d 388, 153 N.W.2d 587 (1967).

14. *Pearson v. Youngstown Sheet & Tube Co.*, 332 F.2d 439 (7th Cir.), *cert. denied*, 379 U.S. 914 (1964).

15. Mont. Code Ann. §39-2-901 (1987).

16. *See, e.g., Pine River State Bank v. Mettille*, 333 N.W.2d 622 (Minn. 1983); *Woolley v. Hoffman-La Roche, Inc.*, 99 N.J. 284, 491 A.2d 1257, *modified*, 101 N.J. 10, 499 A.2d 515 (1985).

17. *See, e.g., Palmateer v. International Harvester Co.*, 85 Ill. 2d 124, 421 N.E.2d 876 (1981); *Frampton v. Central Indiana Gas Co.*, 260 Ind. 249, 297 N.E.2d 425 (1973).

18. *See, e.g., Fortune v. National Cash Register Co.*, 373 Mass. 96, 364 N.E.2d 1251 (1977); *Monge v. Beebe Rubber Co.*, 114 N.H. 130, 316 A.2d 549 (1974).

19. *See* Restatement (Second) of Contracts, §205 (1982).

20. *See, e.g., McKinney v. National Dairy Council*, 491 F. Supp. 1108 (D. Mass. 1980) (employee forced to retire under duress); *Monge v. Beebe Rubber Co.*, 114 N.H. 130, 316 A.2d 549 (1974) (employee discharged for refusing to date her supervisor).

21. *See, e.g., Greco v. Halliburton Co.*, 674 F. Supp. 1447 (D. Wyo. 1987) (drug testing); *Satterfield v. Lockheed Missiles & Space Co.*, 617 F. Supp. 1359 (D.S.C. 1985) (drug testing).

22. *See, e.g., Bruffett v. Warner Communications, Inc.*, 692 F.2d 910 (3d Cir. 1982); *Schactner v. Department of Indus., Labor, & Human Rels.*, 144 Wis. 2d 1, 422 N.W.2d 906 (Ct. App. 1988).

23. 119 Ill. 2d 526, 519 N.E.2d 909 (1988).
24. 119 Ill. 2d at 528, 519 N.E.2d at 911.
25. 109 Ill. 2d 65, 485 N.E.2d 359 (1985).
26. *See, e.g., Lingle v. Norge*, 108 S. Ct. 1877 (1988); *Frampton v. Central Indiana Gas Co.*, 260 Ind. 249, 297 N.E.2d 425 (1973). *See generally* Love, *Retaliatory Discharge for Filing a Workers' Compensation Claim: The Development of a Modern Tort Action*, 37 Hastings L.J. 551 (1986).
27. *See, e.g., Federici v. Mansfield Credit Union*, 399 Mass. 592, 506 N.E.2d 115 (1987); *Clifford v. Cactus Drilling Corp.*, 419 Mich. 356, 353 N.W.2d 469 (1984).
28. 242 Kan. 804, 752 P.2d 645 (1988).
29. 545 S.W.2d 45 (Tex. Civ. App. 1977).
30. *Id.* at 47.
31. 143 Cal. App. 3d 1, 191 Cal. Rptr. 502 (1983).
32. 617 F. Supp. 1359 (D.S.C. 1985).
33. *Greco v. Haliburton Co.*, 674 F. Supp. 1447 (D. Wyo. 1987).
34. *Monroe v. Consolidated Freightways, Inc.*, 654 F. Supp. 661 (E.D. Mo. 1987).
35. 166 Ill. App. 3d 1040, 520 N.E.2d 1227 (1988).
36. 166 Ill. App. 3d at 1042, 520 N.E.2d at 1229.
37. No. 843230 (San Francisco, Cal. Super. Ct., Oct. 30, 1987).
38. The case is summarized in 2 Nat'l Rep. on Substance Abuse, Nov. 11, 1987, at 5–6.
39. 29 U.S.C. §§651–678 (1988).
40. *See generally* M. Rothstein, Occupational Safety and Health Law 11–21 (2d ed. 1983).
41. Section 2(b) of the Act, 29 U.S.C. §651(b) (1988).
42. 599 F.2d 622 (5th Cir. 1979).
43. *Id.* at 625.
44. 647 F.2d 1189 (D.C. Cir. 1980), *cert. denied sub nom. Lead Indus. Ass'n, Inc. v. Donovan*, 453 U.S. 913 (1981).
45. 29 C.F.R. §1910.1017(k)(5) (1988).
46. *Id.* §1910.1001(g)(3)(iv).
47. *Id.* §1910.1025(k).
48. 647 F.2d 1189 (D.C. Cir. 1980), *cert. denied sub. nom. Lead Indus. Ass'n, Inc. v. Donovan*, 453 U.S. 913 (1981).
49. 452 U.S. 490 (1981).
50. *Id.* at 540.
51. *See* Molotsky, *376 Substances in Workplace Put Under New Restrictions*, N.Y. Times, Jan. 14, 1989, at 1, col. 5.
52. *See* Office of Technology Assessment, United States Congress, Preventing Injury and Illness in the Workplace 10–14 (1985).
53. *Farmworker Justice Fund, Inc. v. Brock*, 811 F.2d 613 (D.C. Cir. 1987).
54. 29 U.S.C. §157 (1988).
55. *Id.* §§158(a)(5), (b)(3), and (d).
56. *See NLRB v. Wooster Div. of Borg–Warner Corp.*, 356 U.S. 342 (1958); R. Gorman, Basic Text on Labor Law 498 (1976).
57. 73 N.L.R.B. No. 25 (1984).
58. *See, e.g., OCAW, Local 2-124 v. Amoco Oil Co.*, 651 F. Supp. 1 (D. Wyo. 1986); *Brotherhood of Locomotive Eng'rs v. Burlington N.R.R..*, 620 F. Supp. 163 (D. Mont. 1985), *aff'd*, 838 F.2d 1102 (9th Cir. 1988).

59. *Consolidated Rail Corp. v. Railway Labor Executives Ass'n*, 845 F.2d 1187 (3d Cir. 1987), *cert. granted*, ___ U.S. ___, 109 S. Ct. 52 (1988).

60. *See, e.g., Mor-Flo Indus., Inc.*, 87-2 ARB ¶8486 (King, 1987); *Schafer Bakeries, Inc.*, 87-1 ARB ¶8183 (Lipson, 1987); *Thomas Steel Corp.*, 86-2 ARB ¶8476 (Cox, 1986); *Laclede Gas Co.*, 86-1 ARB ¶8234 (Mikrut, 1986); *Utility Trailer Mfg. Co.*, 85 LA 643 (Brisco, 1985); *Oshkosh Truck Corp.*, 84-2 ARB ¶8315 (Winton, 1984).

61. *See, e.g., Boise Cascade Corp.*, 90 LA 791 (Nicholas, 1988); *Union Plaza Hotel*, 88 LA 528 (McKay, 1986); *Southern Cal. Rapid Transit Dist.*, 76 LA 144 (Sabo, 1980). *See generally* Denenberg & Denenberg, *Drug Testing From the Arbitrator's Perspective*, 11 Nova L. Rev. 371 (1987).

62. *See, e.g., Gulf Atlantic Distrib. Svcs.*, 88 LA 475 (Williams, 1986); *Consolidated Elec. Coop., Inc.*, 84-2 ARB ¶8461 (Heinsz, 1984).

63. *See, e.g., Burns Int'l Security Svcs.*, 86-2 ARB ¶8583 (Cox, 1986); *Jefferson Lines, Inc.*, 84 LA 707 (Gallagher, 1985); *ITT Continental Baking Co.*, 84 LA 41 (Traynor, 1984); *Kansas Gas & Elec.*, 83 LA 916 (Thornell, 1984).

64. *See, e.g., Sanyo Mfg. Corp.*, 87-1 ARB ¶8223 (Nicholas, 1987); *Firestone Tire & Rubber Co.*, 88 LA 217 (Cohen, 1986); *Peabody Coal Co.*, 86-2 ARB ¶8359 (Gibson, 1986); *Molycorp, Inc.*, 82 LA 693 (Sartain, 1984); *Manufacturing Co.*, 82 LA 614 (Ray, 1984).

65. *See, e.g., Armstrong Rubber Co.*, 89 LA 473 (Kindig, 1987); *American Aggregates Corp.*, 86-1 ARB ¶8119 (Dworkin, 1986); *Consolidated Elec. Coop., Inc.*, 85-1 ARB ¶8195 (Heinsz, 1985); *Southern Cal. Edison co.*, 85-2 ARB ¶8520 (Weiss, 1985).

66. *See, e.g., Lever Bros.*, 86-1 ARB ¶8134 (Gentile, 1986); *Van-Dyne-Crotty, Inc.*, 85-2 ARB ¶8332 (Seidman, 1985); *Inland Container Corp.*, 85-2 ARB ¶8381 (Duff, 1985); *Cone Mills Corp.*, 85-1 ARB ¶8244 (Byars, 1985); *Island Creek Coal Co.*, 84-2 ARB ¶8316 (Mittelman, 1984).

67. *Bucklers, Inc.*, 90 LA 937 (Braufman, 1988).

68. *Nursing Home*, 88 LA 681 (Sedwick, 1987).

69. *Arvin Indus.*, 85-2 ARB ¶8509 (Heekin, 1985).

70. *Ohio Dep't of Aging*, 90 LA 423 (Cohen, 1987).

71. *Mead Corp.*, 83-2 ARB. ¶8601 (Heinsz, 1983).

72. *Lone Star Indus.*, 88 LA 879 (Berger, 1987); *Southern Belle Dairy Co.*, 87 LA 245 (Goggin, 1985).

73. *Grand Trunk W. R.R.*, 86-1 ARB ¶8268 (Kovacs, 1985).

74. *General Tel. of Indiana*, 86-1 ARB. ¶8307 (Sinicropi, 1986).

75. *See Kost Bros.*, 86 LA 64 (Berquist, 1986).

76. *Weirton Steel Corp.*, 89 LA 201 (Sherman, 1987).

77. *Transportation Mgmt. of Tenn., Inc.*, 82 LA 671 (Nicholas, 1984).

78. *Whitacre-Greer Fireproofing Co.*, 86-1 ARB ¶8147 (Abrams, 1986); *Southwestern Bell Tel. Co.*, 84-2 ARB ¶8386 (Allen, 1984).

79. *Kaiser Alum. & Chem. Corp.*, 85-2 ARB ¶8497 (Marcus, 1985); *Southwest Forest Indus.*, 83-1 ARB ¶8009 (Cohen, 1982).

80. *Lockheed Missiles & Space Co.*, 89 LA 506 (Wyman, 1987); *Freightlines Corp.*, 85-1 ARB ¶8210 (Peck, 1985).

81. *Phillips's 66 Co.*, 88 LA 617 (Weisbrod, 1987).

82. *Lever Bros.*, 87 LA 260 (Traynor, 1986); *W.R. Grace & Co.*, 85-2 ARB ¶8348 (Flannagan, 1985).

83. *Pacific Power & Light Co.*, 89 LA 283 (Sinicropi, 1987).

84. *United States Steel Corp.*, 82 LA 913 (Tripp, 1984).
85. *American Fed'n of Gov't Employees, Local 1041*, 88-1 ARB ¶8137 (Bard, 1987).
86. *Low Vision Clinic*, 84-1 ARB ¶8013 (Bogue, 1983).
87. *Benzie County Sheriff's Dep't*, 83-2 ARB ¶8583 (Keefe, 1983).
88. *Continental Graphics*, 84-1 ARB ¶8198 (Richman, 1984).
89. *Pro Group, Inc.*, 85-1 ARB ¶8092 (Nicholas, 1984).
90. *Mead Paper*, 84 LA 346 (Ruben, 1985); *Spang & Co.*, 84 LA 342 (Joseph, 1985).
91. *Chevron USA, Inc.*, 88-1 ARB ¶8203 (Smedley, 1987).
92. *Mercy Convalescent Center*, 88-1 ARB ¶8252 (O'Grady, 1988).
93. *Nuodex, Inc.*, 87 LA 256 (Millious, 1986).
94. *Gase Baking Co.*, 86 LA 206 (Block, 1985).
95. *Peabody Coal Co.*, 84 LA 511 (Duda, 1985).
96. *Mueller Co.*, 83-1 ARB ¶8332 (Fish, 1983).
97. *Anaconda Alum. Co.*, 85-1 ARB ¶8059 (Volz, 1983).
98. *Tobin-Arp Mfg. Co.*, 85-2 ARB ¶8516 (Gallagher, 1985).
99. *Union Oil Co.*, 87 LA 612 (Nicholas, 1986).
100. *See, e.g., Allied Corp.*, 87-2 ARB ¶8408 (Clarke, 1987) (restructuring job requirements for employee blind in one eye).
101. 86 LA 65 (Berquist, 1986).
102. *Id.* at 72.
103. 188 Conn. 44, 448 A.2d 801 (1982).
104. *Cf. Beatty v. Chesapeake Center, Inc.*, 835 F.2d 71 (4th Cir. 1987) (en banc) (pregnant applicant who was not hired after she voiced objections to required tuberculin test was not discriminated against on the basis of pregnancy).
105. *See Note, Title VII Discrimination in Biochemical Testing for AIDS and Marijuana*, 1988 Duke L.J. 129.
106. *See Rosenfeld v. Southern Pac. Co.*, 444 F.2d 1219 (9th Cir. 1971).
107. *See Dothard v. Rawlinson*, 433 U.S. 321 (1977).
108. *See Long v. Sapp*, 502 F.2d 34 (5th Cir. 1974); *Weeks v. Southern Bell Tel. Co.*, 408 F.2d 228 (5th Cir.1969).
109. 619 F.2d 611 (6th Cir.), *cert. denied*, 449 U.S. 872 (1980).
110. 619 F.2d at 616.
111. *Compare Berkman v. City of New York*, 812 F.2d 52 (2d Cir.), *cert. denied*, ___ U.S. ___, 108 S. Ct. 146 (1987) (upholding revised regulations of New York Fire Department) *with Evans v. City of Evanston*, 695 F. Supp. 922 (N.D. Ill. 1988) (invalidating firefighter standards for City of Evanston, Ill.).
112. 408 N.W.2d 221 (Minn. App. 1987).
113. *See e.g., Meyer v. Brown & Root Constr. Co.*, 661 F.2d 369 (5th Cir. 1981) (pregnant employee transferred to heavy lifting job).
114. *See, e.g., Cleveland Bd. of Ed. v. La Fleur*, 414 U.S. 632 (1974) (mandatory leave); *Greenspan v. Automobile Club*, 495 F. Supp. 1021 (E.D. Mich. 1980) (pregnant employees forced to quit rather than take leave).
115. 649 F.2d 670 (9th Cir. 1980).
116. *Hayes v. Shelby Mem. Hosp.*, 726 F.2d 1543 (11th Cir.), *reh'g denied*, 732 F.2d 944 (11th Cir. 1984); *Zuniga v. Kleberg County Hosp.*, 692 F.2d 986 (5th Cir. 1982).

117. 479 U.S. 272 (1987).
118. *Id.* at 280.
119. *See* Office of Technology Assessment, United States Congress, The Role of Genetic Testing in the Prevention of Occupational Disease (1983).
120. See Chapter 4 under the heading "Biochemical Genetics: 1963–1983."
121. *See* Winters, *Psychology Tests and Black Police Recruits,* 39 Lab. L.J. 634 (1988).
122. 847 F.2d 718 (11th Cir. 1988).
123. *See Marshall v. Goodyear Tire & Rubber Co.,* 22 FEP Cases 775 (W.D. Tenn. 1979); *Mastie v. Great Lakes Steel Corp.,* 424 F. Supp. 1299 (E.D. Mich. 1976).
124. *See* B. Schlei & P. Grossman, Employment Discrimination Law 506 (2d ed. BNA Books 1983).
125. *See Geller v. Markham,* 635 F.2d 1027 (2d Cir. 1980), *cert. denied,* 451 U.S. 945 (1981) (especially the dissent of Justice Rehnquist, 451 U.S. at 947–49).
126. 531 F.2d 224 (5th Cir. 1976).
127. *Id.* at 238. *But see Hahn v. Buffalo,* 770 F.2d 12 (2d Cir. 1985) (state failed to sustain burden of proving that maximum hiring age of 29 for hiring police officers in New York was a BFOQ).
128. *Compare Murname v. American Airlines, Inc.,* 667 F.2d 98 (D.C. Cir. 1981) (pilot; defense sustained) *with Houghton v. McDonnell Douglas Corp.,* 553 F.2d 561 (8th Cir.), *cert. denied,* 434 U.S. 966 (1977) (pilot; defense rejected).

Chapter 9

1. Federal Employees Compensation Act, 5 U.S.C. §§8101-8193 (1988).
2. Federal Employers Liability Act, 45 U.S.C. §§51-60 (1988).
3. Longshoremen's and Harbor Workers' Compensation Act, 33 U.S.C. §§901–950 (1988).
4. Jones Act, 46 U.S.C. §688 (1988).
5. 1B A. Larson, Workmen's Compensation Law §§41.62, 41.63 (1987).
6. 306 Or. 25, 757 P.2d 410 (1988). *Accord General Motors Corp. v. James,* 74 Md. App. 479, 538 A.2d 782 (1988).
7. *Accord Blue Bell Printing v. Workmen's Comp. App. Bd.,* 539 A.2d 933 (Pa. Commw. Ct. 1988).
8. *See, e.g., Kellogg v. Workers' Comp. App. Bd.,* 26 Cal. 3d 450, 605 P.2d 422, 161 Cal. Rptr. 783 (1980) (all); *Morrison v. Burlington Indus.,* 282 S.E.2d 458 (N.C. 1981) (part).
9. 500 So. 2d 1102 (Ala. App. 1986).
10. *Id.* at 1103–04.
11. *See Yoshida v. General Constr. Co.,* No. AB 86-199 (WH) (9-80-01030) (Haw. Lab. & Indus. App. Bd. 1988), *summarized in* 31 ATLA L. Rep. 266 (1988).
12. *City of New Castle v. Workmen's Comp. App. Bd.,* 546 A.2d 132 (Pa. Commw. Ct. 1988).
13. 78 Or. App. 581, 717 P.2d 1202 (1986).
14. 717 P.2d at 1206. *See also Daniels v. Kalispel Regional Hosp.,* 750 P.2d 455 (Mont. 1988) (nurse sensitized to talc entitled to compensation).

15. 38 Colo. App. 261, 554 P.2d 1357 (1976).
16. *See e.g.*, *Alexander v. Unemployment Ins. App. Bd.*, 104 Cal. App. 3d 97, 163 Cal. Rptr. 411 (1980); *Ellis v. Iowa Dep't of Job Serv.*, 285 N.W.2d 153 (Iowa 1987).
17. 87 Or. App. 152, 741 P.2d 904 (1987).
18. 746 S.W.2d 796 (Tex. App. 1988).
19. La. Rev. Stat. tit. 23, §1601(10)(f) (West Supp. 1988).
20. 539 A.2d 1383 (Pa. Commw. Ct. 1988).
21. 29 U.S.C. §§1001–1461 (1988).
22. *Id.* §1140.
23. 594 F. Supp. 1007 (W.D. Mo. 1982).
24. *See generally* Vogel, *Containing Medical and Disability Costs by Cutting Unhealthy Employees: Does §510 of ERISA Provide a Remedy?*, 62 Notre Dame L. Rev. 1024 (1987).
25. Pub. L. 99-272, §§10001 to –02, 100 Stat. 82, §§222–227 (1986).
26. 26 U.S.C.A. §162(k) (West Supp. 1988).
27. 29 U.S.C.A. §§1161–1166 (West Supp. 1988).
28. *1988 Cobra Survey*, Spencer's Research Reports on Employee Benefits (July 1988), *reported in* Medical Benefits, Aug. 30, 1988, at 8.
29. 26 U.S.C.A. §89 (West Supp. 1988).
30. Pub. L. No. 99-514, §1151(a), 100 Stat. 2085, 2494 (1986).
31. 27 Ohio App. 3d 222, 500 N.E.2d 370 (1985).
32. 86 Or. App. 523, 739 P.2d 1083 (1987). *See Crocker v. Synpol, Inc.*, 732 S.W.2d 429 (Tex. App. 1987) (alleged nonconsensual urine drug test result released).
33. 65 Mich. App. 644, 237 N.W.2d 595 (1975). *Accord Sexton v. Petz*, 428 N.W.2d 715 (Mich. App. 1988).
34. 132 Ariz. 348, 645 P.2d 1262 (Ariz. App. 1982).
35. 785 F.2d 352 (1st Cir. 1986).
36. *Accord Eddy v. Brown*, 715 P.2d 74 (Okla. 1986), discussed in Chapter 1 under the heading "Medical Records."
37. *See Jeffers v. City of Seattle*, 23 Wash. App. 301, 597 P.2d 899 (1979).
38. 672 F. Supp. 473 (D. Kan. 1987).
39. 627 F. Supp. 418 (S.D.W. Va. 1986).
40. *Id.* at 420.
41. 41 FEP Cases 1273 (Mass. Super. Ct. 1986).
42. *Id.* at 1274.
43. *See Benassi v. Georgia Pac. Co.*, 62 Or. App. 698, 662 P.2d 760, *modified*, 63 Or. App. 672, 667 P.2d 532, *review denied*, 295 Or. 730, 670 P.2d 1035 (1983). *But see Eddy v. Brown*, 715 P.2d 74 (Okla. 1986).
44. 81 Mich. App. 279, 265 N.W.2d 124 (1978).
45. 81 Mich. App. at 282; 265 N.W.2d at 127. *See* Larson, *Defamation at the Workplace: Employers Beware*, 5 Hofstra Lab. L.J. 45 (1987).
46. *Welch v. Chicago Tribune Co.*, 34 Ill. App. 3d 1046, 340 N.E.2d 539 (1976).
47. *Hoover v. Peerless Publications, Inc.*, 461 F. Supp. 1206 (E.D. Pa. 1978).
48. 548 S.W.2d 743 (Tex. App. 1976), *appeal dismissed*, 434 U.S. 962 (1977).
49. 548 S.W.2d at 752.
50. 849 F.2d 41 (1st Cir. 1988).

51. *Roane v. Comair, Inc.*, No. 88CI670 (Boone County, Ky. Cir. Ct., Sept. 22, 1988), *reported in* 6 Empl. Rels. Weekly (BNA) 1241 (1988).
52. *See State Charges Comair Executives With Forcible Drug Tests on Employees*, 6 Empl. Rels. Weekly (BNA) 1384 (1988).
53. *See Doe v. Fort Lauderdale Med. Ctr. Mgmt., Inc.*, 522 So. 2d 80 (Fla. App. 1988) (alleged sexual battery during examination).
54. 8 Cal. 3d 551, 503 P.2d 1366, 105 Cal. Rptr. 358 (1972).
55. *Esters v. General Motors Corp.*, 246 Cal. Rptr. 566 (Cal. App. 1988); *Lesavoy v. Harnes*, 127 Misc. 2d 9, 484 N.Y.S.2d 988 (Sup. Ct. 1984); *Frank v. Durkee*, 141 Wis. 2d 172, 413 N.W.2d 667 (Wis. App. 1987); *Unger v. Continental Assurance Co.*, 122 Ill. App. 3d 376, 461 N.E.2d 531 (1984).
56. *LoDico v. Caputi*, 129 A.D.2d 361, 517 N.Y.S.2d 640 (App. Div. 1987).
57. *Davis v. Stover*, 258 Ga. 156, 366 S.E.2d 670 (1988).
58. *Snyder v. Liberty Mutual Ins. Co.*, 686 F. Supp. 525 (E.D. Pa. 1988); *Ray v. District of Columbia*, 535 A.2d 868 (D.C. 1987); *Craddock v. Gross*, 350 Pa. Super. 575, 504 A.2d 1300 (1986).
59. *Nash v. Oberman*, 117 A.D.2d 724, 498 N.Y.S.2d 449 (App. Div. 1986).
60. *Cottone v. County of Schenectady*, 134 Misc. 2d 805, 512 N.Y.S.2d 771 (Sup. Ct. 1987).
61. *See, e.g., Nolan v. Borkowski*, 206 Conn. 495, 538 A.2d 1031 (1988).
62. *See, e.g., Ewing v. St. Louis-Clayton Orthopedic Group, Inc.*, 790 F.2d 682 (8th Cir. 1986).
63. No. 86-L-773 (Will County, Ill. Circuit Ct., Apr. 22, 1988), *reported in* 31 ATLA L. Rep. 370 (1988).
64. Personal communication with Charles J. Reed, attorney for the plaintiff (Nov. 14, 1988).
65. 64 Ohio App. 2d 159, 411 N.E.2d 814 (1978).
66. *Accord Schouest v. Stipelcovich*, 490 So. 2d 294 (La. App.), *writ denied*, 495 So. 2d 304 (La. 1986).
67. *Millison v. E.I. du Pont de Nemours & Co.*, 226 N.J. Super. 572, 545 A.2d 213 (App. Div. 1988); *Johns-Manville Prods. Corp. v. Contra Costa Super. Court*, 27 Cal. 3d 465, 165 Cal. Rptr. 858 (1980).
68. *Downey v. Bexley*, 253 Ga. 125, 317 S.E.2d 523 (1984).
69. *See McGinn v. Valloti*, 363 Pa. Super. 88, 525 A.2d 732, *appeal denied*, 517 Pa. 618, 538 A.2d 500 (1987) (hand injury). *But see Ryherd v. Growmark, Inc.*, 156 Ill. App. 3d 667, 509 N.E.2d 113 (1987) (fraudulent concealment action for lung damage caused by chemicals barred by workers' compensation).
70. *Deller v. Naymick*, 342 S.E.2d 73 (W. Va. 1985).
71. *Kinloch v. Tonsey*, 325 Pa. Super. 476, 473 A.2d 167 (1984).
72. *Panaro v. Electrolux Corp.*, 208 Conn. 589, 545 A.2d 1086 (1988).
73. *Koslop v. Cabot Corp.*, 654 F. Supp. 1271 (M.D. Pa. 1987).
74. *King v. Penrod Drilling Co.*, 652 F. Supp. 1331 (D. Nev. 1987).
75. *Ducote v. Albert*, 521 So. 2d 399 (La. 1988).
76. *Firestein v. Kingsbrook Jewish Med. Center*, 137 A.D.2d 34, 528 N.Y.S.2d 85 (App. Div. 1988).
77. *Sterry v. Bethlehem Steel Corp.*, 64 Md. App. 175, 494 A.2d 748, *cert. denied*, 304 Md. 362, 499 A.2d 191 (1985).

78. *Catherwood v. American Sterilizer Co.*, 130 Misc. 2d 872, 498 N.Y.S.2d 703 (Sup. Ct. 1986).
79. *Security Nat'l Bank. v. Chloride, Inc.*, 602 F. Supp. 294 (D. Kan. 1985).
80. *Gray v. Stillman White Co.*, 522 A.2d 737 (R.I. 1987).
81. *See California Appeals Court Reinstates Negligence Claim in Fathers' DBCP Exposure*, 17 Occup. Safety & Health Rptr. (BNA) 1706 (1988).
82. *Adams v. Denny's, Inc.*, 464 So. 2d 876, *writ denied*, 467 So. 2d 530 (La. 1985) (wrongful death action not barred by workers' compensation).
83. *Fulford v. ITT Raynier, Inc.*, 676 F. Supp. 252 (S.D. Ga. 1987) (denying defendant's motion for summary judgment).
84. *Wharton Transp. Corp. v. Bridges*, 606 S.W.2d 521 (Tenn. 1980), discussed in Chapter 2 under the heading "Mandatory Examinations."
85. *Chesterman v. Barman*, 305 Or. 439, 753 P.2d 404 (1988), discussed in Chapter 6 under the heading "Drugs in the Workplace."
86. 806 F.2d 119 (7th Cir. 1986).
87. *Id.* at 123.

Chapter 10

1. Jain, *Employer-Sponsored Vision Care Brought Into Focus*, Monthly Lab. Rev., Sept. 1988, at 19.
2. Office of Technology Assessment, U.S. Congress, Medical Testing and Health Insurance 3 (1988) [hereinafter cited as Medical Testing].
3. S. Rep. 100-360, 100th Cong., 1st Sess. 20 (1988).
4. *Health Care Priorities in 1988: The Public's View*, Med. Benefits, Apr. 30, 1988, at 6 (reporting study by Gallup Organization, Inc., for the Federation of American Health Systems).
5. *U.S. Industrial Outlook 1988*, Med. Benefits, Feb. 15, 1988, at 1 (citing U.S. Department of Commerce data).
6. A. Foster Higgins & Co., Inc., Foster Higgins Health Care Benefits Survey, 1988, at 11 (1988).
7. *Id.* at 12–13.
8. Medical Testing, *supra* note 2, at 54.
9. A. Foster Higgins & Co., Foster Higgins Health Care Benefits Survey, 1987, at 21 (1987).
10. 471 U.S. 724 (1985).
11. *Id.* at 747 (footnote omitted).
12. *See* Rasmussen, *Mandated Coverage: An Employer Debate*, Bus. & Health, Apr. 1987, at 12; Stipp, *Laws on Health Benefits Raise Firms' Ire*, Wall St. J., Dec. 28, 1988, at B1, col. 3.
13. A. Foster Higgins & Co., Inc., *supra* note 9, at 52.
14. *Id.* at 53.
15. *Id.* at 54.
16. *Id.* at 54–55.
17. DeWitt, *Emerging Facets of Retiree Benefits*, Bus. & Health, Aug. 1988, at 8.
18. *Id.*
19. Bennett, *Firms Stunned by Retiree Health Costs*, Wall St. J., May 24, 1988, at 41, col. 3 (based on data from Tillinghast, Nelson & Warren).
20. *Id.*

21. De Witt, *supra* note 17.
22. *Id.*
23. *Id.* at 10.
24. Bennett, *supra* note 19.
25. Pub. L. 100-334 (1988).
26. *Employers Could Face $402 Billion in Accrued, Future Liabilities, GAO Says*, 6 Empl. Rels. Weekly (BNA) 1203 (1988) (citing testimony of Lawrence H. Thompson, Assistant Comptroller General, U.S. General Accounting Office). *See also* Atkins, *The Game Plan Changes for Retirees*, Bus. & Health, Aug. 1988, at 4, 5.
27. Kramon, *Limits Seen on Retiree Health Care*, N.Y. Times, Aug. 22, 1988, at 21, col. 6 29, col. 1.
28. Schmitt, *Retirees Fight Cuts in Health Benefits*, Wall St. J., Dec. 8, 1988, at B1, col. 3.
29. Noble, *Health Insurance Tied to Life Style*, N.Y. Times, Aug. 6, 1988, at 1, col. 5.
30. *See* Rundle, *Circle K's Effort to Curb AIDS Coverage Provides a Case Study in Bad Planning*, Wall St. J., Aug. 18, 1988, at 25, col. 3.
31. Noble, *Company Suspends Insurance Cutoff*, N.Y. Times, Aug. 12, 1988, at A6, col. 1.
32. *Concern Shifts on Medical Bills of AIDS Victims*, N.Y. Times, Sept. 18, 1988, at 16, col. 2.
33. Rundle, *supra* note 30.
34. *See* Jensen, Morrisey, & Marcus, *Cost Sharing and the Changing Pattern of Employer-Sponsored Health Benefits*, 65 Milbank Q. 521 (1987); Kramon, *Employees Paying Ever-Bigger Share of Medical Costs*, N.Y. Times, Nov. 22, 1988, at 1, col. 6; Short, *Trends in Employee Health Benefits*, 7 Health Affairs 186 (Summer 1988).
35. Rundle, *Insurers Step Up Efforts to Reduce Use of Free-Choice Health Plans*, Wall St. J., May 11, 1988, at 23, col. 4.
36. *See* Gabel, Jajich-Toth, de Lissovoy, et al., *The Changing World of Group Health Insurance*, 7 Health Affairs 48 (Summer 1988).
37. A. Foster Higgins & Co., Inc., *supra* note 9, at 28.
38. *Id.* at 29.
39. *Id.* at 27.
40. *Id.* at 36.
41. *Id.* at 37.
42. *Id.* at 46.
43. Medical Testing, *supra* note 2, at 57.
44. *Id.* at 69.
45. *Id.* at 73.
46. *Id.* at 124.
47. *Id.* at 72.
48. *Id.* at 63.
49. *Id.* at 47-48.
50. *Who Are the High Cost Cases in a Health Benefits Plan?*, Med. Benefits, Sept. 15, 1988, at 7 (study by International Foundation of Employee Benefit Plans, 1988).
51. *See e.g.*, Eakin, Gotay, Rademaker, et al., *Factors Associated With Enrollment in an Employee Fitness Center*, 30 J. Occup. Med. 633 (1988);

Fiedlding & Piserchia, *Frequency of Worksite Health Promotion Activities*, 79 Am. J. Pub. Health 16 (1989); Woodall, Higgins, Dunn, et al., *Characteristics of the Frequent Visitor to the Industrial Medical Department and Implications for Health Promotion*, 29 J. Occup. Med. 660 (1987).

52. *See e.g.*, Harris, Collins & Majure, *The Prevalence of Health Risks in an Employed Population*, 28 J. Occup. Med. 217 (1986); Leviton, *The Yield From Work Site Cardiovascular Risk Reduction*, 29 J. Occup. Med. 931 (1987); Pelletier & Lutz, *Healthy People—Healthy Business: A Critical Review of Stress Management Programs in the Workplace*, Am. J. Health Promotion, Winter 1988, at 5.

53. *See, e.g.*, Baun, Bernacki & Tsai, *A Preliminary Investigation: Effect of a Corporate Fitness Program on Absenteeism and Health Care Cost*, 28 J. Occup. Med. 18 (1986); Bowne, Russell, Morgan, et al., *Reduced Disability and Health Care Costs in an Industrial Fitness Program*, 26 J. Occup. Med. 809 (1984); Tsai, Baun & Bernacki, *Relationship of Employee Turnover to Exercise Adherence in a Corporate Fitness Program*, 29 J. Occup. Med. 572 (1987); Warner, Wickizer, Wolfe, et al., *Economic Implications of Workplace Health Promotion Programs: Review of the Literature*, 30 J. Occup. Med. 106 (1988).

54. *Corporate Wellness Programs: 1987 Biennial Survey Results*, Med. Benefits, Apr. 30, 1988, at 10, 11 (based on data from the Health Research Institute).

55. *Id.*

56. *See* Henderson, *Biomark Program Draws High-Tech Portraits of Employees' Health Risks*, Wash. Post, Mar. 17, 1986, at 1, 11, col. 1.

57. Hollander & Hale, *Worksite Health Promotion Programs: Ethical Issues*, Am. J. Health Promotion, Fall 1987, at 37, 40.

58. James, *Study Lays Groundwork for Tying Health Costs to Workers' Behavior*, Wall St. J., Apr. 14, 1987, at 35, col. 4.

59. *Id.*

60. *See* Kramon, *What's New in Employee Health Plans*, N.Y. Times, July 19, 1987, at F 19, col. 1.

61. S. Rep. 100-360, 100th Cong., 1st Sess., at 20 (1988).

62. *Id.*

63. *Id.*

64. *See* Barnett, *Health Insurers Dropping Small Firms*, Houston Chronicle, Nov. 6, 1988, at 1G, col. 1; Ricklefs, *Health Insurance Becomes a Big Pain for Small Firms*, Wall St. J., Dec. 6, 1988, at B1, col. 3.

65. Hawaii Rev. Stat., tit. 21, §§393-1 to -51 (1985).

66. Southwick, *Despite Law, Many Hawaii Residents Lack Health Benefits*, Health Week, July 5, 1988.

67. Massachusetts Health Security Act of 1988, Mass. Gen. Laws ch. 23 (1988). *See generally* Mazer & Danielson, *A Health Security Program for Massachusetts*, 7 J. Health Pol'y 440 (1986); Sager, *Prices of Equitable Access: The New Massachusetts Health Insurance Law*, Hastings Center Rep., June/July 1988, at 21.

68. Egan, *A State Offers Working Poor Insurance Aid*, N.Y. Times, Jan. 3, 1989, at 1, col. 1.

69. S. 1265, 100th Cong., 1st Sess. (1988).

70. Toner, *Health Insurance and Political Hoopla*, N.Y. Times, Apr. 22, 1988, at A8, col. 4.
71. *Minimum Health Benefits for All Workers Act of 1987*, 100th Cong., 1st Sess., pt. 1, at 24–28 (1987) (statement of Robert L. Crandall, Chairman and President of American Airlines) [hereinafter cited as *Hearings*].
72. *See* Gajda, *Insuring All Employees Could Kill the Company*, Wall St. J., Aug. 14, 1987, at 12, col. 4.
73. *Hearings, supra* note 71, pt. 2, at 28 (statement of Dr. Karen Davis of John Hopkins University).
74. *Kennedy Bill Moves to Full Senate*, Med. Benefits, Mar. 30, 1988, at 1.
75. D. Walsh, Corporate Physicians 196 (1987) (references omitted).

Chapter 11

1. *Drug Testing Upheld, Decried: Physicians Asked to Help Decide*, 259 J.A.M.A. 2341 (1988) (quoting G. Harrison Darby).
2. *Abbye Empl. Agency v. Robinson*, 166 Misc. 820, 824, 2 N.Y.S.2d 947, 952 (App. Div. 1938).
3. *See, e.g.*, Epstein, *In Defense of the Contract at Will*, 51 U. Chi. L. Rev. 947 (1984).
4. Linzer, *The Decline of Assent: At-Will Employment as a Case Study of the Breakdown of Private Law Theory*, 20 Ga. L. Rev. 323, 414–15 (1986). *See also* Finkin, *"In Defense of the Contract at Will"—Some Discussion Comments and Questions*, 50 J. Air. L. & Commerce 727 (1985).
5. *See OCAW v. American Cyanamid Co.*, 741 F.2d 444 (D.C. Cir. 1984).
6. Weiss, *Watch Out: Urine Trouble*, Harper's, June 1986, at 56, 57.
7. *See* Atherly, *Human Rights Versus Occupational Medicine*, 13 Int'l J. Health Servs. 265 (1983).
8. Derr, *Ethical Considerations in Fitness and Risk Evaluations*, 3 Occup. Med.: State of the Art Revs. 193, 196 (1988) (footnote omitted).
9. Fla. Stat. Ann. §448.075 (West 1981) (sickle cell); La. Rev. Stat. Ann. §23:1001–04 (West 1985) (sickle cell); N.J. Stat. Ann. §10:5-5 (y through cc) (West Supp. 1987) (sickle cell, hemoglobin C, thalassemia, Tay-Sachs, cystic fibrosis); N.C. Gen. Stat. §95-28.1 (Michie 1987) (sickle cell and hemoglobin C).
10. Cal. Health & Safety Code §§199.21(f) & 199.38 (West Supp. 1988); Del. H.B. 136 (1988); Fla. Stat. Ann. §381. 606(5) (1985); Iowa H.F. 2344 (1988); Mass. Ann. Laws §70E (Law. Co-op. Supp. 1988); R.I. Pub. L. 88-405 (1988); Tex. Civ. Stat. Ann. art. 4419b-1.5 (Vernon Supp. 1988); Vt. H.B. 239 (1988); Wash. Acts ch. 206 (1988); Wis. Stat. Ann. §§103.15(2)(a), (2)(b), (3) (West Supp. 1987). A number of cities, including Los Angeles, Los Angeles code art. 5.8, §§45.80–45.93 (1987), and San Francisco, San Francisco Police Code §§3801–3816 (1985), also prohibit the use of HIV testing in employment.
11. Conn. Pub. Act. No. 87-551 (West App. Pamph. 1987); Iowa Stat. Ann. §730.5 (West Supp. 1987); Kan. H.B. 1618 (1988); Minn. Stat. Ann. §§181.950–57 (West Supp. 1988); Mont. Code Ann. tit. 39, §2-304 (1987); Neb. Legis. Bill No. 582 (1988); R.I. Gen. Laws §§28-6.5-1 to -2 (1987); Utah Code Ann. §§34-38-1 to -15 (Michie 1987); Vt. Stat. Ann. tit. 21, §§511–520 (1987).

12. S. 2345, H.R. 4498, 100th Cong., 2d Sess. (1988).
13. TRB, *Listen to Your Genes*, New Republic, Aug. 11, 18, 1986, at 4.
14. 29 U.S.C. §206 (1988).
15. 40 U.S.C. §§276a to a-5 (1988).
16. H.R. Rep. No. 88-914, 88th Cong., 2d Sess. (Nov. 20, 1963), in 1964 U.S. Code Cong. & Admin. News 2355, 2513-17.
17. Pub. L. 99-603, 100 Stat. 3359, 1986 U.S. Code Cong. & Admin. News 5649.
18. *See* Reinhardt, *Toward a Fail-Safe Health-Insurance System*, Wall St. J., Jan. 11, 1989, at A16, col. 3.
19. *See, e.g.*, Cyphert & Rohrer, *A National Medical Care Program: Review and Synthesis of Past Proposals,* 9 J. Pub. Health Pol'y 456 (1988); Himmelstein & Woolhandler, *A National Health Program for the United States,* 320 New Eng. J. Med. 102 (1989).
20. *See, e.g,.* Brown, *Canadian, U.S. Systems Face Off*, Med. World News, Aug. 22, 1988, at 76; Evans, *Health Care in Canada: Patterns of Funding and Regulation,* 8 J. Health Politics, Pol'y & L. 1 (1983); Iglehart, *Canada's Health Care System,* 315 New Eng. J. Med. 202 (1986); Relman, *The United States and Canada: Different Approaches to Health Care,* 315 New Eng. J. Med. 1608 (1986).
21. Walker, *Neighborly Advice on Health Care*, Wall St. J., June 8, 1988, at 20, col. 3.
22. Malloy, *Health Canadian Style*, Wall St. J., Apr. 22, 1988, at 21R, col. 1. *See generally* Stevenson, Williams, & Vayda, *Medicare: Professional Response to the Canada Health Act,* 66 Milbank Q. 65 (1988).
23. Iglehart, *supra* note 20, at 205–06.
24. Walker, *supra* note 21.
25. *See generally* Council on Medical Service, American Medical Association, *Protecting the Uninsured: Use of State Risk Pools*, 260 J.A.M.A. 373 (1988); Laudicina, *State Health Risk Pools: Insuring the "Uninsurable,"* 7 Health Affairs 97 (Fall 1988); Tresnowski, *Use of State Risk-Pools in Protecting the Uninsured,* 260 J.A.M.A. 389 (1988).
26. *See generally* Wilensky, *Filling the Gaps in Health Insurance: Impact on Competition,* 7 Health Affairs 133 (Summer 1988).
27. *See, e.g.,* Hayward, Shapiro, Freeman, et al., *Inequities in Health Services Among Insured Americans*, 318 New Eng. J. Med. 1507 (1988).
28. Smith, *The Battle Over Health Insurance*, Fortune, Sept. 26, 1988, at 145 (quoting Sharon Canner, Assistant Vice President of the National Association of Manufacturers).

Glossary of Medical, Scientific, and Health Care Terms

Note: The following are nontechnical definitions for laypersons geared to the context of this book.

absolute risk—the observed or calculated risk of an event in a population under study, as contrasted with the relative risk.

achondroplastic dwarfism—most common type of dwarf; characterized by short limbs, normal trunk, large head with small face, trident hands, and lordosis.

acrophobia—pathological fear or dread of high places.

adult polycystic kidney disease—progressive condition in which the kidneys are enlarged and contain many cysts; eventually may cause kidney failure, uremia, and death.

allele—one of two or more alternative forms of a gene that occupy corresponding places on homologous chromosomes.

alpha$_1$ antitrypsin deficiency—lack of the serum protein that protects the lung from proteolytic enzymes; genetic trait correlated with susceptibility to emphysema.

analgesic—drug that relieves pain; may be narcotic or nonnarcotic.

antihistamine—substance that minimizes effects of histamine, which is a compound released in allergic or inflammatory reactions.

asbestosis—chronic lung disease caused by inhaling asbestos fibers.

ataxia—impaired ability to coordinate voluntary body movements.

atherosclerosis—disorder characterized by formation of plaque on inner layers of artery walls.

AZT—(azidothymidine)—also zidovudine—anti-viral medication used in the treatment of AIDS.

barbiturate—a salt or derivative of barbituric acid, used as a sedative or to deaden pain.

benzodiazepine—any of a group of minor tranquilizers used to treat anxiety, insomnia, and muscle spasms.

bronchitis—acute or chronic inflammation of tracheobronchial tree.

bronchoscopy—examination of the bronchi by use of a tube-like instrument placed down the throat.

cannabinoid—hallucinogenic substance made from the cannabis or hemp plant, including marijuana and hashish.

275

carpal tunnel syndrome—painful disorder of the wrist and hand resulting from compression of the median nerve in the carpal tunnel; often caused by repetitive motion.

chlamydia—intracellular parasite responsible for a variety of diseases, including sexually transmitted diseases.

chorioretinitis—inflammation of the choroid and retina of the eye.

conjunctivitis—inflammation of the lining of the eyelid.

contact dermatitis—skin rash resulting from exposure to an irritant or sensitizing antigen.

Crohn's disease—chronic inflammatory bowel diesease of unknown origin.

cystic fibrosis—cogenital disease characterized by an abnormal increase in the amount of connective tissue in an organ, malfunctioning of the pancreas, and frequent respiratory infections.

cytogenetic—the branch of genetics concerned with the structure and function of the cell, especially the chromosomes, the structures in the cell nucleus that store and transmit genetic information.

DBCP—(dibromochloropropane)—liquid pesticide known to cause sterility, birth defects, and cancer.

DES—(diethylstilbestrol)—synthetic nonsteroidal estrogen associated with increased risk of vaginal and cervical carcinoma.

diabetes mellitus—chronic form of diabetes characterized by excess sugar in blood and urine, resulting from a lack of insulin.

DNA—(deoxyribonucleic acid)—genetic material in the chromosomes of all cells.

DRG—(diagnostic related group)—system used to classify medical services by diagnosis for purpose of reimbursement.

Duchenne muscular dystrophy—congenital condition characterized by progressive, symmetric wasting of leg and pelvic muscles.

dyslexia—impairment of the ability to read.

ELISA—(enzyme-linked immunosorbent assay)—blood screening test used to detect antibodies to HIV.

emphysema—abnormal condition of pulmonary system characterized by over-inflation and destructive changes of alveolar walls.

epicondylitis—"tennis elbow"; inflammation of muscle and tissue surrounding the elbow.

epidemiology—study of the prevalence and spread of disease, especially infectious and epidemic diseases.

epilepsy—chronic disease of nervous system characterized by seizures caused by disturbance of electrical activity of the brain.

femoral—relating to the thigh bone (femur).

GC/MS—(gas chromotography/mass spectrometry)—analytical technique used to identify substances by sorting a stream of charged ions; standard confirmatory test for drug screening.

gene—the fundamental physical and functional unit of heredity; an ordered sequence of nucleotides located in a particular position on a particular chromosome.

genome—all the genetic material in the chromosomes of a particular organism; its size is generally given as its total number of base pairs.

glaucoma—a disease of the eye characterized by increased tension within and hardening of, the eyeball.

G-6-PD deficiency—(glucose-6-phosphate dehydrogenase deficiency)—a genetic red blood cell condition characterized by an enzyme deficiency which can result in anemia.

glutathione (GSH)—enzyme whose deficiency is commonly associated with hemolytic anemia.

hemiplegia—paralysis of one side of the body.

hemolytic—causing or characterized by hemolysis, which is the destruction of red corpuscles.

hemophilia—group of hereditary bleeding disorders in which there is a deficiency of coagulation Factor VIII, necessary for blood coagulation.

HIV—(human immunodeficiency virus)—virus associated with AIDS.

HMO—(health maintenance organization)—group health care practice providing health maintenance and treatment services to voluntary enrollees who prepay a fixed periodic fee.

Huntington's disease—"Huntington's chorea"—hereditary disease characterized by chronic progressive chorea (involuntary, rapid motions) and mental deterioration.

hypercholesterolemia—condition in which greater than normal amounts of cholesterol are present in the blood.

hypersensitivity pneumonitis—lung inflammation triggered by inhalation of antigen (allergen) dust.

hypertension—abnormally high blood pressure or a disease condition of which this is the chief symptom.

immunoassay—analytical technique based on immunological principles.

intertriginous—relating to irritation of opposing skin surfaces caused by friction; common sites include axillae (armpits) and inner aspects of thighs.

Kaposi's sarcoma—rare dermal malignancy often associated with AIDS.

lupus—lupus erythematosus (systemic)—generalized connective tissue disorder affecting skin, blood vessels, kidneys, and other systems of the body.

lymphadenopathy—inflammation of the lymph nodes.

lymphocytic leukemia—acute lymphocytic leukemia—progressive malignant disease of the blood characterized by the appearance in the lymph tissue of excessive numbers of white cells and abnormal cells.

manic-depressive—person with a psychosis characterized by alternating periods of mania and melancholia or depression.

melanoma—a type of skin cancer.

meningococcal septicemia—blood poisoning caused by *Neisseria meningitides*.

mescaline—psychoactive, poisonous alkaloid, which produces hallucinations; also called peyote.

mesothelioma—asbestos-caused cancer, developing from the cells of the pleura (membrane enveloping the lungs), peritoneum (serous sac lining abdominal cavity), or pericardium (membrane around the heart).

methadone—synthetic narcotic analgesic, often used in treatment of heroin addiction.

methamphetamine—"speed"—central nervous system stimulant.

methaqualone—"qualudes"—powerful depressant; a sedative and hypnotic.

methemoglobin—form of hemoglobin in which the iron component has been oxidized and cannot carry oxygen.

multiple myeloma—malignant tumor of the bone marrow.

multiple sclerosis—chronic disease in which there is sclerosis (hardening of body tissues) in various parts of the nervous system; characterized by muscle weakness and tremor.

muscular dystrophy—genetic disease characterized by progressive atrophy of skeletal muscles.

mutagen—substance able to produce mutations or changes in the genetic material of living cells.

neoplasm—a cellular outgrowth characterized by rapid cell multiplication; may be benign or malignant.

neurofibromatosis—congenital condition characterized by numerous fibrous tumors of the nerves and skin.

nucleotide—subunit of DNA or RNA; thousands of nucleotides form DNA or RNA molecules.

opiate—narcotic drug containing or derived from opium.

opportunistic infection—infection caused by normally nonpathogenic organisms in a host whose resistance has been decreased by illness or surgery.

osteoarthritis—noninflammatory degenerative joint disease.

osteophyte—small bony outgrowth.

paranoid schizophrenic—person with a psychotic disorder characterized by persistent delusions, usually of a grandiose, persecutory, or jealous nature.

Parkinson's disease—degenerative disease of later life, characterized by rhythmic tremor and muscular rigidity.

pathology—study of the characteristics, courses, and effects of disease as observed in the structure and function of the body.

PCP—(phencyclidine)—potent analgesic and anesthetic with hallucinogenic properties.

phobia—anxiety disorder characterized by an obsessive, irrational, and intense fear of a specific object, activity, or situation.

PKU—(phenylketonuria)—inborn metabolic disorder caused by the absence or deficiency of the enzyme phenylalanine hydroxylase.

pneumoconiosis—any lung disease caused by chronic inhalation of dust, usually mineral dust of occupational or environmental origin.

polymorphism—difference in DNA sequence among individuals.

PPO—(preferred provider organization)—group of physicians, hospitals, and pharmacists whose members discount their health care services to subscribers.

prophylactic chelation—treatment with a chelating agent to prevent metal poisoning.

pseudofolliculitis barbae—condition caused by ingrown beard stubble; aggravated by shaving.

recombinant DNA—a DNA molecule in which rearrangement of the genes has been artificially induced.

relative risk—the ratio of the risk of disease or death among the exposed to the risk among the unexposed.

renal—relating to the kidney or kidneys.

restriction fragment length polymorphism (RFLP)—variation in DNA fragment sizes cut by restriction enzymes; polymorphic sequences that are responsible for RFLPs are used as markers on genetic linkage maps.

retinitis pigmentosa—hereditary disease of the retina, marked by progressive withering of the nerve cells, a deterioration of blood vessels, and a wasting of the optic disk.

retinoblastoma—hereditary neoplasm arising from retinal germ cells.

sarcoidosis—chronic disorder of unknown origin involving almost any organ or tissue, characterized by the formation of epitheloid cell tubercles.

scoliosis—lateral curvature of the spine.

somatic—all cells of the body except germ cells.

spina bifida—congenital defect characterized by imperfect closure of the spinal column exposing some of the nervous system.

spondylolisthesis—forward displacement of one vertebra over another, usually due to a developmental defect.

spondylolysis—a displacement of the vertebrae due to degenerative joint disease.

strabismus—crossed eyes.

Tay Sachs disease—hereditary condition caused by an enzyme deficiency and characterized by mental retardation, paralysis, and death in early childhood.

teratogen—a drug or other agent that causes abnormal development of the fetus.

thalassemia—any of a group of inherited disorders of hemoglobin metabolism with varying clinical conditions.

varicose vein—vein that is abnormally and irregularly swollen or dilated.

Wasserman test—diagnostic blood test for syphilis.

western blot—confirmatory test used in detecting presence of antibodies to HIV.

Glossary of Legal Terms

Note: *The following are nontechnical definitions for laypersons geared to the context of this book.*

action—legal action or lawsuit.

ADEA—Age Discrimination in Employment Act.

affirmative action—policy or program for correcting effects of past discrimination or for preventing future discrimination.

aggrieved individual—a person whose legal right has been invaded.

amicus curiae—literally friend of the court; a person with a strong interest in or views on an issue before the court who is granted permission to file a brief with the court.

assumption of risk—a defense to a negligence or other tort action; where the plaintiff knowingly assumes the risk of potential injury through the fault of no one or of someone else.

"at-will" doctrine—common law doctrine giving the employer the right to fire employees for any or no reason.

BFOQ—bona fide occupational qualification; statutory defense to Title VII case permitting employers to differentiate on the basis of religion, sex, or national origin when necessary to the normal operation of the business.

business necessity—a defense to an employment discrimination case; a legitimate business purpose so compelling as to override any adverse impact resulting from such practice.

certiorari—a discretionary writ giving a superior court the jurisdiction to review the decision of an inferior court; an appeal.

civil—as distinguished from criminal; relating to the private rights of individuals and to legal actions involving these rights.

common law—body of rules and principles established over time by usage and custom or from the judgments or decrees of the courts.

compensatory damages—money judgment to replace the loss suffered by the plaintiff.

constructive discharge—employer practices making working conditions so intolerable that the employee is forced to quit the job.

contributory negligence—a defense to a negligence or other tort action; act or omission on the part of the complaining party which amounts to lack of ordinary care.

covenant—agreement, convention, or promise; may be expressed or implied by law.

declaratory relief—determination or decision by the court that establishes the legal rights of the parties but that does not order enforcement of those rights.

281

defamation—general term for a communication that tends to injure a person's reputation; includes the torts of libel and slander.

dignitary torts—general term for wrongful acts causing injury to a person's dignity, reputation, or emotional well being; includes the torts of defamation, invasion of privacy, and infliction of emotional distress.

disparate impact—theory of employment discrimination asserting that facially neutral criteria exlude members of a protected group at a disproportionate rate.

disparate treatment—theory of employment discrimination asserting that differences or distinctions in the treatment of individuals in a statutorily protected group are unlawful discrimination.

due process—constitutional guaranty that laws not be unreasonable, arbitrary, or capricious and that legal proceedings be conducted in accordance with established rules and principles.

EEOC—Equal Employment Opportunity Commission; federal agency charged with administering Title VII of the Civil Rights Act of 1964 and the Age Discrimination in Employment Act.

equal protection—constitutional guaranty that equal treatment under the law be afforded to all persons under like circumstances.

false imprisonment—intentional tort of confinement or otherwise interfering with a person's freedom of movement without legal authority.

fellow servant rule—common law rule that the employer is not liable for injuries to an employee caused by the negligence of a fellow employee.

implied contract—contractual relationship by operation of law based on the circumstances and conduct of the parties.

indemnity—an order shifting the entire legal responsibility for a loss from one wrongdoer to another.

informed consent—agreement to allow a medical procedure to be performed, based on full disclosure of facts needed to make the decision.

injunction—a writ or order issued by a court requiring a party to do or refrain from doing a particular thing.

intentional infliction of emotional distress—intentional tort involving extreme and outrageous conduct intended to cause severe emotional distress.

intentional tort—wrongful act performed with desire to injure or with substantial certainty that harm will result.

invasion of privacy—tort of unreasonable interference with a person's solitude or personalty; includes intrusion into seclusion or affairs, public disclosure of private facts, appropriation of name or likeness, and placing a person in false light.

job-relatedness—defense to Title VII cases; use of selection criteria significantly correlated with essential elements of the job.

libel—defamatory statement in writing or some other permanent form.

malpractice—professional negligence.

mandatory subject of bargaining—matter that, by statute, must be negotiated and that may not be changed unilaterally by either an employer or a union prior to bargaining.

Medicaid—program, sponsored jointly by federal and state governments, providing medical aid for low income people.

medical removal protection (MRP)—an employee showing symptoms of adverse effects of exposure to a toxic substance is removed from further exposure until it is medically advisable to return.

Medicare—system of government insurance providing medical and hospital care for the aged and disabled, paid from federal Social Security funds.

negligence—an act which a reasonably prudent person would not perform, or an omission of what a reasonably prudent person would do.

negligent infliction of emotional distress—tort where a negligent act causes mental disturbance in another; generally requires some other independent basis for tort liability.

NIOSH—National Institute for Occupational Safety and Health; part of U.S. Department of Health and Human Services responsible for research on job safety and health matters.

NLRA—National Labor Relations Act.

NLRB—National Labor Relations Board; independent agency charged with enforcement and adjudication under the NLRA.

OFCCP—Office of Federal Contract Compliance Programs; part of U.S. Department of Labor charged with enforcing legal obligations of government contractors, including section 503 of the Rehabilitation Act.

OSHA—Occupational Safety and Health Administration; federal agency charged with administering the Occupational Safety and Health Act of 1970.

otherwise qualified—able to perform the essential requirements of a job despite handicap.

perjury—false statement made willfully under oath.

private action—lawsuit brought by a nongovernmental entity or individual.

privilege—exemptions from tort liability when the action taken was in performance of political, judicial, social, public, or personal duty.

products liability—area of torts concerning the liability of a supplier of products or goods to one injured by the products or goods.

public policy exception to the at-will rule—allows an at-will employee to bring a tort action where his or her discharge violates a clearly expressed public policy.

punitive damages—exemplary damages; increased damages awarded for extreme actions by the defendant to punish the wrongdoer and to deter future misconduct.

rate retention (RR)—maintenance of wage benefit levels during a period of medical removal.

reasonable accommodation—affirmative obligation imposed by handicap discrimination laws to accommodate the physical and mental limitations of employees and applicants unless it would impose an undue burden on the conduct of the business.

regulation—guidelines or rules issued by various governmental departments or agencies to carry out the intent of the law.

rulemaking—legal process by which administrative rules are promulgated.

slander—defamatory statement by spoken word.

standard (OSHA)—regulation specifying required methods of eliminating workplace safety or health hazard.

strict liability—tort liability not based on negligence or fault; legal theory permitting injured party to recover from responsible party for personal injury and property damage caused by wild animals, ultrahazardous activities (e.g., blasting), and defective products based on the fair and efficient allocation of risks and other policies.

summary judgment—motion granted when movant can demonstrate that there is no genuine issue (dispute) of material fact and that movant is entitled to prevail as a matter of law.

Title VII—part of the Civil Rights Act of 1964 prohibiting discrimination in employment based on race, color, religion, sex, or national origin.

tort—a private or civil wrong, independent of a contract, arising from a violation of a duty.

Table of Cases
Mentioned in Text

A

American Motors Corp. v. Labor & Industry Review Commission, 119 Wis. 2d 706, 350 N.W.2d 120 (1984) 157

American National Insurance Co. v. Fair Employment & Housing Commission, 32 Cal. 3d 603, 651 P.2d 1151, 186 Cal. Rptr. 345 (1982) 153

American Textile Manufacturers' Institute, Inc. v. Donovan, 452 U.S. 490 (1981) 169

Armstrong v. Morgan, 545 S.W.2d 45 (Tex. Civ. App. 1977) 165

B

Barnes v. Barbosa, 144 Ill. App. 3d 860, 494 N.E.2d 619 (1986) 156

Bayport-Blue Point School District v. State Division of Human Rights, 131 A.D.2d 849, 517 N.Y.S.2d 209 (App. Div. 1987) 154

Becker v. R.E. Cooper Corp., No. 86-L-773 (Will County, Ill. Circuit Ct., April 22, 1988), *reported in* 31 ATLA L. Rep. 370 (1988) 192

Bentivegna v. United States Department of Labor, 694 F.2d 619 (9th Cir. 1982) 150

Blitz v. Northwest Airlines, Inc., 363 N.W.2d 94 (Minn. App. 1985) 146

Board of Trustees v. Human Rights Commission, 138 Ill. App. 3d 71, 485 N.E.2d 33 (1985) 146

Boynton Cab Co. v. Department Of Industry, Labor & Human Relations, 96 Wis. 2d 396, 291 N.W.2d 850 (1980) 146

Bratt v. International Business Machines Corp., 785 F.3d 352 (1st Cir. 1986) 188

Brown v. City of Portland, 80 Or. App. 464, 722 P.2d 1282 (1986), *rev. denied*, 302 Or. 460, 730 P.2d 1250 (1986) 130

Burka v. New York City Transit Authority, 680 F. Supp. 59 (S.D.N.Y. 1988) 115

C

California Federal Savings & Loan Association v. Guerra, 479 U.S. 272 (1987) 177

Carr v. General Motors Corp., 425 Mich. 313, 389 N.W.2d 686 (1986) 133

Carrero v. New York City Housing Authority, 116 A.D.2d 141, 500 N.Y.S.2d 246 (App. Div. 1986) 156

Carter v. Casa Central, 849 F.2d 1048 (7th Cir. 1988) 154

Casias v. Industrial Commission, 30 Colo. App. 261, 554 P.2d 1357 (1976) 183

Chalk v. United States District Court, 840 F.2d 701 (9th Cir. 1988) 88

Chaney v. Southern Railway, 847 F.2d 718 (11th Cir. 1988) 178

Chesterman v. Barman, 305 Or. 439, 753 P.2d 404 (1988) 100

Chevron Corp. v. Redmon, 745 S.W.2d 314 (Tex. 1987) 131

Chrysler Outboard Corp. v. Department of Industry, Labor & Human Relations, 14 FEP Cases 344 (Wis. Cir. Ct. 1976) 143, 149

Clarke v. Shoreline School District,
106 Wash. 2d 560, 720 P.2d 793
(1986)   158

Coffee v. McDonnell-Douglas Corp.,
8 Cal. 3d 551, 503 P.2d 1366, 105
Cal. Rptr. 358 (1972)   191

Coleman v. Safeway Stores, Inc., 242
Kan. 804, 752 P.2d 645
(1988)   165

Commonwealth v. Pennsylvania
Human Relations Commission,
512 Pa. 534, 517 A.2d 1253
(1986)   215

Consolidation Coal Co. v. Ohio Civil
Rights Commission, 473 N.E.2d
325 (Ohio C.P. 1981)   141

Crane v. Dole, 617 F. Supp. 156
(D.D.C. 1985)   134

Cronan v. New England Telephone
Co., 41 FEP Cases 1273 (Mass.
Super. Ct. 1986)   189

D

Dauten v. County of Muskegon, 128
Mich. App. 435, 340 N.W.2d 117
(1983)   142

Davidson v. United States
Department of Energy, 838 F.2d
850 (6th Cir. 1988)   40

Davis v. Monsanto, 627 F. Supp. 418
(S.D.W. Va. 1986)   188

Davis v. United States Postal Service,
675 F. Supp. 225 (M.D. Pa.
1987)   152

Delamotte v. Unitcast Division of
Midland Ross & Co., 64 Ohio
App. 2d 159, 411 N.E.2d 814
(1978)   192

de la Torres v. Bolger, 781 F.2d 1134
(5th Cir. 1986)   159

Dexler v. Tisch, 660 F. Supp. 1418
(D. Conn. 1987)   157

E

Eddy v. Brown, 715 P.2d 74 (Okla.
1986)   19

F

Father Flanagan's Boys' Home v.
Goerke, 224 Neb. 731, 401
N.W.2d 461 (1987)   142

Fitzgerald v. Green Valley Area
Education Agency, 589 F. Supp.
1130 (S.D. Iowa 1984)   154

Folz v. Marriott Corp., 594 F. Supp.
1007 (W.D. Mo. 1982)   185

Foods, Inc. v. Iowa Civil Rights
Commission, 318 N.W.2d 162
(Iowa 1982)   151

Forrisi v. Bowen, 794 F.2d 931 (4th
Cir. 1986)   131

G

Gargiul v. Tompkins, 704 F.2d 661
(2d Cir. 1983), *vacated and
remanded on other grounds*, 465
U.S. 1016 (1984)   161

Glide Lumber Products Co. v.
Employment Division, 87 Or.
App. 152, 741 P.2d 904
(1987)   183

Grusendorf v. City of Oklahoma City,
816 F.2d 539 (10th Cir. 1987)
64, 161

Gurmankin v. Costanzo, 556 F.2d 184
(3d Cir. 1977), *cert. denied*, 450
U.S. 923 (1981)   158

H

Halsey v. Coca-Cola Bottling Co., 410
N.W.2d 250 (Iowa 1987)   133

Harless v. Duck, 619 F.2d 611 (6th
Cir.), *cert. denied*, 449 U.S. 877
(1980)   170

Harriss v. Pan American World
Airways, Inc., 649 F.2d 670 (9th
Cir. 1980)   177

Higgins v. Maine Central Railroad,
471 A.2d 288 (Me. 1984)   143

Hinthorn v. Roland's of Bloomington,
Inc., 119 Ill. 2d 526, 519 N.E.2d
909 (1988)   164

Homer v. Pabst Brewing Co., 806
F.2d 119 (7th Cir. 1986)   194

Houston Belt & Terminal Railway v.
    Wherry, 548 S.W.2d 743 (Tex.
    App. 1976), *appeal dismissed*, 434
    U.S. 962 (1977)   190

I

International Paper Co. v. Rogers, 500
    So. 2d 1102 (Ala. App.
    1986)   182

J

Jansen v. Food Circus Supermarkets,
    Inc., 110 N.J. 363, 541 A.2d 682
    (1988)   135, 142

K

Kelley v. Bechtel Power Corp., 633
    F. Supp. 927 (S.D. Fla.
    1986)   150
Kelly v. Schlumberger Technology
    Corp., 849 F.2d 41 (1st Cir.
    1988)   190
Khalifa v. G.X. Corp., 408 N.W.2d
    221 (Minn. App. 1987)   176
Kost Brothers, Inc., 86 LA 65
    (Berquist, 1986)   173

L

Laclede Cab Co. v. Missouri
    Commission on Human Rights,
    748 S.W.2d 390 (Mo. App.
    1988)   143, 146
LaCross, City of, Police & Fire
    Commission v. Labor & Industry
    Review Commission, 139 Wis. 2d
    740, 407 N.W.2d 510 (1987)   147
Leggett v. First Interstate Bank, 86
    Or. App. 523, 739 P.2d 1083
    (1987)   187
Levias v. United Airlines, 27 Ohio
    App. 3d 222, 500 N.E.2d 370
    (1985)   19, 187
Lockheed Shipbuilding &
    Construction Co., 73 N.L.R.B.
    No. 25 (1984)   170

Luck v. Southern Pacific
    Transportation Co., No. 843230
    (San Francisco, Cal. Super. Ct.,
    October 30, 1987)   166

M

McCleod v. City of Detroit, 9 FEP
    Cases 225 (E.D. Mich.
    1985)   115
Maine Human Rights Commission v.
    Canadian Pacific, Ltd., 458 A.2d
    1225 (Me. 1983)   152
Mass Transit Administration v.
    Maryland Commission on Human
    Relations, 68 Md. App. 703, 515
    A.2d 781 (1986)   153
Merritt v. Detroit Memorial Hospital,
    81 Mich. App. 279, 265 N.W.2d
    124 (1978)   189
Metropolitan Life Insurance Co. v.
    Massachusetts, 471 U.S. 724
    (1985)   198
Micu v. City of Warren, 147 Mich.
    App. 573, 382 N.W.2d 823
    (1985)   133
Moreland v. Department of
    Corrections, 166 Ill. App. 3d
    1040, 520 N.E.2d 1227
    (1988)   166

N

Nelson v. Thornburgh, 567 F. Supp.
    369 (E.D. Pa. 1983), *aff'd*, 732
    F.2d 146 (3d Cir. 1984), *cert.
    denied*, 469 U.S. 1188
    (1985)   138, 158

O

Oesterling v. Walters, 760 F.2d 859
    (8th Cir. 1985)   158
OFCCP v. E.E. Black, Ltd., 19 FEP
    Cases 1624 (U.S. Dep't of Labor
    1979)   128
Olson v. Western Airlines, Inc., 143
    Cal. App. 3d 1, 191 Cal. Rptr.
    502 (1983)   165

P

Pearson Candy Co. v. Huyen, 373
N.W.2d 377 (Minn. App.
1985)   137

Prewitt v. United States Postal
Service, 662 F.2d 292 (5th Cir.
1981)   139

Price v. Carmack Datsun, Inc., 109
Ill. 2d 65, 485 N.E.2d 359
(1985)   164

Q

Quinn v. Southern Pacific
Transportation Co., 76 Or. App.
617, 711 P.2d 139 (1985)   134

R

Rezza v. United States Department of
Justice, 46 FEP Cases 1366 (E.D.
Pa. 1988)   156

Redmond v. City of Overland Park,
672 F. Supp. 473 (D. Kan.
1987)   188

Robinson v. SAIF Corp., 78 Or. App.
581, 717 P.2d 1202 (1986)   182

Rogers v. Horvath, 65 Mich. App.
644, 237 N.W.2d 595 (1975)   187

Ross v. Beaumont Hospital, 687
F. Supp. 1115 (Mich. 1988)   141

Rozanski v. A-P-A Transport, 47 FEP
Cases 179 (Me. 1986)   137

S

Satterfield v. Lockheed Missiles &
Space Co., 617 F. Supp. 1359
(D.S.C. 1985)   165

Schmerber v. California, 384 U.S. 757
(1966)   110

School Board v. Arline, 480 U.S. 273
(1987)   87, 114, 139, 153

Shaw v. Unemployment
Compensation Board of Review,
539 A.2d 1383 (Pa. Commw. Ct.
1988)   184

Shelby Township Fire Department v.
Shields, 115 Mich. App. 98, 320
N.W.2d 306 (1982)   149

Smith v. National Railroad Passenger
Co., 856 F.2d 467 (2d Cir.
1988)   31

In re State Division of Human Rights
(Granelle), 70 N.Y.2d 100, 510
N.E.2d 799, 517 N.Y.S.2d 715
(1987)   136

State Division of Human Rights
—v. Leroy Central School
District, 107 A.D.2d 153, 485
N.Y.S.2d 907 (App. Div.
1985)   153
—v. Xerox Corp., 65 N.Y.2d 213,
480 N.E.2d 695, 491 N.Y.S.2d
106 (1985)   143, 155

State ex rel. Gomez-Bethke v.
Metropolitan Airport
Commission, 358 N.W.2d 432
(Minn. App. 1984)   135

Steele v. B.F. Goodrich Chemical
Co., 9 Ill. Hum. Rts. Comm'n
Rep. 5 (1983)   54

Sterling Transit Co. v. Fair
Employment Practice
Commission, 121 Cal. App. 3d
791, 175 Cal. Rptr. 548
(1981)   148

Stutts v. Freeman, 694 F.2d 666 (11th
Cir. 1983)   138, 153

Stepp v. Review Board, 521 N.E.2d
350 (Ind. App. 1988)   89

Stovall v. Sally Salmon Seafood, 306
Or. 25, 757 P.2d 410 (1988)   181

T

Taylor Diving & Salvage Co. v.
United States Department of
Labor, 599 F.2d 622 (5th Cir.
1979)   167

Texas Employment Commission v.
Hughes Drilling Fluids, 746
S.W.2d 796 (Tex. App.
1988)   184

Tudyman v. United Airlines, 608
F. Supp. 739 (C.D. Cal.
1984)   157

U

United Steelworkers of America v.
Marshall, 647 F.2d 1189 (D.C.
Cir. 1980), *cert. denied, sub nom*

Lead Indus. Ass'n, Inc. v.
Donovan, 453 U.S. 913
(1981)   167, 168
Usery v. Tamiami Trail Tours, Inc.,
531 F.2d 224 (5th Cir. 1976)

V

Valencia v. Duval Corp., 132 Ariz.
348, 645 P.2d 1262 (Ariz. App.
1982)   188
Vickers v. Veterans Administration,
549 F. Supp. 85 (W.D. Wash.
1982)   138

W

Wallace v. Veterans Administration,
803 F.2d 67 (2d Cir. 1986)   115

Westinghouse Electric Corp. v. State
Division of Human Rights, 63
A.D.2d 170, 406 N.Y.S.2d 912
(1978), *aff'd*, 425 N.Y.S.2d 74
(1980)   149

Wharton Transport Corp. v. Bridges,
606 S.W.2d 521 (Tenn. 1980)   43

Whitlock v. Donovan, 598 F. Supp.
126 (D.D.C. 1984), *aff'd mem.*
sub nom Whitlock v. Brock, 790
F.2d 964 (D.C. Cir. 1986)   145

Wright v. Olin Corp., 697 F.2d 1172
(4th Cir. 1982)   53

Wroblewski v. Lexington Gardens,
Inc., 188 Conn. 44, 448 A.2d 801
(1982)   174

Index

A

A. Foster Higgins & Company   2
ACGIH (*see* American Conference of
    Governmental Industrial
    Hygienists)
Acquired immune deficiency
    syndrome   56, 59, 80 81–94,
    172, 202
ADEA (*see* Age Discrimination in
    Employment Act)
Adolph Coors   63
Affirmative action   114, 126
Age Discrimination in Employment
    Act   174, 178–179
AIDS-related complex   81, 83, 92
AIDS (*see* Acquired immune
    deficiency syndrome)
Alcohol or alcoholism   95–97, 99,
    114–116, 145–146
Allied Chemical   51
AMA (*see* American Medical
    Association)
American Academy of Forensic
    Sciences   105
American Board of Preventive
    Medicine   7
American College of Obstetricians and
    Gynecologists   28–29
American College of Occupational
    Medicine   7
American Conference of
    Governmental Industrial
    Hygienists   70
American Cyanamid Company   51,
    219
American Medical Association   21,
    88, 94, 104, 117
American Occupational Medical
    Association   7, 11, 69, 92, 120
Americans with Disabilities Act   221
Ames, Bruce   56
Amputations   146–147
AOMA (*see* American Occupational
    Medical Association)

AOMA Code of Ethics   13, 16
Applied genetics   76–80
Arbitration   170–174
ARC (*see* AIDS-related complex)
Arthritis   147
Asbestos   2, 7, 8, 46, 59, 62
Ash, Philip   35
AT&T   63, 94
At-will rule   163

B

B.F. Goodrich   51
Back conditions   147–148
Benzene   7, 55
Berkowitz, Edward   126
BFOQ (*see* Bona fide occupational
    qualification)
Biochemical genetics   70–72
Boeing   63
Bona fide occupational
    qualification   86, 140–141
Brown, Michael   73
Business necessity   54, 140

C

Califano, Joseph A., Jr.   195
California Confidentiality of Medical
    Information Act   20
California Workers' Compensation
    Institute   31
Campbell Soup   63
Canada   226–227
Caplan, Arthur   80
Carcinogens   56–58
Centers for Disease Control
    (CDC)   29, 81–83, 85, 89, 92
Charles D. Spencer &
    Associates   186
Chrysler Corporation   195
Circle K Corporation   201–202
Citizens Commission on AIDS   93
Civil Rights Act of 1964   80, 127,
    140, 149, 174–178, 223

Civil Rights Restoration Act of
    1988   88
Clinical Laboratory Improvement
    Amendments of 1988   29–30
Coal dust   62
Consolidated Omnibus Budget
    Reconciliation Act of 1985
    (COBRA)   185–186
Collective bargaining   170–174
College of American Pathologists   29
Common law   19, 163–166
Comprehensive Alcohol Abuse and
    Alcoholism Prevention,
    Treatment, and Rehabilitation
    Act   145
Conflict of interest   9–10
Constitutional issues   110–112,
    160–162, 175
Continental Airlines   215
Controlled Substances Act   102
Cotton dust   62
Crandall, Robert L.   215
Crick, Francis H.C.   76
Curtis, E. Carroll   13
Cystic fibrosis   74, 76, 79
Cytogenetic tests   71

D

Davis, Karen   216
Davis-Bacon Act   223
Defamation   189–190
Department of Defense   101
Department of Health and Human
    Services   2, 102–103, 210
Department of
    Transportation   40–43, 118
Derr, Patrick G.   11–12
Diabetes   15, 149–150, 172, 178
Diagnostic screening   21–43
Dignitary torts   187–191
Disability   21–22
Disparate impact   175–176, 178
Disparate treatment   175
DOT (see Department of
    Transportation)
Dow Chemical   51
Drug abuse   65, 95–100, 114–115
Drug testing   2, 14, 16–17, 65,
    95–124, 165–166, 183–184

Due process   111–112
Dukakis, Michael   214–215, 225
DuPont   51, 71

E

EAP (see Employee assistance
    program)
Eastern Airlines   55
EEOC (see Equal Employment
    Opportunity Commission)
ELISA (see Enzyme-linked
    immunosorbent assay)
EMIT (see Enzyme-multiplied
    immunoassay technique)
Emphysema   15, 59
Employee assistance program   7,
    101–102, 104, 124
Employee benefits   184–187
Employee Polygraph Protection Act of
    1988   35
Employee Retirement Income
    Security Act of 1974   184–187,
    198
Environmental Protection Act   48
Enzyme-linked immunosorbent
    assay   83
Enzyme-multiplied immunoassay
    technique   66–68, 105–107
EPA (see Environmental Protection
    Agency)
Epilepsy   15, 150–151, 172–173
Equal Employment Opportunity
    Commission   54, 174
Equitable Life Assurance
    Society   211
ERISA (see Employee Retirement
    Income Security Act of 1974)
Executive Order 12,564   101–102

F

FAA (see Federal Aviation
    Administration)
Fair Labor Standards Act   223
FDA (see Food and Drug
    Administration)
Federal Aviation Administration   40
Female exclusionary policies   51–54

Fetal protection policy 53–54
Financial Accounting Standards
    Board 201
Firestone 51
Focus Technologies 211
Food and Drug Administration 83
Future risks 128–131

G

Gas chromatography/mass
    spectrometry (GC/MS) 106–108
General Motors 51
Genetic testing 56, 70–80, 177–178
Georgia Power Company 219
Gilbert, Walter 78
Glucose-6-phosphate
    dehydrogenase 70–72, 177
Goldman, Rose 23
Goldstein, Joseph 73
Goodyear 51
Gore, Albert, Jr. 71
Gulf Oil 51
Gusella, James 72
G-6-PD (see Glucose-6-phosphate
    dehydrogenase)

H

Haldane, J.B.S. 70
Handicap 15, 21–22, 79–80, 87–90,
    92, 113–117, 125–159
Handwriting analysis 33
Hanks, Thrift G. 14
Harkin, Tom 89
Hatch, Orrin 216
Hayden, Mike 112–113
Hazard communication standard 9
Health insurance 6, 195–217
Health Insurance Association of
    America 203
Health insurance
    underwriting 205–210
Health maintenance
    organizations 29, 91, 203–204
Health Resources Institute 211
Hearing 151, 172
Heart disease 151–152, 172
Hemophilia 76, 82, 152

High Risk Occupational Disease
    Notification Act 9
Hirschhorn, Kurt 77
HIV (see Human immunodeficiency
    virus)
HMOs (see Health maintenance
    organizations)
Home Office Reference
    Laboratory 210
Honesty tests 33–36
Honeywell 63
Human immunodeficiency virus 2,
    14, 19, 56, 81–86, 90–94
Humphrey, Gordon 89
Huntington's disease 72, 74, 76
Hypersensitivity 46
Hypertension 153

I

IBM 63, 94
Ilka, Richard 12–13
Immigration Reform and Control Act
    of 1986 224
Immunoassays 7, 105
Impairment 21–22
Infante, Peter F. 48
Informed consent 30
Invasion of privacy 187–190

J

Job relatedness 133–134, 140–141
Johnson Controls 51
Johnson & Johnson 94

K

Kaposi's sarcoma 82
Kennedy, Edward 214
Kristein, Marvin M. 61

L

Lead 2, 7
Leukemia 55
Levinson, David 213
Lundberg, George D. 27–28

M

Magee, W. Edwin   64
Mandatory medical
    examinations   36–43
Manville Corporation   63
Matthew Bender & Company   112
Medical history   22–26, 30
Medical Information Bureau   18, 210
Medical questionnaires   22
Medical records   18–20
Medical removal protection and rate
    retention   167–169
Medicare   200
Meese, Edwin   119
Metropolitan Life Insurance   201
Michigan State University   29
Milles, Saul   10
Mine Safety and Health Act   39
Mine Safety and Health
    Administration   98
Minimum Health Benefits for All
    Workers Act   214–216
Minnesota Multiphasic Personality
    Inventory (MMPI)   32–33
Mock, Harry E.   1
Monsanto   51
Morson, Alan   226
MRP and RR (see Medical removal
    protection and rate retention)
MSHA (see Mine Safety and Health
    Administration)
Multiple physician review   167–168
Multiple sclerosis   154
Mutagens   52–53

N

National Academy of Sciences   8, 94,
    215
National Institute on Drug Abuse   95
National Institute for Occupational
    Safety and Health   2, 48, 98
National Labor Relations
    Act   170–174
National Labor Relations Board   170
Negligence   165, 191–192, 194
Neurological conditions   154–155
New York City Human Rights
    Commission   89

NIDA (see National Institute on Drug
    Abuse)
NIOSH (see National Institute for
    Occupational Safety and
    Health)
NLRA (see National Labor Relations
    Act)
NLRB (see National Labor Relations
    Board)
Nonoccupational illnesses   55–58
Non-Smokers Inn   65
Nuclear Regulatory Commission
    (NRC)   33

O

Obesity   155, 172
Occupational health history   22–26
Occupational illness   44–47
Occupational medicine or
    physicians   6–13, 22
Occupational Safety and Health
    Act   4, 7, 38–39, 166–170
Occupational Safety and Health
    Administration   9, 18, 36–39, 48,
    166–170
Office of Federal Contract Compliance
    Programs (OFCCP)   126–127
Office of Technology
    Assessment   34–35, 71–72,
    206–210
Olin   51
Orthopedic conditions   155–156
OSHA (see Occupational Safety and
    Health Act/Administration)
OTA (see Office of Technology
    Assessment)

P

PCR test (see Polymerase chain
    reaction test)
PDA (see Pregnancy Disability Act)
Personal injury   191–194
Personality tests   32–33
Physician-patient relationship   10–12,
    19
Pillsbury   55
Polygraphs   33–36, 68–69
Polymerase chain reaction test   83–84

PPOs (*see* Preferred provider
    organizations)
Predictive screening   44–69, 128, 147
Predictive value   66–69, 107
Preemployment and preplacement
    screening   2–3, 31–32, 40,
    147–148
Preferred provider
    organizations   203–204
Pregnancy   176–177
Pregnancy Disability Act   176–177
President's Commission on Organized
    Crime   101
Preventive Plus   6
Privacy   19, 47, 111
Productivity   97–99, 119
Prudential Insurance Company   94,
    212
Psychiatric conditions   156, 172
Psychological screening   31–36

Q

Quaker Oats   55

R

Ralston Purina   64
Reagan, Ronald   100–101
Reasonable accommodation   137–139,
    145, 168–169
Recombinant DNA   72–76
Rehabilitation Act of 1973   87–89,
    113–117, 125–128, 143, 145, 147,
    149, 152
Reinhardt, Charles   71
Reinhardt, Uwe   228
Renal disease   156–157
Reproductive hazards   47–55,
    193–194
Respiratory conditions   157
Retiree Benefits Bankruptcy
    Protection Act   200–201
Risk factors   44–47, 58
Rothman, Barbara Katz   76

S

Scheel, L.D.   70
Schilling, Richard   26–27
Schroeder, Elinor P.   103

Sears, Roebuck & Company   1
Self-insurance   197–198
Sensitivity   66–69
Severo, Richard   71
Sickle cell   71–73, 76, 79, 177
Singer   201
Smoking   46, 59–65, 181–182
Specificity   66–69
St. Joe's Minerals   51
Stature   157–158
Stokinger, Herbert E.   70
Sun Oil   51
Synergistic effects   62–63
Syva Corporation   66, 105

T

Tax Reform Act of 1986   186–187
Tay Sachs disease   73, 79
Tenneco, Inc.   31
Teratogens   52
Thalassemia   73, 76, 79
Theft   99, 119
Title VII (*see* Civil Rights Act of 1964)
Torts   19, 187–194
Toxic Substances Control Act   48
TRW, Inc.   201

U

Unemployment insurance   183–184
U.S. Customs Service   118
USG Acoustical Products
    Company   63
Utah Drug and Alcohol Testing
    Act   113

V

Vascular conditions   158
Vision   135, 158–159, 173

W

Waivers   17
Walker, Michael A.   226–227
Walsh, Diana Chapman   216–217
Walters, LeRoy   79
Watkins, James   94
Watson, James D.   76

Waxman, Henry   214
Wellness programs   210–213
Western Blot   83
Wexler, Nancy   80
Workers' compensation   4, 31, 55,
    63, 180–183, 191
Wrongful discharge   163–166

X

Xerox   94

Z

Zito, Dominick S.   6

About the Author

Mark A. Rothstein is Professor of Law and Director of the Health Law Institute at the University of Houston. He is also Adjunct Professor of Public Health at The University of Texas School of Public Health.

Professor Rothstein received his B.A. from the University of Pittsburgh and his J.D. from Georgetown University. Before assuming his present position in 1985, he was Professor of Law and Adjunct Professor of Medicine at West Virginia University, where he was the Director of the Occupational Health Law Program.

Professor Rothstein has concentrated his research on employment and occupational health law. He has written over thirty articles on these subjects as well as three other books: *Cases and Materials on Employment Law* (with Knapp and Liebman) (Foundation Press 1987), widely used in law school courses on the rights of nonunion employees; *Medical Screening of Workers* (BNA Books 1984), the first book to explore the medical, legal, and social implications of increased medical testing in the employment setting; and *Occupational Safety and Health Law* (West Publishing Co., 2d ed. 1983), a standard reference book for lawyers on OSHA law.

Professor Rothstein has lectured widely on issues such as medical screening of workers, AIDS, reproductive hazards, drug abuse, genetic testing, and OSHA. He has served as a consultant to the Office of Technology Assessment of the United States Congress, National Academy of Sciences, American Medical Association, American Hospital Association, and other organizations.